Respiratory System and Artificial Ventilation

AF666970

Umberto Lucangelo • Paolo Pelosi
Walter A. Zin • Andrea Aliverti

Respiratory System and Artificial Ventilation

Springer

Editors
Umberto Lucangelo
Department of Perioperative Medicine
Intensive Care and Emergency
Cattinara Hospital
Trieste University School of Medicine
Trieste, Italy

Paolo Pelosi
Department of Clinical Science
University of Insubria
Varese, Italy

Walter A. Zin
Laboratory of Respiration Physiology
Carlos Chagas Filho Institute of Biophysics
Federal University of Rio de Janeiro
Rio de Janeiro, Brazil

Andrea Aliverti
TMB Laboratory
Department of Bioengineering
Politecnico di Milano
Milan, Italy

Library of Congress Control Number: 2007939294

Milan Heidelberg New York
ISBN 978-88-470-0764-2 ISBN 978-88-470-0765-9 (eBook)
DOI 10.1007/978-88-470-0765-9

Springer is a part of Springer Science+Business Media
springer.com
© Springer-Verlag Italia 2008

This work is subject to copyright. All rights are reserved, whether the whole or part of the material is concerned, specifically the rights of translation, reprinting, reuse of illustrations, recitation, broadcasting, reproduction on microfilm or in any other way, and storage in data banks. Duplication of this publication or parts thereof is permitted only under the provisions of the Italian Copyright Law in its current version, and permission for use must always be obtained from Springer. Violations are liable to prosecution under the Italian Copyright Law.

The use of general descriptive names, registered names, trademarks, etc. in this publication does not imply, even in the absence of a specific statement, that such names are exempt from the relevant protective laws and regulations and therefore free for general use.
Product liability: the publisher cannot guarantee the accuracy of any information about dosage and application contained in this book. In every individual case the user must check such information by consulting the relevant literature.

Cover design: Simona Colombo, Milan, Italy
Typesetting: Graphostudio, Milan, Italy

Springer-Verlag Italia S.r.l., Via Decembrio 28, I-20137 Milan

Preface

Intellectual undertakings, such as publishing a medical book—in this case, one concerning the respiratory tract and artificial support techniques—offer an important incentive for experts in a particular field, in that, as authors, they have the opportunity to share research results, whether their own or those of the working group they represent. Such books provide challenging and qualified updates to young researchers, who are thereby able to enhance their knowledge and working methods, for example, with the aim of improving the treatment standards of intensive-care patients.

The purpose of this book is to pursue the mission undertaken for the past thirty years by the Trieste University School of Anaesthesia and Intensive Care and, more recently, by the School of Anaesthesia and Intensive Care of Catania University.

The editors' task was made easier through a project promoted by the University of Catania, which involved the presence in Catania of my colleague Walter Zin, from Rio de Janeiro, who held a series of lectures and seminars on respiratory pathophysiology, aimed at teachers and students alike. Furthermore, important contributions by my colleagues Paolo Pelosi, from Varese; Andrea Aliverti, from Milan; and Umberto Lucangelo, from Trieste, must also be acknowledged. Their valuable co-operation and support contributed to achieving the high quality of this book.

The 18 chapters that make up this volume were written by highly regarded and internationally known clinical experts and researchers. To facilitate access to the information provided in the chapters, the volume has been subdivided into the following sections: Properties of the Respiratory System; Interaction Between the Pulmonary Circulation and Ventilation; Monitoring of Respiratory Mechanics, Acute Lung Injury–ARDS, Controlled Mechanical Ventilation in ARDS and the Open-Lung Concept; Nosocomial Pneumonia; Prone Ventilation;

Old and New Artificial Ventilation Techniques; Non-invasive Ventilation. 'Respiratory System and Artificial Ventilation' serves as a valuable tool for continuing medical education and for updating one's state-of-the-art clinical knowledge.

Venice, November 9, 2007

Antonino Gullo
Head and Chairman,
Department and School of Anaesthesia and Intensive Care,
University of Catania - Italy
Council, World Federation of Societies of Intensive and Critical Care Medicine (WFSICCM)

Contents

Contributors

Aliverti A.
TMB Laboratory, Department of Bioengineering, Politecnico di Milano, Milan, Italy

Antonaglia V.
Biomechanics Laboratory, Department of Perioperative Medicine, Intensive Care and Emergency, Azienda Ospedaliera-Universitaria, Trieste, Italy

Bacer B.
Department of Perioperative Medicine, Intensive Care and Emergency, Trieste University School of Medicine, Cattinara Hospital, Trieste, Italy

Beuret P.
Intensive Care Unit, Centre Hospitalier, Roanne, France

Blanch L.
Critical Care Center, Hospital de Sabadell, Institut Universitari Fundació Parc Taulí, Universitat Autònoma de Barcelona, Barcelona, Spain

Broccard A.F.
University of Minnesota, Medical Intensive Care Unit and Critical Care Division, Regions Hospital, St Paul, USA

Cagido V.R.
Laboratory of Respiration Physiology, Carlos Chagas Filho Institute of Biophysics, Federal University of Rio de Janeiro, Rio de Janeiro, Brazil

Calderini E.
Pediatric Intensive Care Unit, Department of Anesthesia and Critical Care, Fondazione Policlinico Mangiagalli Regina Elena IRCCS, Milan, Italy

Chidini G.
Pediatric Intensive Care Unit, Department of Anesthesia and Critical Care, Fondazione Policlinico Mangiagalli Regina Elena IRCCS, Milan, Italy

Chiumello D.
Institute of Anaesthesia and Critical Care, University of Milan, Policlinico IRCCS Hospital, Milan, Italy

Crimi E.
Interdepartmental Division of Critical Care Medicine, Division of Respirology, St. Michael's Hospital, University of Toronto, Canada

Del Sorbo L.
Interdepartmental Division of Critical Care Medicine, Division of Respirology, St. Michael's Hospital, University of Toronto, Canada

d'Onofrio D.
Department of Environment, Health and Safety, University of Insubria, Varese, Italy

Feihl F.
Division of Clinical Pathophysiology, Lausanne University Hospital (CHUV), Lausanne, Switzerland

Fontanesi L.
Department of Perioperative Medicine, Intensive Care and Emergency, Trieste University School of Medicine, Cattinara Hospital, Trieste, Italy

Gommers D.
Department of Anaesthesiology and Department of Intensive Care, Erasmus-MC, Rotterdam, The Netherlands

Gramaticopolo S.
Department of Perioperative Medicine, Intensive Care and Emergency, Trieste University School of Medicine, Cattinara Hospital, Trieste, Italy

Gruson D.
Department of Medical Intensive Care, University Hospital of Bordeaux, Bordeaux, France

Hilbert G.
Department of Medical Intensive Care, University Hospital of Bordeaux, Bordeaux, France

Lachmann B.
Department of Anaesthesiology, Erasmus-MC, Rotterdam, The Netherlands

Liapikou A.
Respiratory Intensive Care Unit, Pulmonology Department, Hospital Clinic of Barcelona, Barcelona, Spain

Lucangelo U.
Department of Perioperative Medicine, Intensive Care and Emergency, Cattinara Hospital, Trieste University School of Medicine, Trieste, Italy

Nagato L.K.S.
Laboratory of Respiration Physiology, Carlos Chagas Filho Institute of Biophysics, Federal University of Rio de Janeiro, Rio de Janeiro, Brazil

Pascotto S.
Biomechanics Laboratory, Department of Perioperative Medicine, Intensive Care and Emergency, Azienda Ospedaliera-Universitaria, Trieste, Italy

Pelosi P.
Department of Clinical Science, University of Insubria, Varese, Italy

Piller F.
Biomechanics Laboratory, Department of Perioperative Medicine, Intensive Care and Emergency, Azienda Ospedaliera-Universitaria, Trieste, Italy

Preis C.
Department of Anaesthesiology, Erasmus-MC, Rotterdam, The Netherlands

Ranieri V.M.
Department of Anaesthesia and Intensive Care Medicine, S. Giovanni Battista – Molinette Hospital, University of Turin, Turin, Italy

Santos F.B.
Laboratory of Respiration Physiology, Carlos Chagas Filho Institute of Biophysics, Federal University of Rio de Janeiro, Rio de Janeiro, Brazil

Torres A.
Respiratory Intensive Care Unit, Pulmonology Department, Hospital Clinic of Barcelona, Barcelona, Spain

Valencia M.
Respiratory Intensive Care Unit, Pulmonology Department, Hospital Clinic of Barcelona, Barcelona, Spain

Valente Barbas C.S.
Departamento de Cardio-Pneumologia e Patologia da Faculdade de Medicina da Universidade de São Paulo, Brazil

Vargas F.
Department of Medical Intensive Care, University Hospital of Bordeaux, Bordeaux, France

Voggenreiter G.
Department of Orthopaedic and Trauma Surgery, Hospitals in the Natural Parc Altmühltal, Eichstätt, Germany

Zin W.A.
Laboratory of Respiration Physiology, Carlos Chagas Filho Institute of Biophysics, Federal University of Rio de Janeiro, Rio de Janeiro, Brazil

List of Abbreviations

ALI	Acute lung injury
APCV	Adaptive pressure control ventilation
ARDS	Acute respiratory distress syndrome
ARDSexp	Extrapulmonary acute respiratory distress syndrome
ARDSp	Pulmonary acute respiratory distress syndrome
ARF	Acute respiratory failure
BAL	Bronchoalveolar lavage
BALF	Bronchoalveolar lavage fluid
BBS	Blind bronchial sampling
BiPAP	Bilevel positive airway pressure
BPD	Bronchopulmonary dysplasia
C	Compliance
CABG	Coronary artery bypass grafting
CHF	Congestive heart failure
CNAP	Continuous negative airway pressure
COPD	Chronic obstructive pulmonary disease
COX	Cyclooxygenase
CPAP	Continuous positive airway pressure
CPB	Cardiopulmonary bypass
CPG	Central pattern generator
CPIP	Chronic pulmonary insufficiency of prematurity
CPIS	Clinical pulmonary infection score
CPP	Cerebral perfusion pressure
CSA	Central sleep apnoea
CSF	Cerebrospinal fluid
CSR	Cheyne-Stokes respiration
CT	Computed tomography
CV	Conventional ventilation
DRG	Dorsal respiratory group
E	Elastance
ECMO	Extracorporeal membrane oxygenation
EELV	End-expiratory lung volume
EFL	Expiratory flow limitation
EHFO	External high-frequency oscillation

EIC	Electrical impedance tomography
ETA	Endotracheal aspiration
ETT	Endotracheal tube
FOT	Forced oscillation technique
FRC	Functional residual capacity
GGT	Galactosyl-hydroxylysylglucosyltransferase
HAP	Hospital-acquired pneumonia
HCAP	Health-care-associated pneumonia
HFOV	High-frequency oscillation ventilation
HFPV	High-frequency percussive ventilation
HFV	High-frequency ventilation
IAPV	Intermittent abdominal positive ventilation
ICP	Intracranial pressure
ICU	Intensive care unit
IL	Interleukin
iNOS	Inducible nitric oxide synthase
INPV	Intermittent negative-pressure ventilation
IPPV	Invasive positive-pressure ventilation
LAP	Left atrial pressure
LT	Leucotriene
MAP	Mean arterial pressure
MIP	Maximal inspiratory pressure
MIP-2	Macrophage inflammatory protein-2
MOD	Multi-organ dysfunction
MRSA	Methicillin-resistant *Staphylococcus aureus*
MS	Multiple sclerosis
NEEP	Negative end-expiratory pressure
NEP	Negative expiratory pressure
NICU	Neonatal intensive care unit
NIPPV	Non-invasive positive-pressure ventilation
NIV	Non-invasive ventilation
NO	Nitric oxide
NP	Nosocomial pneumonia
NPV	Negative-pressure ventilation
OEP	Optoelectronic plethysmography
OLC	Open lung concept
PAI	Plasminogen activator inhibitor
PAV	Proportional assist ventilation
PCV	Pressure control ventilation
PEEP	Positive end-expiratory pressure
PEEPi	Intrinsic positive end-expiratory pressure
Pga	Gastric pressure
PIP	Peak inspiratory pressure
P_L	Transpulmonary pressure
PMM	Potentially multiresistant microorganism

Poes	Oesophageal pressure
PPV	Positive-pressure ventilation
PRG	Pontine respiratory group
PS	Pressure support
PSB	Protected telescopic catheter
P_{TM}	Transmural airway pressure
PVR	Pulmonary vascular resistance
Pw	Abdominal wall pressure
R	Resistance
RARs	Rapidly adapting stretch receptors
RV	Residual volume
SARs	Slowly adapting stretch receptors
SIDS	Sudden infant death syndrome
SIRS	Systemic inflammatory response syndrome
sNIPPV	Synchronised nasal intermittent positive-pressure ventilation
TLC	Total lung capacity
TNF	Tumour necrosis factor
TREM	Triggering receptor expressed on myeloid cells
TTA	Transthoracic needle aspiration
VALI	Ventilator-associated lung injury
VAT	Ventilator-associated tracheobronchitis
V_E	Minute ventilation
VILI	Ventilator-induced lung injury
VMR	Ventilatory muscle rest
VRG	Ventrolateral respiratory group
V_T	Tidal volume
ZEEP	Zero end-expiratory pressure

Properties of the Respiratory System

Control of Breathing

F.B. Santos, L.K.S. Nagato, W.A. Zin

Introduction

The physiological control of the respiratory system is unique among organ systems. Breathing is essential to life and must occur 24 h a day, 365 days a year, in the conscious or unconscious state, awake or asleep. At the same time, humans and other mammals need to be able to temporarily interrupt the normal pattern of breathing to perform other functions, such as eating and vocalising [1]. The voluntary and involuntary control of the respiratory system is unequalled and a very complex process. This chapter will appraise some relevant issues to improve clinicians' understanding of the normal mechanism of breathing and its possible disorders in disease.

Respiratory Control Components

Ventilation is constantly monitored and adjusted to maintain appropriate arterial pH and PaO_2. This homeostatic control system requires a set of sensors, a central controlling mechanism and an effector arm to carry out its commands (Fig. 1). Afferent information from sensors modulates the central command of respiratory muscles [2]. The brain constantly receives information from the upper airways, lungs and chest wall and decides how the ventilatory pump will respond.

Respiratory Sensors

Afferent input into the central system is provided primarily by groups of neural receptors, either mechanoreceptors or chemoreceptors. The latter respond to alterations in PaO_2, $PaCO_2$ and pH.

U. Lucangelo, P. Pelosi, W.A. Zin, A. Aliverti (eds.) *Respiratory System and Artificial Ventilation.* © Springer 2008

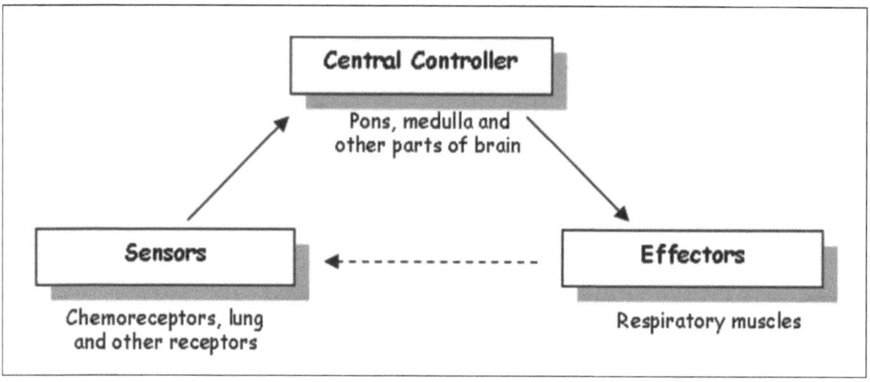

Fig. 1 The control of breathing: basic elements. Sensors transmit information to the central controller. Subsequently, stimuli are sent to the effectors–the respiratory muscles–to adjust ventilatory responses. Adapted from [3]

Peripheral Chemoreceptors

From their location in the carotid and aortic bodies, peripheral chemoreceptors direct the response to changes in PaO_2, $PaCO_2$ and pH. The carotid bodies are found at the bifurcation of the common carotid artery into the internal and external carotid arteries (Fig. 2) and their sensory supply reaches the brain via the glossopharyngeal nerve. The aortic bodies are located around the ascending aorta and send their afferent stimuli via the vagal nerves to the central nervous system. Since the arterial blood supply of these bodies amounts to approximately 2 l/min/100 g tissue (they are located on the outside of the main arteries and receive their own perfusion), they are one of the most highly perfused tissues in the human body [4,5]. The carotid and aortic bodies consist of two different cell types, glomus cells (type I) and sheath cells (type II). Afferent neurons terminate on glomus cells. There is also an unmyelinated supply to the sheath cells.

It is not clear how the carotid and aortic bodies sense hypoxaemia, but is clear that the stimulus for increased ventilation is PaO_2, not the oxygen content of the blood [1]. At normal levels of PaO_2, some neural activity arises from these chemosensors. At hyperoxic levels, this activity is only slightly reduced in normal people whereas in arterial hypoxaemia the intensity of the response varies in a non-linear manner according to the severity of the condition [7]. The greatest increase in activity in response to hypoxaemia occurs when PaO_2 falls to ≤ 60 mmHg or an $F_IO_2 \leq 0.1$ [1,7]. This increase in ventilation is manifested primarily by an increase in the depth of breathing (tidal volume or V_T) but an increased respiratory rate is also observed. These responses vary according to the degree of hypoxaemia.

In mammals, the carotid bodies account for about 90% of the ventilatory response to hypoxaemia; the remaining 10% arises from the aortic bodies. The former are also responsible for 20–50% of the response to arterial hypercapnia and acidaemia, with the remaining 50–80% of the response mediated by central brainstem receptors [8].

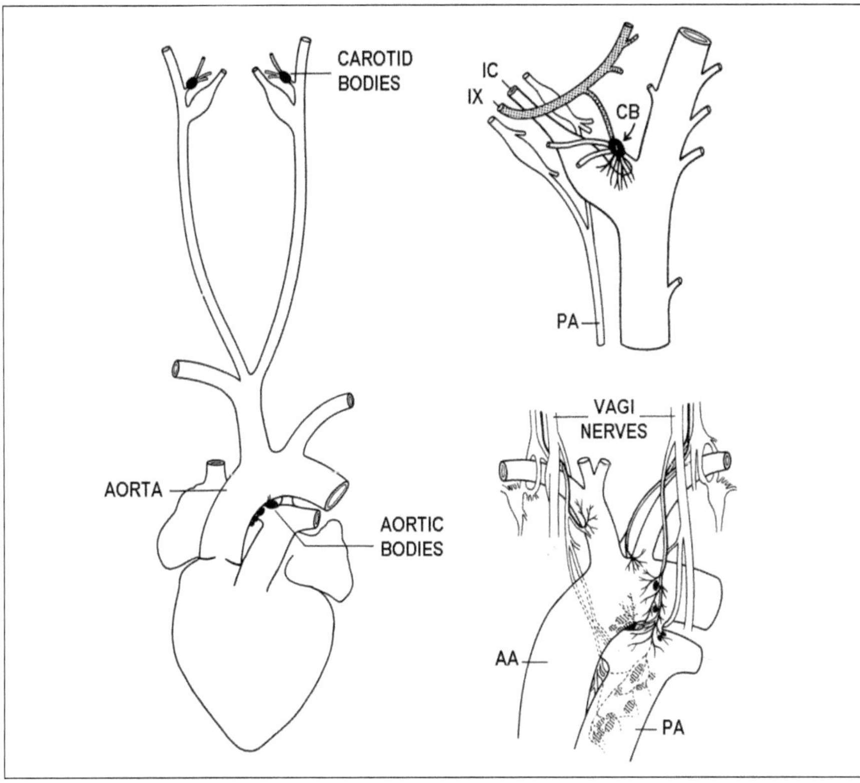

Fig. 2 Sites where carotid and aortic bodies are located. *Left* Anatomical positioning of the carotid and aortic chemoreceptors. *Right, top* The sensory output of the carotid bodies (*CB*) reaches the brain via the glossopharyngeal nerve (*IX*); *X*, Vagus nerve; *IC*, internal carotid. *Right, bottom* Aortic chemoreceptors. *PA*, Pulmonary artery; *AA*, ascending aorta. Adapted from [6]

The activity of the peripheral chemoreceptors also increases with high levels of $PaCO_2$ and reduced levels of arterial pH, leading to increased ventilation. It is not immediately evident whether $PaCO_2$ and/or pH represent the stimulus under conditions of acute hypercapnia. Although responsive to changes in oxygen and carbon dioxide levels, the chemoreceptor is much more sensitive to acute hypercapnia than to hypoxaemia [7].

Central Chemoreceptors

The fact that a ventilatory response to additional CO_2 persists in experimental animals despite peripheral chemoreceptor denervation suggests that there are chemoreceptors in the brain that are sensitive to CO_2 or hydrogen ions [9]. These receptors respond to changes in $PaCO_2$ (by increasing ventilation in response to increased PCO_2 and vice versa) and pH (by increasing ventilation to a decreased pH and vice versa). Although no definite chemoreceptors have been defined anatomically, results of experiments involving the local application of chemical, electrical and thermal stimuli suggest that central chemoreceptors are located at or near the ventral surface of the medulla [9]. This location may facilitate the ability of the central chemoreceptors to monitor changes in $PaCO_2$ and pH levels in the cerebrospinal fluid (CSF). Hydrogen ions enter and are found in the CSF and extracellular fluid in the vicinity of the central chemoreceptors. The presence of these ions is a result of CO_2 dissociation and direct diffusion into and out of the bloodstream. Elevated arterial CO_2 easily crosses the blood–brain barrier because this gas is highly membrane-permeable, is converted to carbonic acid (H_2CO_3) and rapidly dissociates into H^+ and HCO_3^- ions. As a result, H^+ rises in the CSF and interstitium in parallel with $PaCO_2$. This increased H^+ stimulates respiration by a direct action on the central chemoreceptors [1,10].

There is an interaction between the responses of the peripheral and central chemoreceptors. The blood–brain barrier exhibits different permeabilities to ions, such as H^+ (low permeability), and lipid-soluble molecules, such as carbon dioxide (high permeability). In an acidic environment, the peripheral chemoreceptors would trigger an increase in ventilation before the local environment in the fluid bathing the medulla reflected the acid pH in the blood. As ventilation increases owing to stimulation of peripheral chemoreceptors, $PaCO_2$ decreases. The environment of central chemoreceptors would rapidly reflect the lower $PaCO_2$, but only later sense the elevated H^+ concentration of the blood (because of the extra time needed for the H^+ ions to cross the blood–brain barrier) [10]. However, when $PaCO_2$ level is chronically elevated, as might occur in a patient with severe COPD, the activities of the peripheral and central chemoreceptors decrease within a few days, as pH normalises. At extremely high levels of carbon dioxide ($PaCO_2$>80–100 mmHg) an anaesthetic effect may be produced and ventilation decreases rather than increases. This occurs because a chronically elevated $PaCO_2$ results in renal compensation and consequent retention of HCO_3^-. This HCO_3^- gradually diffuses through the blood–brain barrier and into the CSF, where it binds to the excess H^+ produced by the elevated $PaCO_2$, which balances the stimuli on ventilatory drive [10].

At moderate degrees of hypoxaemia—between 45 and 60 mmHg—ventilation rises moderately to about twice its normal level. Only when PaO_2 falls below 40 mmHg is there a sharp increase in ventilation. When hypercapnia occurs simultaneously with acute hypoxaemia, a synergistic effect results and ventilation rises substantially.

Pulmonary Receptors

Pulmonary receptors can be found in the airways and lung parenchyma and are innervated by the vagus nerves.

– *Pulmonary stretch receptors* are slowly adapting stretch receptors (SARs) located among smooth muscle cells within the intra- and extra-thoracic airways. These receptors are stimulated by pulmonary inflation and may play a role in the early termination of inspiration when tidal volume increases—Breuer-Hering inflation reflex [11]. In humans, this reflex is manifest only at a V_T >3 l and seems to play a protective role in preventing excessive lung inflation. The SARs do not accommodate to a persistent stimulus, such as prolonged distension [12].

- *Irritant receptors* are also called rapidly adapting stretch receptors (RARs) and are located among the airway epithelial cells. RARs respond to noxious stimuli, such as dust, cigarette smoke and histamine [13]. They are concentrated in the carina and primary bronchi and are also believed to trigger cough [12]. During normal quiet breathing, their discharge does not depend on the phases of the breathing cycle (inspiration and expiration); therefore, these receptors do not seem to influence to any great extent the baseline breathing pattern at rest [14]. RARs also seem to trigger the augmented ventilation and sighs occurring sporadically during normal breathing, which help to prevent atelectasis of the air spaces [15]. They have also been described as taking part in the dyspnoea, bronchoconstriction and rapid and shallow breathing that occur in asthma [13,16,17].
- *C fibres* are unmyelinated fibres that carry information from a variety of receptors whose function is not totally understood [1]. Located within the airways, these receptors respond to either mechanical or chemical factors.
- *Chest-wall and muscle mechanoreceptors* respond to changes in length, tension or movement. The primary mechanoreceptors in the chest are the muscle spindles, tendon organs of the respiratory muscles and the joint proprioceptors. Afferent information from these receptors reaches the respiratory centres in the medulla [7]. Mechanoreceptors may also contribute to the increase in ventilation that occurs during the early stages of exercise [18]. Muscle spindles and tendon organs sense changes in the force of contraction of the respiratory muscles. While muscle spindles regulate muscle tonus, tendon organs have an inhibiting effect on inspiration. Joint proprioceptors sense the degree of chest-wall movement and may also influence the level and timing of respiratory activity [19].

Central Respiratory Controllers

The central respiratory controllers are divided into the brainstem group (involuntary) and the cerebral cortex group (voluntary). The neural structures responsible for the automatic control of breathing are found in the medulla and pons. Two aggregates of neurons, termed the dorsal respiratory group (DRG) and the ventrolateral respiratory group (VRG), contain both inspiratory and expiratory neurons. The DRG seems to play an important role in processing information from receptors in the lungs, chest wall and chemoreceptors that modulate breathing. Neural activity from the DRG is important to activate the diaphragm and the VRG. The DRG also exhibits a role in determining breathing rhythm and in regulating the changes in diameter of the upper airway that occur with breathing by stimulating the muscles to expand the upper airway during inspiration [1,2,7]. The DRG is located in the nucleus of the tractus solitarius in the medulla and apparently represents the site of origin of the normal rhythmic respiratory drive, which consists of repetitive bursts of inspiratory action potentials [20]. The exact mechanism by which this rhythm is generated remains unknown. The VRG is located within the nucleus ambiguus (rostrally) and nucleus retroambiguus (caudally). It innervates respiratory effector muscles by the phrenic, intercostal and abdominal respiratory motoneurons [20].

In the pons, the pontine respiratory group (PRG) contains neurons that may contribute to the transitions or switching from inspiration to expiration. Damage to the respiratory neurons in the pons leads to an increase in inspiratory time, a decrease in respiratory frequency and an increase in tidal volume [1,2,7]. Nuclei so far located in the pons are the parabrachialis medialis and Kölliker-Fuse.

The breathing rhythm of the central pattern generator (CPG) has been explained as follows. Inspiration begins by the abrupt removal of inhibitory impulses to the DRG. An increased inspiratory motoneuron activity ensues in the form of a slowly augmenting ramp of signals that is suddenly terminated by an off-switch mechanism. During expiration, another burst of inspiratory neuronal activity takes place [21]. In fact, so many different bursting patterns can be detected in the respiratory neurons in the medulla and pons that, so far, any model or hypothesis of the triggering or interaction among the structures remains speculative.

The cerebral cortex may temporarily influence or bypass the central respiratory control mechanism in order to accomplish behaviour-related respiratory activity, such as cough, speech, singing and voluntary breath-holding [22,23]. Discomfort and anxiety may also influence the respiratory rhythm. When experiencing pain or shortness of breath, most people increase their respiratory rate, and total ventilation increases. The pattern of breathing may also reflect attempts to reduce the discomfort associated with ventilation. Patients with significantly reduced respiratory system compliance tend to breath with a rapid, shallow pattern. For patients with increased airway resistance, on the other hand, the high flow required for rapid, shallow breathing requires considerable work. These patients tend to adopt a slower breathing pattern with large tidal volumes [1].

Neural Control of Smooth Muscle in the Airways

The autonomous nervous system importantly participates in the regulation of the calibre of the airways both in normal individuals and in those with pulmonary illness.

Cholinergic fibres (parasympathetic) penetrate between the muscle fibres of the bronchi and their stimulation results in the contraction of airway smooth muscle. Evidence for such an action stems from fact of that bronchodilatation ensues after sectioning of the vagus nerves and after the administration of anticholinergic drugs. The cholinergic system participates in the maintenance of the bronchial tonus at rest and in the majority of bronchoconstriction cases. In contrast, the smooth muscle fibres in the airways present adrenergic innervation. While the amount of α-adrenoreceptors is reduced and their role seems insignificant, β-adrenoreceptors antagonise bronchoconstriction in asthmatic patients, by promoting the relaxation of airway smooth muscle [23].

Evidences show that the airways contain a system of innervation in which the neurotransmitters are neither adrenergic nor cholinergic. This system is known as non-adrenergic non-cholinergic innervation (NANC). Its location cannot be distinguished morphologically from those of the classic sympathetic and parasympathetic ways, but its stimulation can result in an excitatory response but its stimulation can result in a non-adrenergic non-cholinergic excitatory or inhibitory response. Among the neurotransmitters of this system, neuropeptides, such as substance P and neurokinin A, among others, can be found [24].

Effector System

The pathways and muscles involved in the actual performance of inspiration and expiration make up the effector system. The spinal descending pathways connect the DRG and VRG to the ventrolateral columns of the spinal cord; finally, the stimuli reach the α-motoneurons leading to the diaphragm, intercostal and abdominal muscles, and to other muscles promoting respiratory movements.

The respiratory muscles encompass the diaphragm and the intercostal, abdominal and accessory muscles of respiration. The diaphragm is responsible for the majority (75%) of gas movement during quiet inspiration, while the parasternal internal intercostals and scalenes account for the remainder [25].

Control of Breathing in Disease

Chronic Obstructive Pulmonary disease

The patient with chronic obstructive pulmonary disease (COPD) presents altered V'/Q' distribution with hypoxaemia, with or without CO_2 accumulation. Airflow obstruction could be the most important fact to explain the hypercapnia in COPD patients. Inspiratory muscle dysfunction and the coexistence of nocturnal hypoventilation may worsen the hypercapnia. However, the true reason that some patients present with CO_2 retention while others do not, despite the same degree of obstruction, remains unknown. The native ventilatory response to $PaCO_2$ might constitute an inter-individual factor contributing to the variable hypercapnia in COPD patients. This concept of inherent differences in the ventilatory response to CO_2 arose from observations of the considerable variability in the magnitude of the ventilatory response to experimentally induced increases in arterial PCO_2 in normal subjects. According to this paradigm, COPD patients have been classified into those with high ventilatory responses to abnormal blood gases ('pink puffers') and those with low responses ('blue bloaters') [26].

Another factor that may contribute to the variable arterial CO_2 retention in severe COPD patients is a corresponding coincidence of sleep-related hypoventilation: patients with a larger amount of sleep-disordered breathing have daytime hypoventilation and those with normal ventilation during sleep only slight hypoventilation. Additionally, patients with obstructive sleep apnoea syndrome and concurrent COPD have higher daytime $PaCO_2$ values than patients without COPD [27].

The effects of a high inspiratory oxygen fraction are still controversial. Some patients with CO_2 retention worsen their respiratory acidosis when they inhale high O_2 concentrations. This effect is usually explained by the loss of the hypoxic stimulus to breathing. However, a reduction in the hypoxic ventilatory drive may not be the only mechanism inducing hypercapnia in these patients. The worst V'/Q' mismatch results in a significantly increased dead space; this is another explanation for the arterial hypercapnia associated with supplemental oxygen administration. Prior to the use of supplemental oxygen, areas of local alveolar hypoxia produce pulmonary hypoxic vasoconstriction, thereby diverting the flow of CO_2-rich blood from poorly ventilated to better aerated lung segments. When supplemental oxygen reverses local hypoxaemia, pulmonary hypoxic vasoconstriction nullifies and allows the perfusion of very poorly ventilated lung segments, increasing the dead space and reducing the effective alveolar ventilation. As a result, arterial CO_2 rises. Finally, $PaCO_2$ may increase in the face of supplemental oxygen administration because of a concurrent decrease in the CO_2 carrying capacity of the haemoglobin molecule secondary to the increasing oxygenation. This results in an altered steady-state relationship between carbaminohaemoglobin and $PaCO_2$, which raises the latter by several millimetres of mercury. This is known as the Haldane effect [28].

COPD patients exhibit an increased neural drive to their respiratory muscles that seems to be larger in hypercapnic COPD patients than in normocapnic patients. This increased respiratory drive is probably needed to overcome both increased airway resistance and mechanically disadvantaged respiratory muscles [26,29].

Neurological Diseases

Respiratory dysfunction may constitute an early and relatively major manifestation of several neurological disorders, including structural or degenerative ailments of the central or peripheral nervous system or metabolic encephalopathies [30]. Neuromuscular diseases are often associated with abnormalities of ventilatory control and their associated hypoventilation, particularly during sleep, and with a reduced ventilatory response to CO_2 and O_2 [30,31]. Such patients increase their respiratory rate rather than V_T in response to hypercapnia and hypoxaemia. This rapid and shallow breathing response is thought to be an attempted compensation aimed at increasing ventilation with minimal increase in the work of breathing. Tachypnoea may then worsen respiratory muscle fatigue, leading to a further reduction in tidal volume. Respiratory failure typically complicates advanced neuromuscular disease by compromising effective respiratory muscle function. Death in these patients is usually due to progressive respiratory failure and superimposed infections secondary to aspiration resulting from pharyngeal dysfunction [30,31].

Respiratory control may be affected acutely or subacutely, as in stroke or multiple sclerosis. Lesions affecting the PRG, DRG, VRG or chemoreceptors may express an abnormal respiratory rhythm, central alveolar hypoventilation or both. A unilateral lesion of the lateral medulla, including the VRG, leads to blunting of the ventilatory response to CO_2 and sleep apnoea syndrome, particularly when there is another predisposing factor such as nasal septum deviation. Cheyne-Stokes respiration typically accompanies bilateral infarcts of the cerebral hemispheres, but also occurs in infratentorial ischaemic stroke [30,31].

Multiple sclerosis (MS) may yield respiratory dysfunction, in general associated with large lesions involving the upper cervical cord or medulla. Acute demyelinating lesions involving the dorsolateral medulla may result in loss of automatic breathing, usually associated with impaired swallowing and cough reflex. Thus, there ensues a risk of aspiration pneumonia [30,31]. Paroxysmal hyperventilation may occur as a manifestation of an acute lesion in the upper brainstem. Bulbar weakness, leading to aspiration followed by bronchopneumonia, is common in the terminal stages of MS. More rarely, loss of response to CO_2 and hypercapnic respiratory insufficiency may occur early in the course of the disease [30,31].

Brainstem tumours may produce central neurogenic hyperventilation, central sleep apnoea, irregular breathing, short breath-holding time and apneustic breathing. Occasionally, abnormalities of respiratory control are the only manifestations of the tumour and resolve after its resection. Patients with severe traumatic brainstem or high cervical-cord injury may lose both voluntary and autonomic control of breathing. These patients require ventilatory support, which is given via a tracheostomy through which tracheal suction can also be performed [30,31].

Sudden Infant Death Syndrome

Sudden infant death syndrome (SIDS) is, according to the newly proposed definition: 'The sudden unexpected death of an infant <1 year of age, with onset of the fatal episode apparently occurring during sleep, that remains unexplained after a thorough investigation, including performance of a complete autopsy and review of the circumstances of death and the clinical history' [32]. Despite the fact that the diagnosis of SIDS originates from the exclusion of known causes of death, there are common features in most cases. These observations have led to the introduction of a triple-risk model for the understanding of SIDS. The model proposed in 1993 implies that SIDS only occurs if three conditions occur simultaneously: a vulnerable developmental stage of the CNS and the immune system;

predisposing factors, including a certain genetic pattern; and trigger events, such as sleeping position, maternal smoking, or infection [32]. Despite many studies in this area, the real aetiology of SIDS remains unknown.

Abnormal functioning of the central chemoreceptors represents one of the possible mechanisms generating SIDS. The recently born with apparently lethal episodes and the victims of SIDS studied before death presented a ventilatory pattern that was depressed with respect to the hypercapnic stimulus. Additionally, infants with episodes of apnoea in infancy present a slightly higher $PaCO_2$ as well as a lower sensibility to CO_2 as a trigger alert during sleep. The arcuate nuclei in the ventral medulla oblongata have been closely studied in SIDS victims. They are integrative sites for vital autonomic functions, including breathing and arousal, and are integrated with other regions that regulate arousal and autonomic chemosensory function. Quantitative three-dimensional anatomical studies indicated that some SIDS victims show hypoplasia of the arcuate nuclei, and as many as 56% of SIDS victims exhibit histopathological evidence of less extensive bilateral or unilateral hypoplasia. Studies on neurotransmission in the arcuate nuclei have also identified receptor abnormalities in some SIDS victims that involve several receptor types relevant to state-dependent autonomic control overall and to ventilatory and arousal responsiveness in particular. These deficits include significant decreases in binding to muscarinic, cholinergic and serotonergic receptors [33].

Cheyne-Stokes Respiration

Cheyne-Stokes respiration (CSR) with central sleep apnoea (CSA) is a breathing disorder seen in patients with advanced congestive heart failure (CHF). It is characterised by central apnoeas and hypopnoeas that alternate with periods of increasing-decreasing tidal volume. CSR-CSA has been associated with increases in sympathetic nervous activity in CHF patients, which is an important predictor of CHF progression, arrhythmias and mortality. Indeed, CSR-CSA, independent of other risk factors, elevates the risk of mortality in CHF by two- to three-fold. Successful treatment of CSR by continuous positive airway pressure (CPAP) leads to a significant reduction in sympathetic nervous activity and may reduce mortality by up to 40% in patients with CHF and CSR-CSA. Since CPAP has salutary effects on cardiac function (independent of its effect on CSR), it remains uncertain whether CSR-CSA is a mere phenomenon of a failing heart or a major contributor to poor outcomes in patients with CHF. Supplemental oxygen may be used as treatment and tends to eliminate or decrease CSR in CHF by eliminating hypoxaemia, which contributes to respiratory cycling [34]. The classic cases of CSR are caused by CNS dysfunction, such as a cerebrovascular accident. In this setting, CSR is usually associated with bilateral supramedullary damage in conjunction with a depressed level of consciousness, such as occurs during sleep, sedation or diffuse cortical injury [35].

References

1. Schwartzstein RM, Paker MJ (2006) Respiratory physiology. A clinical approach. Lippincott Williams & Wilkins, Philadelphia
2. Gallego J, Nsegbe E, Durand E (2001) Learning in respiratory control. Behav Modif 25:495–512
3. West JB (2000) Respiration physiology. 6th edition. Lippincott Williams & Wilkins, Philadelphia
4. Ganong WF (1993) Regulation of respiration. In: Review of medical physiology, 16th edition. Appleton & Lange, Norwalk, pp 611–619
5. Bee DH (1993) The carotid body: a review of its anatomy, physiology and clinical importance. Monaldi Arch Chest Dis 48:48–53
6. Comroe JH (1974) Physiology of respiration: an introductory text. 2nd Edition. Chicago: Yearbook Publishers, Chicago
7. Montaldo-Caruana B, Gleeson K, Zwillich CW (2000) The control of breathing in clinical practice. Chest 117:205–225
8. Gonzales C, Almara L, Obeso A et al (1192) Oxygen and acid chemoreception in the carotid body receptors. Trends Neurosci 15:146–153
9. Bruce EN, Cherniak NS (1987) Central chemoreceptors. J Appl Physiol 62:389–402
10. Bledsoe SW, Hornbein TF (1981) Central chemoreceptors and the regulation of their chemical environment. In: Hornbein TF (ed) Regulation of breathing (part I). Marcel Dekker, New York, pp 347–428
11. Manning HL, Schwartzstein RM (1995) Pathophysiology of dyspnea. N Engl J Med 333:547–553
12. Sant'Ambrogio G (1987) Nervous receptors of the tracheobronchial tree. Ann Rev Physiol 49:611–627
13. Widdicombe J (2006) Reflexes from the lungs and airways: historical perspective. J Appl Physiol 101:628–634
14. Sampson SR, Vidruk EH (1975) Properties of 'irritant' receptors in canine lungs. Respir Physiol 25:9–22
15. Sant'Ambrogio G (1982) Information arising from the tracheobronchial tree of mammals. Physiol Rev 62:531–569
16. Schwartzstein R, Lilly J, Israel E et al (1991) Breathlessness of asthma differs from that of external resistive loading. Am Rev Respir Dis 143(suppl):A596
17. Widdicombe, J (2001) Airway receptors. Respir Physiol 125:3–15
18. Mitchell RA, Berger AJ (1981) Neural regulation of respiration. In: Hornbein TF (ed) Regulation of breathing (part I). Marcel Dekker, New York, pp 541–620
19. Duron B (1981) Intercostal and diaphragmatic muscle endings and afferents. In: Hornbein TF (ed) Regulation of breathing (part I). Marcel Dekker, New York, pp 473–540
20. Berger AJ, Mitchell RA, Severinghaus JW (1977) Regulation of respiration, Part II. N Engl J Med 297:138–143
21. von Euler C (1983) On the central pattern generator for the basic breathing rhythmicity. J Appl Physiol 55:1647–1659
22. Mithoeffer JC (1964) Breath holding. In: Handbook of physiology: respiration (section 3, vol II). American Physiology Society, Washington, DC 38:1011–1025
23. Ramirez JM, Viemari JC (2005) Determinants of inspiratory activity. Respir Physiol Neurobiol 147:145–157
24. Adriaensen D, Brouns I, Pintelon I et al (2006) Evidence for a role of neuroepithelial bodies as complex airway sensors: Comparison with smooth muscle-associated airway receptors. J Appl Physiol 101:960–970
25. Ganong WF (1993) Pulmonary function. In: Review of medical physiology. 16th ed. Appleton & Lange, Norwalk, pp 587–603
26. Mountain R, Zwillich CW, Weil JV (1978) Hypoventilation in obstructive lung disease. N Engl J Med 298:521–525

27. Chan CS, Bye PTP, Woolcock AJ et al (1990) Eucapnia and hypercapnia in patients with chronic airflow limitation. Am Rev Respir Dis 141:861–866
28. Kalhoff H, Werkmiester F, Kiwull-Schone L et al (1994) The Haldane effect under different acid-base conditions in premature and adult humans. Adv Exp Med Biol 361:353–361
29. Gorini M, Spinelli A, Ginanni R et al (1990) Neural respiratory drive and neuromuscular coupling in patients with chronic obstructive pulmonary disease. Chest 98:1179–1186
30. Nogués MA, Roncoroni AJ, Benarroch E (2002) Breathing control in neurological diseases. Clin Auton Res 12:440–449
31. Johnson DC, Homeyoun K (1994) Central control of ventilation in neuromuscular disease. Clin Chest Med 15:607–615
32. Opdal SH, Rognum TO (2004) New insight into sudden infant-death syndrome. Lancet 364:825–826
33. Hunt CE (2005) Gene-environment interactions: implications for sudden unexpected deaths in infancy. Arch Dis Child 90:48–53
34. Sin DD, Man GCW (2003) Cheyne-Stokes respiration. A consequence of a broken heart? Chest 124:1627–1628
35. Hanly PJ, Zuberi-Khokhar S (1996) Increased mortality associated with Cheyne-Stokes respiration in patients with congestive heart failure. Am J Respir Crit Care Med 153:272–276

Elastic and Resistive Properties of the Respiratory System

W.A. Zin

Introduction

This chapter will consider basic aspects of respiratory-system mechanics in order to provide a background for the analysis of the most common disorders related to the elastic and resistive components of the lung and chest wall. Excellent reviews articles can be consulted, if further details are desired [1–9b].

The movements of the lungs are entirely passive. Forces must be applied to the respiratory system to move it from its resting position at the end of expiration. In spontaneous breathing, the respiratory muscles provide the external forces, whereas artificial ventilation moves the relaxed respiratory system. In either situation, movement depends on the impedance of the lung and chest wall, the two components of the respiratory system. This impedance stems mainly from the elastic and resistive mechanical properties that are found in the lung and in the chest wall. The inertial component of gas and tissue is usually negligible [10].

Elastic Properties

Both the lungs and the chest wall can be considered as elastic structures, with transmural pressure gradients corresponding to stress and lung volume to strain. Over a certain range of volumes and pressures, lung and chest-wall structures obey Hooke's law, and the change in lung and chest-wall volumes divided by the transmural pressures required to produce them defines the compliance (C). Elastance (E) is the reciprocal of compliance, i.e. $\Delta P/\Delta V$, and is usually expressed in cmH_2O per litre. Stiff structures present a high elastance. Respiratory-system elastance equals the sum of lung plus chest wall elastances (Ers=EL+Ew, respectively), whereas respiratory-system compliance is more complex: 1/Crs=1/CL+1/Cw.

U. Lucangelo, P. Pelosi, W.A. Zin, A. Aliverti (eds.) *Respiratory System and Artificial Ventilation*. © Springer 2008

Pleural Pressure

Since variations in lung and chest wall volumes are virtually identical, the compliances of the respiratory system, lung and chest wall vary according to the change in the transmural pressure (i.e. inside minus outside pressures) across these structures. Under static conditions, the distending pressure of the respiratory system (Prs), lung (PL) and chest wall (Pw) are (Fig. 1):

$$PL = Palv - Ppl \qquad \text{(Eq. 1)}$$

where Palv represents the alveolar pressure [which is equal to the airway pressure (Paw) or pressure at the airway opening (Pao) under static conditions and in the face of an open glottis] and Ppl stands for intrapleural pressure. PL is commonly referred to as the transpulmonary pressure:

$$Pw = Ppl - Pbs \qquad \text{(Eq. 2)}$$

where Pw represents the transthoracic or chest-wall pressure, and Pbs the pressure at the body surface (usually barometric pressure);

$$Prs = PL + Pw \qquad \text{(Eq. 3)}$$

or

$$Prs = Palv - Ppl + Ppl - Pbs = Palv - Pbs \qquad \text{(Eq. 4)}$$

As can be easily understood, precise determination of swings in intrapleural pressure is of paramount importance when it is necessary to divide respiratory

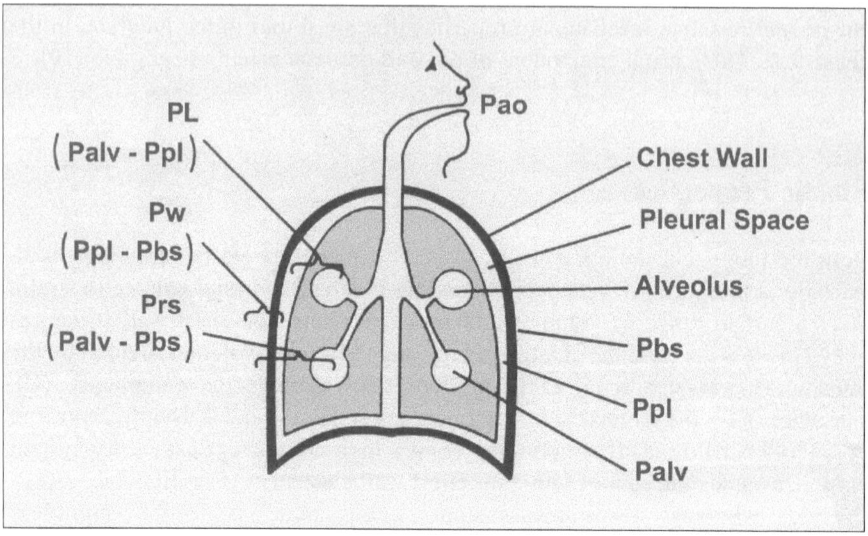

Fig. 1 Schematic representation of the structures and pressures involved in breathing. *Pao*, Pressure at the airway opening; *Pbs*, pressure at the body surface; *Ppl*, intrapleural pressure; *Palv*, alveolar pressure; *PL*, transpulmonary pressure; *Pw*, chest-wall pressure; *Prs*, pressure difference across the respiratory system

system mechanics into their lung and chest-wall components. However, in clinical practice, pleural pressure is rarely measured because of all the risks involved in the procedure. Instead, variations in oesophageal pressure (Poes) are determined as these reflect quite accurately the changes in pleural pressure. Usually a latex balloon or a liquid-filled catheter is placed in the lower third of the oesophagus and its correct positioning must be accomplished to achieve a perfect reading of the changes in intrathoracic pressure [11]. Complete descriptions of the techniques used to measure Poes can be found in the literature [12–14].

Elastic Recoil of the Lungs

The elastic recoil of the lungs tends to bring them down to their minimum volume. Accordingly, the elastic component (Pel,rs) of the total pressure applied to the respiratory system during inspiration is restored during expiration to promote expiration. In other words, the potential energy stored during inspiration returns to the system as kinetic energy. The passive volume–pressure curve of the lung is almost linear (constant compliance) up to volumes around 80% of the total lung volume. Beyond this point the curve flattens (compliance decreases) mainly because the elastic limit of the lung is approached and the structures stiffen. If transpulmonary pressure rises above 30 cmH_2O, the danger of tissue rupture may ensue.

Tissue Recoil

Two components account for the elastic recoil of the lungs [15]. One of them is represented by the elastic components of lung tissue (mainly collagenous and elastic fibres). It is believed that the elastic behaviour of the lung does not depend strongly on the elongation of these fibres, but mainly on their geometric arrangement. The network of pulmonary connective tissue interconnects all pulmonary structures (vessels, bronchioles, alveoli, and so forth) and, as a result, they dilate during inspiration. This phenomenon is known as interdependence and contributes to keep the alveoli open, since if some of them collapsed, their neighbours would tether their walls, tending to reopen them. In addition to their tissue elastic properties, the lungs present another component that contributes importantly to their elastic characteristics: the surface tension of the liquid lining the alveoli and distal air spaces.

Surface Tension

The air-liquid interface of the thin film of liquid that covers the surface of terminal respiratory units and probably also lines the luminal surface of terminal bronchioles displays surface tension, i.e. the molecules in the film attract each other along its surface. This component must also be overcome during inspiration:

energy is stored throughout inspiration and returned during expiration. Pure liquids and solutions present a constant surface tension and obey Laplace's law:

$$P = K \times T/R \qquad \text{(Eq. 5)}$$

where P corresponds to the pressure inside a sphere, T represents the tension on its wall, and R equals its radius. K corresponds to a constant. Thus, if two soap (constant T) bubbles with different radii are connected, the one with the shorter radius (and higher internal pressure) will empty into the one with a larger radius (with a smaller internal pressure) until the two pressures become equal. If the same behaviour were found in the lung, one would expect that a great deal of its 300 million alveoli would discharge their gas content into the larger ones, yielding massive atelectasis.

The liquid lining the terminal air spaces, however, is not a simple saline solution (constant T). Type II pneumocytes constantly secrete into this liquid layer a mixture of lipids (90%) and proteins (10%). As a result, the surface tension decreases well below that of a simple saline solution, both in large and in small alveoli [16,17], as shown in Fig. 2. Furthermore, the surface tension varies remarkably as the area of the surface layer changes, so that T and R in Laplace's equation vary proportionately and P remains equal in all alveoli. Larger alveoli have a higher surface tension than their smaller neighbours and the danger of

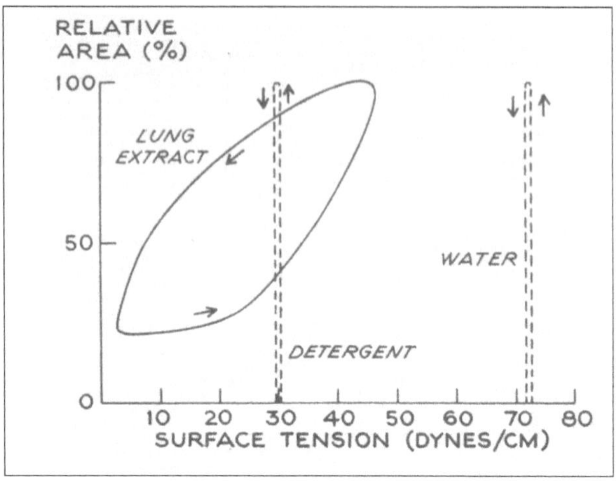

Fig. 2 Relative area of liquid films plotted against surface tension during a cycle of compression and expansion of the film. The surface tension of water is constant and approximates 72 dynes/cm, whereas detergent exhibits the same behaviour but a lower surface tension, circa 30 dynes/cm. The liquid obtained after rinsing the lung with warm (37°C) saline solution (0.9% NaCl) has a surface tensions that varies from about 5 to 45 dynes/cm during the compression-decompression cycle. Note that (1) at any relative area the surface tension of the lung extract is smaller than that of the water; (2) the lung extract shows a positive association between area and tension and (3) the lung extract displays hysteresis, i.e. the expansion and compression limbs are not superimposable

atelectasis is avoided [18], as can be inferred from Fig. 2. Pulmonary hysteresis constitutes the third phenomenon resulting from the presence of the surfactant lining the alveoli, i.e. if the lung is slowly inflated from its degassed volume up to total lung capacity and subsequently deflated, two diverse limbs will result: an inspiratory limb, which is lower and to the right of the expiratory one (Fig. 2).

The lung is known to be active in the synthesis of fatty acids, lipid esterification, hydrolysis of lipid-ester bonds and the oxidation of fatty acids [19]. Type II pneumocytes represent the main site of release of surfactant, which they otherwise store in their lamellar bodies. Surfactant undergoes a constant turnover, with some molecules leaving the surface film and other recently synthesised ones added to it.

The role of surfactant can be easily appreciated by means of a simple experiment. Excised and degassed lungs are stepwise inflated with known gas volumes. At each step, airway pressure is also measured. After the total lung capacity is reached, known gas volumes are removed while the pressures continue to be determined. In the end, the V-P curve 2 in Fig. 3 results. Note that the inspiratory and expiratory limbs are not superimposable, thereby characterising the pulmonary hysteresis. After this step in the experiment, the lungs are filled with warm (37°C) saline solution (0.9% NaCl) and the aforementioned inflation and deflation manoeuvres are repeated. In this case, the hysteresis results are practically negligible. Furthermore, a smaller pressure is required to totally inflate the lung (Fig. 3, curve 1). It should be kept in mind that when the lungs are inflated

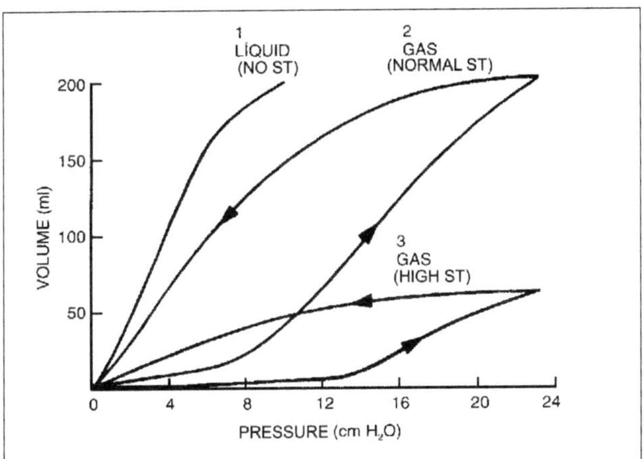

Fig. 3 Static volume-pressure relationships in isolated lungs. The curves comprise points from the minimum volume up to the total lung capacity during inflation and deflation. *Curve 2* represents the V-P relationship gathered from a normal lung (normal surface tension of the liquid lining the alveoli). If the same lung is filled and deflated with warm (37°C) saline solution (0.9% NaCl), surface tension disappears because the air-liquid interface does not exist, and hysteresis tends to minute values (*curve 1*). Finally, if the lung is rinsed with warm saline solution (surfactant removal) and submitted to the same cycle, the surface tension increases and many alveoli collapse, as displayed by the small volume achieved at total lung capacity

with a liquid, surface tension disappears as a consequence of the absence of the air-liquid interface. Some conclusions stem from these experiments: (1) in the absence of surface tension lung compliance is higher than in the aerated normal lung; (2) pulmonary hysteresis is almost exclusively due to the surface tension of the air-liquid interface; (3) the pressure required to overcome tissue tension at any lung volume corresponds to the horizontal distance between the ordinate and curve 1 (Fig. 3); and (4) at any lung volume additional energy is required to overcome surface tension (distance between curves 1 and 2 in Fig. 3). In order to stress the importance of the surfactant, curve 3 (Fig. 3) represents a condition in which the lung is filled with air, but no surfactant lines the alveoli. It can be seen that the end-inspiratory lung volume in this case lies well below that obtained in the normal lung, because of a large amount of atelectatic alveoli.

In summary, the lung component of the elastic pressure (part of the total applied pressure) developed by the respiratory muscles or by a ventilator during inspiration overcomes two pulmonary elastic components: tissue forces and surface forces.

Elastic Recoil of the Chest Wall

The chest wall comprises all the structures that move during the breathing cycle except the lungs. Thus, it includes the diaphragm, the abdominal wall and the mediastinum, in addition to the thorax. A simple experiment can clarify this assertion: a person lies in the supine position and to inspire his/her diaphragm must produce some force (work) to push caudally the abdominal contents and outwards the abdominal wall. If a 10-kg weight is placed on the top of the abdominal wall, the neuromuscular drive to the diaphragm will increase in order to cope with the added elastic load. Hence, any change in the abdominal wall will induce mechanical modifications in the respiratory system.

Naturally, the chest wall also exhibits elastic properties. It can be depicted for schematic purposes as a compressible and distensible structure that contains an appreciable volume in its resting state [20]. While the lung always tends to retract to its minimum volume, the elastic properties of the chest wall expand it from its residual volume up to about 75% of vital capacity. From this point onwards, the elastic forces of the chest wall change direction and favour its closure [20]. To calculate chest-wall elastance (Ew), transthoracic pressure (= Ppl – Pbs) is divided by the change in lung volume. As in the case of lung compliance, there is an elastic limit to the chest wall. From total lung capacity down to approximately 20% of the vital capacity, chest-wall compliance (Cw) is fairly constant. Below this point, it decreases progressively with the fall in lung volume.

The ability to determine elastance/compliance yields important clinical information, since the elastic behaviour of the chest wall can be affected by a series of pathological conditions, e.g. ascites, obesity, extremely voluminous breasts, vertebral ankylosis and severe kyphoscoliosis.

Elastic Recoil of the Respiratory System

For didactic purposes it is useful to describe the recoil characteristics of the lungs and chest wall separately, but obviously they have to be appraised together. The two structures are in series with each other and, therefore, the elastic pressure of the total respiratory system (Pel,rs) constitutes the sum of the elastic pressures of the lung and chest wall (Pel,L and Pel,w, respectively). Thus, the respiratory system volume-pressure curve has an S-shaped profile: it is limited at high lung volumes by the fall in lung compliance and at low lung volumes by the smaller compliance of the chest wall. In a normal adult, the expanding tendency of the chest wall exactly counterbalances lung recoil at a lung volume approximating 35% of its vital capacity. This point on the V-P curve of the respiratory system represents the functional residual capacity and the system is said to be at its elastic equilibrium point. In other words, to inflate the lung above FRC an inspiratory force must be applied, whereas exhalation below FRC demands an expiratory force.

Since the lungs and chest wall recoil in opposite directions, forces tending to separate the visceral from the parietal pleura result. If the pleural surface is considered as a continuum, a virtual closed space (pleural space) is formed. A small amount of liquid exists in this space, which allows not only the coupling of visceral and parietal pleurae, thus yielding the transmission of forces between the two structures, but also generates a lubricated system that allow the free and rapid movement of the lung in relation to the chest wall. Measurement of the intrapleural pressure at the elastic equilibrium point of the respiratory system (FRC) yields a sub-atmospheric value, normally around -4 cmH_2O. This 'negative' pressure reflects the net result of the forces acting on the pleurae (lung recoil and chest-wall expansion). During spontaneous inspiration, muscle contraction expands the chest wall and the parietal pleura pulls away from the visceral leaflet. As a result, Ppl becomes more negative, reaching values around -7 or -8 cmH_2O during resting tidal breathing. Naturally, during expiration it returns to its resting value. Intrapleural pressure may, however, become positive; for instance, it may increase during the augmented ventilation resulting from physical exertion or during cough. Under these conditions, muscle force is directed to quickly diminish lung volume and the parietal pleura compresses the visceral one. Intrapleural pressure can also increase and become positive during artificial ventilation, as the positive pressure in the airways pushes the visceral pleura against the parietal leaflet.

Intrapleural pressure should not be confounded with alveolar pressure. During spontaneous tidal breathing, Palv can reach -2 cmH_2O at mid-inspiration and rise to +2 cmH_2O at mid-expiration. When airflow is null (end-inspiration and end-expiration), Palv equals Pbs. Palv is generated during inspiration as a result of inspiratory muscle contraction and the ensuing dilatation of air spaces. However, there is a resistance opposing the fast inlet of gas, and, hence, Palv decreases. During expiration the process is inverted.

Resistive Properties

So far we have dealt with pressures related solely to the elastic properties of the respiratory system, hence depending on the gas volume and the elastance of each component of the system, i.e., lung and chest wall. Pressure gradients generated by pure elastic forces are static and, thus, independent of the existence of airflow.

When the respiratory system moves an additional mechanical element must be overcome by the driving force of the system: resistance or resistive pressure. Respiratory system resistance (Rrs) can be measured by dividing Pres,rs by airflow, where Pres,rs represents the respiratory system resistive pressure, or, in other words, the pressure used to overcome its resistive elements. Airway resistance and the resistance offered by the lung and chest wall tissues contribute to Rrs. Rrs can be divided into RL (pulmonary resistance) and Rw (chest wall resistance).

Pulmonary Resistance

Pulmonary resistance can be subdivided into airway resistance and lung tissue resistance.

Airway resistance

Airway resistance (Raw) depends on the airflow in the lungs. Since air is a fluid, the concepts of fluid dynamics can be directly applied to Raw. Thus, Raw can be defined as the ratio between the pressure gradient necessary to move gas from room air to the alveoli and airflow.

If air flows in a tube, there is a pressure difference (ΔP) between the two extremities of the tube. This pressure gradient will depend on the airflow (V') and its characteristics. In the face of low airflows, the gas molecules move smoothly along the entire length of the tube with different velocities. This constitutes the laminar flow and can be depicted as a series of parallel ring-like sheets of fluid sliding past each other. The more external fluid sheet has a longer perimeter (and surface) and, as a consequence, a higher shear force; its velocity will be small. In contrast, the central sheet has a minute area and, thus, a higher velocity of the fluid. In the face of laminar flow resistance equals ΔP/V'.

According to Hagen-Poiseuille's law:

$$\Delta P = (V' \times 8 \times \eta \times L)/(\pi \times r^4) \qquad \text{(Eq. 6)}$$

and

$$R = (8 \times \eta \times L)/(\pi \times r^4) \qquad \text{(Eq. 7)}$$

where η represents the gas viscosity, L is the length of the tube, and r corresponds to the tube radius. It can be readily appreciated that the radius of the airways represents the main component of airway resistance since it is raised to the power of 4. Accordingly, if the radius of the tube is halved, ΔP should be multiplied by 16 ($=2^4$), if the same airflow is to be maintained.

If airflow increases, the gas molecules lose their laminar arrangement and turbulence ensues. This random movement of the gas molecules is called turbulent flow. The pressure required to maintain this flow is substantially larger than that necessary to maintain a laminar flow. Under these conditions, the driving pressure is proportional to the square of the flow:

$$\Delta P = K_2 \times V'^2 \quad \text{(Eq. 8)}$$

Turbulent flow depends on the density of the gas but not on its viscosity.

The tracheobronchial tree represents a complicated system of tubes with many branching points, changes in diameter and irregular surfaces. In a system, such as the lung, that branches out quite rapidly, laminar flow occurs solely in the small airways. Over the major portion of the tree, flow is transitional, and Rohrer's equation, in which resistive pressure is determined by flow and also by its square, should be employed:

$$Pres = K_1 \times V' + K_2 \times V'^2 \quad \text{(Eq. 9)}$$

where K_1 relates to the laminar flow and K_2 to the turbulent component. Thus, for the same driving pressure, if no turbulence occurs, the second component of the equation becomes null, and all the pressure produces airflow. However, in the presence of turbulence, the same pressure must be split between the two components and less energy is available to generate airflow, since part of it will be spent as heat by the turbulent flow [21].

Since the radius constitutes the most important factor determining resistance through a tube, the cross-sectional area of each branching generation of the tracheobronchial tree was thoroughly measured. Interestingly, the narrower segment of the tree occurs in the central airways, somewhere around the segmental–subsegmental bronchi [22]. As a result, Raw is much higher in the central bronchi than at the lung periphery, which explains the difficulty in measuring peripheral airway resistance.

Pulmonary Tissue Resistance

Pulmonary tissue resistance results from the energy loss generated by the viscosity pertaining to the movement of lung tissue itself. In other words, the molecules that constitute the tissue burn energy as heat as they move past each other. Previously, tissue resistance was regarded as negligible, but it is now known to be highly dependent on inspiratory duration [23], volume and flow [24–26].

Chest-Wall Resistance

The shear forces that develop during movement of the chest-wall tissues determine chest-wall resistance. Similar to pulmonary tissue resistance, chest-wall tissue resistance depends on volume and airflow [26–28]. Chest-wall resistance is not negligible in normal subjects and may account for a substantial amount of energy expenditure in pathological conditions that compromise the unhindered movement of the chest wall.

Respiratory-System Resistance

Respiratory-system resistance is the net result of the pulmonary plus chest-wall resistances. It thus follows that the simple measurement of Rrs may blunt the diagnosis of an important condition that could be localised in the abdomen, for instance.

Work of Breathing

Work may be defined as the cumulative result (till end-inspiration, for example) of the product volume × pressure measured at every instant during the breathing cycle ($W = \int P \times dV$). In the respiratory system there are two kinds of work: elastic and resistive. The former always stores potential energy in the elastic pulmonary and chest-wall tissues, whereas the latter dissipates energy as heat.

Elastic Work

The amount of work done to overcome the elastic recoil of the chest wall, lung parenchyma and alveolar surface tension is evaluated as elastic work. It is not burned during inspiration but rather stored as potential energy that will provide the kinetic energy to promote expiration. The elastic work of the respiratory system (Wel,rs) can be defined as:

$$Wel,rs = \int Pel,rs \times dV \qquad \text{(Eq. 10)}$$

It can also be calculated more simply by recording a static V-P curve. As the lung inflates, the V-P curve draws the hypotenuse of a triangle that lies on the ordinate and whose area represents elastic work (Fig. 4). Naturally Wel,L (pulmonary elastic work) and Wel,w (chest wall elastic work) can also be measured.

Resistive Work

Respiratory-system resistive work (Wres,rs) can be defined as:

$$Wres,rs = \int Pres,rs \times dV \qquad \text{(Eq. 11)}$$

Wres can be calculated using the dynamic V-P curve of the respiratory system or its pulmonary and chest-wall components. The dynamic V-P curve is spindle-shaped and Wres corresponds to the area to the right of the elastic work, as depicted in Fig. 4. The total work of breathing equals the sum of the elastic work and the resistive work (areas 1 plus area 2, Fig. 4).

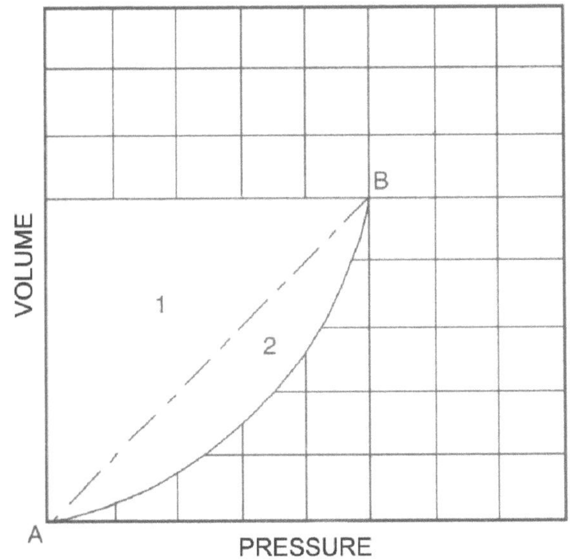

Fig. 4 Volume-pressure curve during inspiration. The triangular area *1* corresponds to elastic work and area *2* to inspiratory resistive work

References

1. Mead J (1961) Mechanical properties of lungs. Physiol Rev 41:281–330
2. Fenn WO, Rahn H (eds) (1964) Handbook of physiology, Section 3, Respiration, Volume 1. American Physiological Society, Washington, DC, pp 357–476
3. Campbell EJM, Agostoni E, Davis JN (eds) (1970) The respiratory muscles: mechanics and neural control. Lloyd-Luke, London
4. Hoppin Jr FG, Hildebrandt J (1977) Mechanical properties of the lung. In: West JB (ed) Bioengineering aspects of the lung. Marcel Dekker, Inc, New York, pp 83–162
5. McFadded Jr ER, Ingram Jr RH (1980) Clinical application and interpretation of airway physiology. In: Nadel JA (ed) Physiology and pharmacology of the airways. Marcel Dekker, New York, pp 297–324
6. Forster II RE, DuBois AB, Briscoe WA, Fisher AB (eds) (1986) The lung: physiologic basis of pulmonary function tests. Year Book Medical Publishers, Chicago, pp 65–114
7. Macklem PT, Mead J (eds) (1986) Handbook of physiology, Section 3, The respiratory system, Volume III. American Physiological Society, Bethesda, pp 113–461
8. Milic-Emili J (eds) (1999) Respiratory mechanics. European Respiratory Society, Leeds
9a. Milic-Emili J, Lucangelo U, Pesenti A, Zin WA (eds) (1999) Basics of respiratory mechanics and artificial ventilation. Springer, Milan
9b. Hamid Q, Shannon J, Martin J (eds) (2005) Physiologic basis of respiratory disease. BC Dekker, Inc, Hamilton, pp 15–131
10. Rodarte JR, Rehder K (1986) Dynamics of respiration. In: Macklem PT, Mead J (eds) Handbook of physiology, Section 3, The respiratory system, Volume III. American Physiological Society, Bethesda, pp 131–144

11. Baydur A, Behrakis PK, Zin WA et al (1982) Simple method for assessing the validity of the esophageal balloon technique. Am Rev Respir Dis 126:788–791
12. Milic-Emili J, Mead J, Turner JM, Glauser EM (1964) Improved technique for estimating pleural pressure from esophageal balloons. J Appl Physiol 19:207–211
13. Zin WA, Milic-Emili J (1998) Esophageal pressure measurement. In: Tobin MJ (ed) Principles and practice of intensive care monitoring. McGraw-Hill, New York, pp 545–552
14. Zin WA, Milic-Emili (2005) Esophageal pressure measurement. In: Hamid Q, Shannon J, Martin J (eds) Physiologic basis of respiratory disease. BC Dekker, Hamilton, pp 639–647
15. von Neergaard K (1929) Neue Auffassungen über einen Grundbegriff der Atemmechanik. Die Retraktionskraft der Lunge, abhängig von der Oberflächenspannung in den Alveolen. Z Ges Exp Med 66:373–394
16. Pattle RE (1955) Properties, function and origin of the alveolar lining fluid. Nature 175:1125–1126
17. Brown ES, Johnson RP, Clements JA (1959) Pulmonary surface tension. J Appl Physiol 14:717–720
18. Schurch S, Goerke J, Clements JA (1976) Direct determination of surface tension in the lung. Prof Natl Acad Sci USA 73:4698–4708
19. King RJ, Clements JA (1985) Lipid synthesis and surfactant turnover in the lungs. In: Fishman AP, Fisher AB (eds) Handbook of physiology, Section 3, The respiratory system, Volume I. American Physiological Society, Bethesda, pp 309–336
20. Rahn H, Otis AB, Chadwick LE, Fenn WO (1946) The pressure–volume diagram of the thorax and lung. Am J Physiol 146:161–178
21. Rohrer F (1915) Der Strömungswiderstand der unregelmässigen Verzweigung des Bronchialsystems auf den Atmungsverlauf in verschiedenen Lungenbezirken. Pfluegers Arch 162:225–299
21. Rocco PRM, Zin WA (1995) Modelling the mechanical effects of tracheal tubes on normal subjects. Eur Respir J 8:121–126
22. Pedley TJ, Schroter RC, Sudlow MF (1970) The prediction of pressure drop and variation of resistance within the human bronchial airways. Respir Physiol 9:387–405
23. Similowski T, Levy P, Corbeil C et al (1989) Viscoelastic behavior of lung and chest wall in dogs determined by flow interruption. J Appl Physiol 67:2219–2229
24. Kochi T, Okubo S, Zin WA, Milic-Emili J (1988) Flow and volume dependence of pulmonary mechanics in anesthetized cats. J Appl Physiol 64:441–450
25. Auler Jr JOC, Saldiva PHN, Carvalho CR et al (1990) Flow and volume dependence of respiratory system mechanics during constant flow ventilation in normal subjects and in adult respiratory distress syndrome. Crit Care Med 18:1080–1086
26. D'Angelo E, Robatto FM, Calderini E et al (1991) Pulmonary and chest wall mechanics in anesthetized paralyzed humans. J Appl Physiol 70:2602–2610
27. Kochi T, Okubo S, Zin WA, Milic-Emili J (1988) Chest wall and respiratory system mechanics in cats: effects of flow and volume. J Appl Physiol 64:2636–2646
28. D'Angelo E, Prandi E, Tavola M et al (1994) Chest wall interrupter resistance in anesthetized paralyzed humans. J Appl Physiol 77:883–887

Flow Limitation and its Determination

W.A. Zin, V.R. Cagido

The Maximum Expiratory Flow-Volume Relation

During expiration, there is a maximum limit to the gas flow rate that can be achieved; once this limit is attained, greater muscular effort does not further augment flow. This phenomenon, known as expiratory flow limitation (EFL), has been identified from flow-volume curves. The key documentation was made by Fry and co-workers [1,2], who identified EFL from iso-volume pressure-flow relationships. To obtain such curves, flow, volume and oesophageal pressure (i.e. pleural pressure) were simultaneously measured in subjects seated in a volume displacement plethysmograph, which corrects for gas compression. The subjects were instructed to perform repeated vital capacity manoeuvres with varying amounts of effort. The highest flow obtained at each lung volume was then plotted against pleural pressure, as shown in Fig. 1 (left). It can be seen that at high lung volumes (e.g. 90% of vital capacity) expiratory flow is not limited; however, at volumes <80–85%, vital capacity plateaus occur, indicating maximum flow limitation. A maximum expiratory flow–volume curve (Fig. 1, right) can be easily constructed from the iso-volume flow-pressure curves depicted in the left panel of Fig. 1. After peak flow is achieved, flow decreases with volume but it always reflects the maximum attainable flow at that particular lung volume. If the expiratory flow generated during tidal respiration represents the maximal possible flow someone can generate at that volume, this subject is said to be flow limited [3].

Mechanics of Expiratory Flow Limitation

The explanation behind the occurrence of EFL involves airways compliance [4,5]. The basic mechanism is a coupling between airway wall compression and the pressure drop that occurs along the airways. The first attempt to explain EFL

U. Lucangelo, P. Pelosi, W.A. Zin, A. Aliverti (eds.) *Respiratory System and Artificial Ventilation*. © Springer 2008

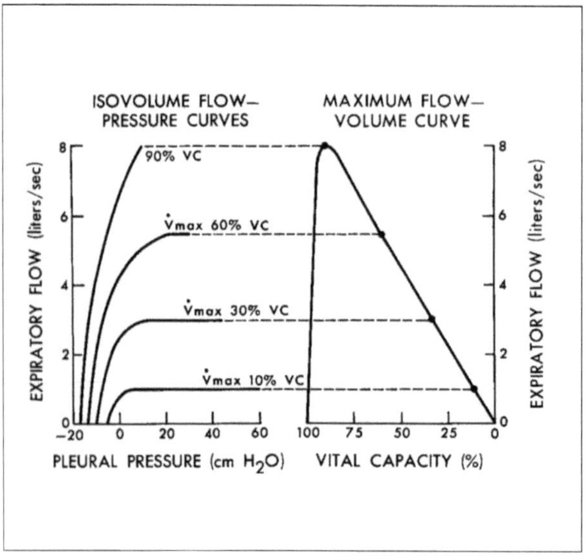

Fig. 1 *Left* Iso-volume pressure-flow relationships. Flow, volume, and oesophageal pressure were simultaneously measured in subjects seated in a volume-displacement plethysmograph. Repeated vital capacity manoeuvres with varying amounts of effort were performed. The highest flow obtained at each lung volume was then plotted against pleural pressure. *Right* Maximum expiratory flow-volume curve constructed from the iso-volume flow-pressure curves depicted on the *left*

derived from two simultaneously proposed models: the equal pressure point model [6] and the Starling resistor model [7].

Equal Pressure Point Theory

The driving pressure for expiration is the sum of the lung elastic recoil pressure, P_L, (e.g. 10 cmH_2O) and the pleural pressure, which is augmented during forced expiration (e.g. +10 cmH_2O), adding up to an elevated alveolar pressure (i.e. +20 cmH_2O). Progressive dissipation of the total pressure to overcome flow resistance occurs along the airways up to their opening (where pressure is null). Thus, it follows that there must exist a point (or points) somewhere along the intrathoracic airway at which the airway intraluminal pressure equals the pleural pressure (assuming that peribronchial and pleural pressures are very similar)–this is the equal pressure point. When expiratory flow increases to levels at which EFL occurs and the expiratory muscles generate a transpulmonary pressure exceeding the minimal pressure necessary to produce maximal flow, the airways undergo dynamic compression downstream to the equal pressure point, since extraluminal pressure surpasses its intraluminal counterpart [8,9]. Under these conditions, maximum flow at a given volume is reached, and the driving pressure of the upstream segment is the elastic recoil pressure of the lung. In addition, the resistance to flow is generated in the airway segment that leads from the alveoli to the equal pressure point (Fig. 2).

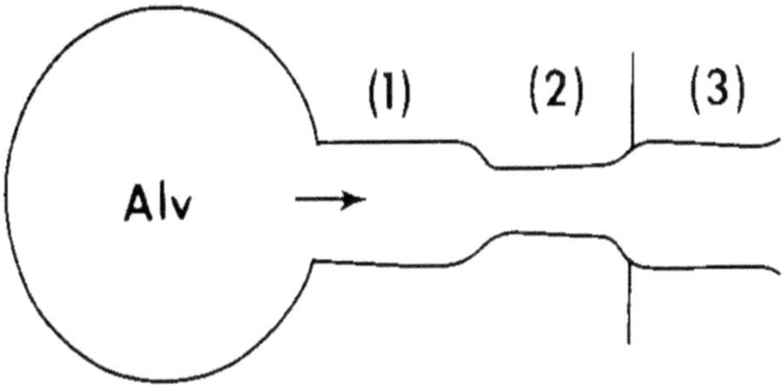

Fig. 2 The airways within the respiratory system. A progressive dissipation of the total pressure occurs along the airways to overcome flow resistance up to their opening. Distal airways are sustained by the tethering of the surrounding tissue (interdependence) and are thus stable (region 1). Somewhere along the intrathoracic airways, the airway intraluminal pressure equals the pleural pressure (region 2)—this is the equal pressure point. Downstream from this point, the airways undergo dynamic compression and the maximum flow at a given volume is reached. In addition, the resistance to flow is generated in the airway segment that leads from the alveoli to the equal pressure point. The intracranial airways cannot be compressed because of their anatomical location (region 3)

Starling Resistor Theory

In this case, flow limitation is likened to the behaviour of a Starling resistor, with the upstream driving pressure being the lung elastic recoil pressure plus a critical transmural pressure (i.e. the difference between internal lateral and external pressures). Note that if this critical pressure is nil, the model reduces to the equal pressure point one. Mechanisms influencing the decrease of transmural pressure in quasi-static conditions (i.e. loss of pressure due to frictional and turbulent dissipation of gas energy, convective acceleration, and flow velocity approaching wave-speed propagation along the airway) will result in a drop of internal pressure and then narrowing of the elastic airway [10–12]. The Starling resistor theory stresses the importance of the compressibility and tone of the flow-limiting segment.

Hence, both theories consider that: (1) towards the mouth, the intrathoracic airways become narrowed distally to a given point according to the transmural pressure compressing them; (2) the principal driving pressure at maximal flow is the lung elastic recoil pressure.

Convective Acceleration

The equal pressure point and the Starling resistor theories, although providing very important insights into the phenomenon, do not fully explain EFL [13]. Fry, in 1968 [14], pointed out that if the total cross-sectional area of the bronchial tree (A) could be defined as a function of transpulmonary pressure (PL) and position along the tree (x), then:

$$A = f(PL,x) \qquad \text{(Eq. 1)}$$

And if the pressure gradient (dP/dx) in the airways could be described as a function of area, position, and flow (V'):

$$dP/dx = f(A,x,V') \qquad \text{(Eq. 2)}$$

then for a given flow this coupled set of equations could, in principle, be integrated from the alveoli to the trachea.

Attention was then directed to the possibility that there might be localised mechanisms that were dominant in producing flow limitation. It was thus postulated that most of the frictional pressure loss occurs in the periphery and the convective acceleration pressure drop take place mainly in the central airways [15–17].

Positive convective acceleration occurs when the cross-sectional area of a tube decreases and the volume flow rate remains constant. Thus, in the narrower segment the fluid velocity rises and is accelerated; hence (from Bernoulli's theorem) the kinetic energy rises at the expense of a decrease in pressure (potential energy).

The transmural airway pressure (P_{TM}) can then be expressed as:

$$P_{TM} = PL - \Delta P_f - \rho(/A)^2/2 \qquad \text{(Eq. 3)}$$

where ΔP_f is the frictional pressure loss, ρ is gas density and the third term on the right is the pressure loss at the junction between two generations due to convective acceleration, i.e. the Bernoulli effect. If there is no flow, transmural pressure equals recoil pressure and the airway is expanded. However, the existence of airflow implies a condition in which transmural pressure is less than recoil pressure and therefore the area of the airway diminishes.

The approach described by Eq. 3 was tested in excised human lungs. A very good agreement between measured maximal flows and those predicted by this equation was found over two-thirds of the vital capacity but was weak at low lung volumes [18]. Indeed, it is now accepted that there are two basic flow-limiting mechanisms: (1) the wave-speed mechanism resulting from the coupling between airway compliance and the pressure drop due to the convective acceleration of the flow and (2) the coupling between airway compliance and viscous flow losses.

Wave-Speed Limitation

The airways are most compliant at transmural pressures near zero and become progressively stiffer at large positive transmural pressures. It has been recognised that the lung, like other systems, cannot present a greater flow velocity than the speed at which a mechanical disturbance travels along the walls of a compliant tube [10,19]. Thus, a maximal expiratory flow is reached when the velocity of air matches the speed of wave propagation at some point in the intrathoracic airways [20]. This flow-limiting site is the critical or choke point. A very recent work using a model-based method to analyse flow limitation in the heterogeneous human lung supported the hypothesis that the most probable locations of the choke points in the bronchial tree are the regions of the airway junctions [12]. Wave speed decreases with an increase in the density of the fluid, a decrease in the cross-sectional area of the tubes and an increase in the compliance of their walls. When the wave speed no longer exceeds the speed of expiratory flow, the system operates like a Starling resistor, and flow becomes independent of downstream pressure.

According to Mead's analysis [21], there are three features that contribute to a gradient of decreasing wave-speed during expiration, as the gas travels from the alveoli to the airway opening: (1) decreasing transmural pressure, (2) decreasing cross-sectional area and (3) a mechanical interdependence that stiffens intrapulmonary airways more than extrapulmonary ones.

Viscous Flow Limitation

At low lung volumes, the driving pressure is small, the viscosity dependence of maximal flow predominates over density dependence and the wave-speed concept is less applicable. A purely viscous flow limitation in a compliant tube has been reported [11]: if the cross-sectional area of the airways remained circular and flow were small, the pressure drop in the airways could be described by Hagen-Poiseuille's equation. It could thus be demonstrated that if upstream pressure is held constant while downstream pressure falls, V' approaches a limiting value. In conclusion, a wave-speed mechanism is responsible for flow limitation for most of vital capacity and viscous pressure dissipation for the last part of the forced expiration [12]

Determination of Airflow Limitation

Direct assessment of EFL requires the determination of iso-volume relationships between flow and transpulmonary pressure, an approach that is technically complex, time-consuming and invasive, because it requires measurement of oesophageal pressure [22,23]. As a result, detection of flow limitation is generally based on comparison of tidal and maximal flow-volume curves [22]. In this approach, a flow-volume loop of a tidal breath is accurately superimposed within a maximal flow-volume loop. If tidal flow meets or exceeds the expiratory boundary of the maximal flow-volume curve, then a flow limitation is characterised [24]. However, apart from the fact that flow-volume curves should actually be measured with a body plethysmograph [25], there are additional factors that make assessment of flow limitation based on comparison of tidal and maximal flow-volume curves problematic. It remains controversial how to best define the maximal expiratory flow compared with the tidal flow-volume loop, since the former is influenced by: (1) changes in airway resistance and static lung recoil owing to the maximal inspiration prior to the forced vital capacity manoeuvre [26]; and (2) time-dependent lung emptying due to time-constant inequality [27] and (3) viscoelastic forces [28] within the lung.

An alternative technique to detect EFL is the negative expiratory pressure (NEP) method [29,30], which does not require forced vital capacity manoeuvres or a body plethysmograph. It consists in applying a negative pressure to the mouth during expiration and comparing the ensuing flow-volume curve with that of the previous control expiration. The increase in the expiratory driving pressure owing to the application of NEP enhances expiratory flow if the subject is not flow limited, whereas in flow-limited patients flow does not change, independently of the NEP value (typically set at -3 to -10 cmH_2O) [24]. The technique has been applied to spontaneously breathing COPD patients at rest [30] and during exercise [31], after lung transplantation [32], in asthma [33], restrictive respiratory disorders [34], infants [35] and elderly patients [36], and to evaluate the relationship between chronic dyspnoea and EFL [37]. NEP was also valuable in detecting EFL during the mechanical ventilation of patients with acute ventilatory failure [29]. Application of pulses of negative pressure has been shown to be a simple method for on-line recognition of whether a forced vital capacity manoeuvre is performed with sufficient effort to achieve flow limitation [38].

There is a potential limitation of NEP concerning normal snorers and patients with obstructive sleep apnoea-hypopnoea syndromes since the technique may cause upper airway collapse, resulting in a false comparison with spontaneous expiration [39,40]. Other limitations of the NEP method are the inability to detect changes in end-expiratory lung volume and the ‘all or none’ quantification of EFL [24,39].

Another non-invasive test to detect EFL at rest and during exercise is manual compression of the abdomen concomitantly with the onset of expiration [41]. As in the NEP technique, the resulting expiratory flow-volume loop recorded at the mouth is superimposed on the preceding tidal breath. This method has not been widely applied despite its relative simplicity [42].

Recently, the forced oscillation technique has been used in the detection of EFL [43]. Normally, oscillatory pressures generated by a loudspeaker system at the mouth are transmitted throughout the respiratory system and, by studying the resulting pressures that are in and out of phase with the signal, both the respiratory system resistance and reactance can be computed. In the presence of EFL, the oscillatory pressure will no longer reach the alveoli and the reactance will reflect the mechanical properties of the airway wall rather than those of the whole respiratory system. As a result, reactance becomes much more negative and there is a clear difference between within-breath inspiration and expiration [42,43].

Finally, theoretical and mathematical models derived from the symmetrical lung description of Weibel [44], or the asymmetric structure of the bronchial tree reported by Horsfield et al. [45] were recently proposed [12,46,47]. These non-linear morphological models of respiratory mechanics include both the wave-speed and viscous mechanisms limiting expiratory flow. They have been used to simulate EFL conditions, especially under mechanical ventilation [48], to track the locations of the choke points, to identify flow limitation degree and regime as well as to investigate the arrangement of the flow-limiting sites [12] and to simulate different pathophysiological conditions [49,50].

References

1. Fry DL, Ebert RV, Stead WW et al (1954) The mechanics of pulmonary ventilation in normal subjects and in patients with emphysema. Am J Med 16:80–97
2. Fry DL, Hyatt RE (1960) Pulmonary mechanics: a unified analysis of the relationship between pressure, volume and gas flow in the lungs of normal and diseased human subjects. Am J Med 29:672–689
3. O'Donnell DE, Parker CM (2006) COPD exacerbations 3: pathophysiology. Thorax 61:354–361
4. Dayman H (1951) Mechanics of airflow in health and in emphysema. J Clin Invest 30:1175–1190
5. Fry DL (1958) Theoretical considerations of the bronchial pressure-flow-volume relationships with particular reference to the maximum expiratory flow-volume curve. Phys Med Biol 3:174–194
6. Mead J, Turner JM, Macklem PT et al (1967) Significance of the relationship between lung recoil and maximum expiratory flow. J Appl Physiol 22:95–108
7. Pride NB, Permutt S, Riley RL et al (1967) Determinants of maximal expiratory flow from the lungs. J Appl Physiol 23:646–662
8. Olafsson S, Hyatt RE (1969) Ventilatory mechanics and expiratory flow limitation during exercise in normal subjects. J Clin Invest 48:564–573
9. Guenette JA, Sheel AW (2007). Physiological consequences of a high work of breathing during exercise in humans. J Sci Med Sport [Epub ahead of printing, doi:10.1016/j.jsams.2007.02.003]
10. Dawson SV, Elliott EA (1977) Wave-speed limitation on expiratory flow–a unifying concept. J Appl Physiol 43:498–515
11. Shapiro AH (1977) Steady flow in collapsible tubes. J Biomech Eng 99:126–147
12. Polak AG (2007) A model-based method for flow limitation analysis in the heterogeneous human lung. Comput Methods Pograms Biomed [Epub ahead of printing, doi:10.1016/j.cmpb.2007.03.009]
13. Hyatt RE (1983) Expiratory flow limitation. J Appl Physiol 55:1–8
14. Fry DL (1968) A preliminary model for simulating the aerodynamics of the bronchial tree. Comput Biomed Res 2:111–134
15. Lambert RK, Wilson TA (1973) A model for the elastic properties of the lung and their effect on expiratory flow. J Appl Physiol 34:34–48
16. Pardaens J, Van de Woestijne KP, Clement J (1972) A physical model of expiration. J Appl Physiol 33:479–490
17. Pedersen OF, Thiessen B, Lyager S (1982) Airway compliance and flow limitation during forced expiration in dogs. J Appl Physiol 52:357–369

18. Hyatt RE, Wilson TA, Bar-Yishay E (1980) Prediction of maximal expiratory flow in excised human lungs. J Appl Physiol 48:991–998
19. Elliot EA, Dawson SV (1977) Test of wave-speed theory of flow limitation in elastic tubes. J Appl Physiol 43:516–522
20. Pellegrino R, Brusasco V (1997) On the causes of lung hyperinflation during bronchoconstriction. Eur Respir J 10:468–475
21. Mead J (1980) Expiratory flow limitation: a physiologist's point of view. Fed Proc 39:2771–2775
22. Hyatt RE (1961) The interrelationship of pressure, flow and volume during various respiratory maneuvers in normal and emphysematous patients. Am Rev Respir Dis 83:676–683
23. Potter WA, Olafsson S, Hyatt R (1971) Ventilatory mechanics and expiratory flow limitation during exercise in patients with obstructive lung disease. J Clin Invest 50:910–919
24. Johnson BD, Beck KC, Zeballos et al (1999) Advances in pulmonary laboratory testing. Chest 116(5):1377–1387
25. Ingram RH Jr, Schilder DP (1966) Effect of gas compression on pulmonary pressure, flow, and volume relationship. J Appl Physiol 21:1821–1826
26. Fairshter RD (1985) Airway hysteresis in normal subjects and individuals with chronic airflow obstruction. J Appl Physiol 58:1505–1510
27. Melissinos CG, Webster P, Tien YK et al (1979) Time dependence of maximum flow as an index of nonuniform emptying. J Appl Physiol 47:1043–1050
28. D'Angelo E, Prandi E, Marazzini L et al (1994) Dependence of maximal flow-volume curves on time course of preceding inspiration in patients with chronic obstructive lung disease. Am J Respir Crit Care Med 150:1581–1586
29. Valta P, Corbeil C, Lavoie A et al (1994) Detection of expiratory flow limitation during mechanical ventilation. Am J Respir Crit Care Med 150:1311–1317
30. Koulouris NG, Valta P, Lavoie A et al (1995) A simple method to detect expiratory flow limitation during spontaneous breathing. Eur Respir J 8:306–313
31. Koulouris NG, Dimopoulou I, Valta P et al (1997) Detection of expiratory flow limitation during exercise in COPD patients. J Appl Physiol 82:723–731
32. Murciano D, Pichot M-H, Boczkowski J et al (1997) Expiratory flow limitation in COPD patients after single lung transplantation. Am J Respir Crit Care Med 155:1036–1041
33. Boczkowski J, Murciano D, Pichot MH et al (1997) Expiratory flow limitation in stable asthmatic patients during resting breathing. Am J Respir Crit Care Med 156(3Pt1):752–757
34. Baydur A, Milic-Emili J (1997) Expiratory flow limitation during spontaneous breathing: comparison of patients with restrictive and obstructive respiratory disorders. Chest 112:1017–1023
35. Tauber E, Fazekas T, Eichler I et al (2003) Negative expiratory pressure: a new tool for evaluating lung function in children? Pediatr Pulmonol 35:162–168
36. Vanpee D, Swine CH, Delwich JP, Delanois L (2002) Evaluation of flow limitation in elderly patients unable to perform a forced expiratory maneuver. Aging Clin Exp Res 14:208–211
37. Eltayara L, Becklake MR, Volta CA et al (1996) Relationship between chronic dyspnea and expiratory flow limitation in patients with chronic obstructive pulmonary disease. Am J Respir Crit Care Med 154:1726–1734
38. Volta CA, Ploysongsang Y, Eltayara L et al (1996) A simple method to monitor performance of forced vital capacity. J Appl Physiol 80:693–698
39. Tantucci C, Duguet A, Ferretti A et al (1999) Effect of negative expiratory flow limitation on respiratory system flow resistence in awake snorers and nonsnorers. J Appl Physiol 87:969–976
40. Baydur A, Wilkinson L, Mehdian R et al (2004) Extrathoracic expiratory flow limitation in obesity and obstructive and restrictive disorders: effects of increasing negative expiratory pressure. Chest 35:162–168
41. Ninane V, Leduc D, Kafi SA et al (2001) Detection of expiratory flow limitation by manual compression of the abdominal wall. Am J Respir Crit Care Med 163:1326–1330
42. Calverley PM, Koulouris NG (2005) Flow limitation and dynamic hyperinflation: key con-

cepts in modern respiratory physiology. Eur Respir J 25(1):186–199
43. Dellaca RL, Santus P, Aliverti A et al (2004) Detection of expiratory flow limitation in COPD using the forced oscillation technique. Eur Respir J 23:232–340
44. Weibel ER (1963) Morphometry of human lung. Springer Verlag, Heidelberg-Berlin
45. Horsfield K, Dart G, Olso DE et al (1971) Models of the human bronchial tree. J Appl Physiol 31:207–217
46. Barbini P, Brighenti C, Cevenini G et al (2005) A dynamic morphometric model of the normal lung for studying expiratory flow limitation in mechanical ventilation. Ann Biomed Eng 33:518–530
47. Polak AG, Mroczka J (2006) Nonlinear model for mechanical ventilation of human lungs. Comput Biol Med 36:41–58
48. Barbini P, Brighenti C, Gnudi G (2006) A simulation study of expiratory flow limitation in obstructive patients during mechanical ventilation. Ann Biomed Eng 4:1879–1889
49. Brighenti C, Barbini P, Gnudi G et al (2007) Helium-oxygen ventilation in the presence of expiratory flow-limitation: a model study. Respir Physiol Neurobiol 157:326–334
50. Liu CH, Niranjan SC, Clark Jr et al (1998). Airway mechanics, gas exchange, and blood flow in a nonlinear model of the normal human lung. J Appl Physiol 84:1447–1469

Intrinsic PEEP and its Determination

W.A. Zin, V.R. Cagido

Introduction

Facing a patient who presents with respiratory functional impairment, the physician is left with the task of conducting tests to determine whether there is a mechanical component to the illness. One abnormality that must be considered is intrinsic positive end-expiratory pressure (PEEPi). PEEPi [1,2] is the difference between alveolar pressure and the pressure at the airway opening at the end of expiration. It has also been termed auto-PEEP [3], occult PEEP [3], inadvertent PEEP [4], endogenous PEEP, and internal PEEP. Although not difficult to accomplish, precise determination of PEEPi and subsequent interpretation of the results demand a thorough awareness of the pertinent theoretical and methodological concepts [5,6].

Aetiology

Intrinsic PEEP can result from dynamic hyperinflation, expiratory muscle activity or dynamic hyperinflation associated with expiratory muscle activity [6,7].

Until recently, PEEPi was considered to be a result of dynamic hyperinflation owing to expiratory flow limitation. With airways collapse, a supra-atmospheric pressure is maintained inside the alveoli and airways. Later on, the concept of PEEPi promoted by expiratory muscles contraction was proposed. In this case, the muscle activity increases the pressure inside the lungs, and the subsequent respiratory cycle shows a difference between alveolar and airway opening pressures. That these two phenomena (dynamic hyperinflation and expiratory muscle activity) can occur concomitantly is a more recent consideration, and although it is a very common situation, the contribution of muscle activity to PEEPi has proved difficult to measure.

U. Lucangelo, P. Pelosi, W.A. Zin, A. Aliverti (eds.) *Respiratory System and Artificial Ventilation*. © Springer 2008

Dynamic Hyperinflation

In the presence of high expiratory resistance or expiratory flow limitation, the expiratory time during spontaneous breathing is often insufficient to allow a return of lung volume to its natural relaxation volume, at which elastic recoil equals external PEEP [8]. In such patients, the inability of lung volume to return to its functional residual capacity (FRC) before the subsequent inspiration takes place determines an alveolar pressure that is greater than extrinsic PEEP throughout expiration, and implies that dynamic hyperinflation will result [9]. Thus, dynamic hyperinflation and the ensuing PEEPi can be characterised by expiratory flow detected up to the beginning of the subsequent inspiration, unless airways collapse is present. The occurrence of this scenario is influenced by respiratory system compliance, lung volume at the beginning of expiration and the duration of the expiratory phase.

Clinical experience, especially with COPD patients, suggests that hyperinflation can develop slowly over many years. Thus, the negative results of this so-called static hyperinflation may not be perceived because the respiratory system adapts to the mechanical disadvantages caused by hyperinflation. The chest wall reconfigures to accommodate the overdistended lungs, and the diaphragm partially preserves its ability to generate pressure during resting breathing despite its shortened operating length [10]. In these patients, dynamic hyperinflation can be superimposed on static hyperinflation during exercise [11] and on COPD exacerbations (due to bronchospasm, mucosal oedema and sputum) [8].

Dynamic hyperinflation is most frequently caused by either slow pulmonary emptying or an inadequate ventilator setting. In the former case, the patient's mechanical characteristics, for instance, high expiratory resistance can slow down expiration. Another cause of slow pulmonary emptying rests on the physical characteristics of the ventilation tubing: a narrow tracheal tube, kinking along the expiratory circuit and fluid accumulation in the tubing, connectors and valves. The ventilator setting can contribute to dynamic hyperinflation to the extent that a high respiratory frequency and the use of an elevated inspiratory:expiratory (I:E) ratio may yield a too-short expiratory duration, thus impairing lung emptying. In this same context, if tidal volume is high, the clinician should bear in mind the need to adjust expiratory duration accordingly [5–7,9,12].

The consequences of dynamic hyperinflation include: increased tidal inspiratory effort, since the inspiratory muscles must first overcome PEEPi before inspiratory flow can be initiated [8]; overestimation of the pressure gradient required to generate tidal breathing, thus leading to underestimation of respiratory system compliance [1,6]; cycling of the respiratory system at volumes closer to total lung capacity (TLC), at which compliance is decreased [13]; interference with ventilator triggering in assisted and pressure support modes [12,13]; an increase in respiratory work during weaning attempts [14,15] and alterations of haemodynamics as if external PEEP were the causal factor [16,17].

Expiratory Muscle Activity

Alveolar pressure results from the interaction between the elastic recoil pressure of the respiratory system and the pressure generated by the active expiratory muscles. Thus, only the active patient can generate PEEPi under these circumstances. It is important to note that under these conditions PEEPi can occur at FRC, or even at smaller lung volumes. If the patient contracts his or her expiratory muscles until the end of expiration, the next breath can begin at lung volumes below FRC. Concomitant dynamic hyperinflation is not mandatory, and the magnitude of PEEPi generated by expiratory muscle activity does not represent the amount of dynamic hyperinflation. Expiratory muscle activity frequently occurs in the face of increased respiratory neuromuscular drive and/or expiratory resistance.

As a consequence of expiratory muscle activity, the respiratory system will not cycle near TLC. In this case, lung volume may be smaller than FRC, with a possible decrease in inspiratory muscle work. The compliance will not be underestimated, but may be overestimated instead. In this case, ventilator triggering will not be jeopardised and the use of external PEEP is not recommended because it may thwart expiratory muscle function.

Dynamic Hyperinflation Associated with Expiratory Muscle Activity

When the two aforementioned conditions are associated, their characteristics intermingle. For instance, expiratory muscle activity may worsen expiratory flow limitation such that the use of external PEEP is not recommended because it may add an extra load to the system. Hence, the magnitude of the resulting PEEPi represents the addition of the effects of both dynamic hyperinflation and expiratory muscle activity. As a consequence of this complex interaction, a consensus has yet to be reached on the optimal method to correct for the effect of expiratory muscle activity, in order to arrive at a more accurate estimate of the true elastic recoil pressure of the respiratory system [6].

Measurement of Intrinsic PEEP

Intrinsic PEEP can be determined under static and dynamic conditions: Static PEEPi is measured when no movement can be detected; it is thought that this measurement provides an average of all pulmonary PEEPi values [3]. Dynamic PEEPi is determined during respiratory movement and may represent the smallest PEEPi that could be found in the uneven lung [1,18]. In the presence of dynamic hyperinflation or expiratory muscle activity, PEEPi can be determined under passive breathing as well as during active ventilation.

Passive Ventilation

Under passive ventilation, PEEPi can be determined using one of five methods:

1. End-expiratory airway occlusion: the airways are occluded at end expiration, and the pressure difference obtained from the values taken before and during the occlusion equals PEEPi, as shown in Fig. 1 [3].
2. Plateau pressures: initially, the airways are occluded at end inspiration during a regular breathing cycle, and the plateau pressure is determined. Then, ventilation is interrupted for 20 s. In the following inspiration, the plateau pressure is measured again. The difference between the two plateau pressure values equals PEEPi.
3. Apnoea: inspiration is initially impeded for 20–30 s, while the volume of the exhaled gas (previously dynamically withheld in the lungs) is measured. Thereafter, this volume is divided by the respiratory system compliance. The resulting pressure value equals PEEPi [19–21].
4. Extrinsic PEEP: starting from zero end-expiratory pressure (ZEEP), extrinsic PEEP is progressively augmented up to a point at which an increase in lung volume and/or peak airway pressure can be detected. This PEEP value repre-

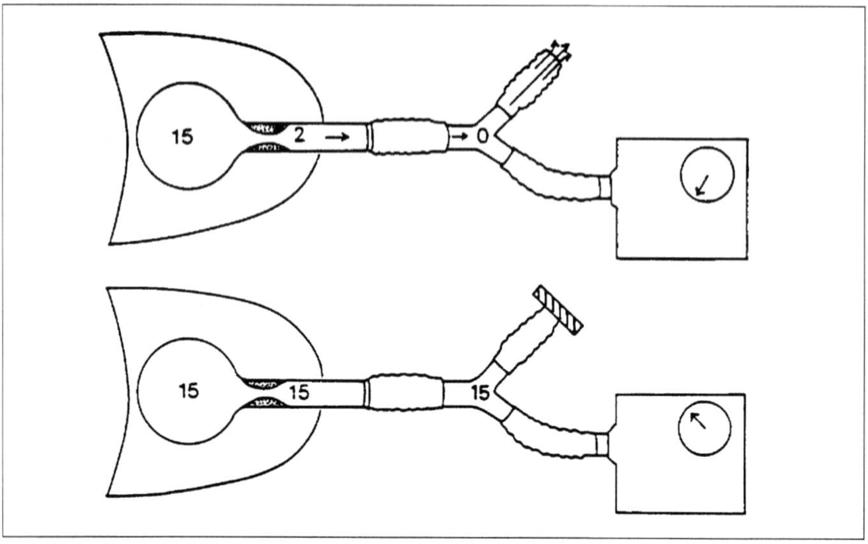

Fig. 1 End-expiratory airway occlusion. *Top* Alveolar pressure corresponds to 15 cmH_2O, but immediately after airway narrowing it falls to 2 cmH_2O, becoming null (0 cmH_2O) in the expiratory branch. Note the difference, amounting to 15 cmH_2O, between alveolar pressure and the pressure at the airway opening (PEEPi). *Bottom* The airways are occluded at end expiration, resulting in the distribution of alveolar pressure along the airways, since there is no flow (Pascal's principle). At that moment, the ventilator manometer will show a pressure of 15 cmH_2O

sents PEEPi. This method is valid solely in the presence of dynamic compression of the airway and thus cannot be used when a simple increase in expiratory resistance occurs [22].

5. Optoelectronic plethysmography (OEP): this non-invasive method is based on computation of the chest-wall volume from a network of points that are identified by shining infrared light at a series of reflective markers attached to the ribcage and abdomen [23,24]. With this technique, changes in regional chest-wall volume can be detected and any modification in PEEPi will be determined. OEP is an excellent tool for measuring chest-wall volume changes in ICU patients and may be used to study different ventilatory conditions [25].

Active Ventilation

During active ventilation, four methods can be employed to quantify PEEPi:

1. End-expiratory airway occlusion: the airways are occluded at the end of a spontaneous expiration. Occlusion is maintained for one to three inspiratory efforts. The difference between the pressure values obtained before the occlusion and after inspiratory muscle relaxation equals PEEPi, as shown in Fig. 2 [3,18].

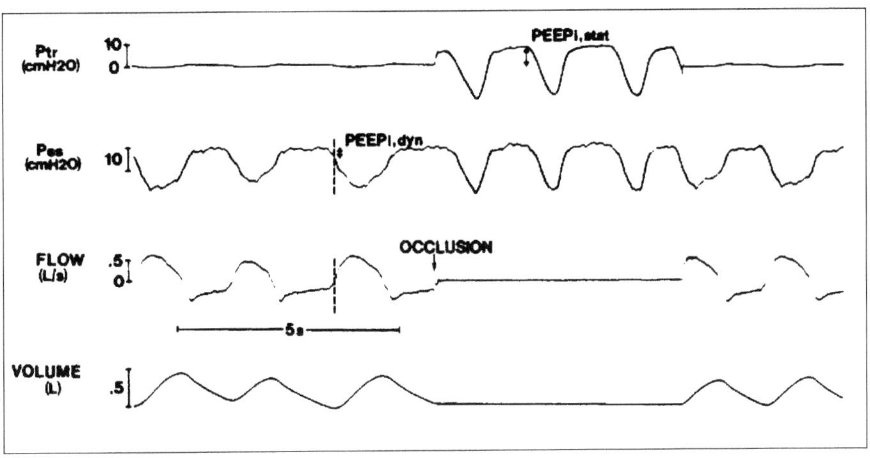

Fig. 2 From *top* to *bottom*: tracheal pressure (*Ptr*), oesophageal pressure (*Poes*), flow and lung volume in a COPD patient. The end-expiratory airway occlusion is represented by the *arrow* on the flow signal. Static PEEPi (*PEEPi,stat*) can be determined by the difference between pressures before end-expiratory airway occlusion and after muscle relaxation is achieved during the respiratory efforts against occluded airways. Dynamic PEEPi (*PEEPi,dyn*) is measured by the negative deflection of Poes from the beginning of the inspiratory effort until the point at which flow is null (transition between inspiration and expiration), indicated by the *dashed lines*. There is an important difference between PEEPi,stat and PEEPi,dyn. Note that the Poes value at the end of expiration is the same in the presence or absence of occlusion, indicating that the expiratory muscles were relaxed. Adapted from [18]

2. Pressure variation between the onsets of inspiratory effort and flow: airflow and pressure (oesophageal or transpulmonary) are recorded. Pressure is read both at the onset of the inspiratory effort and when flow is nil, at the beginning of inspiration. This pressure gradient represents PEEPi (Fig. 2) [1].
3. Recording of inspiratory capacity: this method has been used to estimate changes in end-expiratory lung volume (EELV) during exercise in patients with COPD [26]. If a constant TLC is assumed, a decrease in inspiratory capacity after exercise compared to that determined during baseline breathing indicates a similar increase in EELV. The variation between rest and post-exercise EELV equals the increase in PEEPi.
4. OEP: good results were obtained with this technique (described above) in healthy subjects [27] and in those with COPD at rest and during exercise [28].

Dynamic Hyperinflation and Expiratory Muscle Activity

Expiratory muscle activity may add its effects to those pertaining to dynamic hyperinflation [29,30] in generating PEEPi. This association leads to a less accurate measurement of the elastic recoil pressure of the lung and, consequently, of PEEPi.

The first approach to estimating elastic recoil pressure from recordings of PEEPi was introduced in 1994 [31]. The negative deflection in gastric pressure (Pga) is subtracted from the negative deflection in oesophageal pressure (Poes) during the interval between the onset of an increase in transdiaphragmatic pressure (Pdi) and the onset of inspiratory flow.

In 1995, two methods were proposed to correct for the contribution of expiratory muscle activity to measured values of PEEPi, as determined by the pressure variation between the onsets of inspiratory effort and flow [30]. The first approach is to subtract the total fall in Pga from the initial decrease in Poes, based on the assumption that the former is solely due to abdominal muscle relaxation. However, a fall in Pga could also result from some degree of diaphragmatic dysfunction associated with excessive accessory muscle recruitment. This method also ignores possible contributions from the expiratory muscles of the rib cage. The second approach subtracts the rise in Pga (from the end-inspiratory value to the peak end-expiratory value) from the initial decrease in Poes. This method assumes that the diaphragm has no phasic activity during expiration and functions as a passive membrane. It ignores the post-inspiratory activity of the diaphragm and may also underestimate the activity of the expiratory intercostal muscles.

Conclusions

In conclusion, although simple to be identified and measured under certain conditions, PEEPi may prove to be an elusive mechanical parameter whose presence can impair patients' respiratory and cardiovascular function.

References

1. Rossi A, Gottfried SB, Zocchi L et al (1985) Measurement of static compliance of the total respiratory system in patients with acute respiratory failure during mechanical ventilation. The effect of 'intrinsic' PEEP. Am Rev Respir Dis 131:672–767
2. Rossi A, Polese G, Brandi G et al (1995) The intrinsic positive end expiratory pressure (PEEPi): physiology, implications, measurement, and treatment. Intens Care Med 21:522–536
3. Pepe PE, Marini JJ (1982) Occult positive end-expiratory pressure in mechanically ventilated patients with airflow obstruction: the auto-PEEP effect. Am Rev Respir Dis 126:166–170
4. Bancalari E (1986) Inadvertent positive end-expiratory pressure during mechanical ventilation. J Pediatr 108:567–569
5. Rossi A, Polese G, Milic-Emili J (1997) Monitoring respiratory mechanics in ventilator-dependent patients. In: Tobin MJ (ed) Principles and practice of intensive care monitoring. McGraw-Hill, New York, pp 553–596
6. Tobin MJ (1997) Monitoring respiratory mechanics in spontaneously breathing patients. In: Tobin MJ (ed) Principles and practice of intensive care monitoring. McGraw-Hill, New York, pp 617–654
7. Marini JJ (1988) Monitoring during mechanical ventilation. Clin Chest Med 9:73–100
8. O'Donnell DE, Parker CM (2006) COPD exacerbations 3: pathophysiology. Thorax 61:354–361
9. Marcy TW, Marini JJ (1994) Respiratory distress in the ventilated patient. Clin Chest Med 15:55–73
10. O'Donnell DE (2006) Hyperinflation, dyspnea, and exercise intolerance in chronic obstructive pulmonary disease. Proc Am Thorac Soc 3(2):180–184
11. Cooper CB (2006) The connection between chronic obstructive pulmonary disease symptoms and hyperinflation and its impact on exercise and function. Am J Med 119(10 Suppl 1):21–31
12. Marcy TW, Marini JJ (1992) Modes of mechanical ventilation. Curr Pulmonol 13:43–90
13. Amato MBP, Barbas CSV, Bonassa J et al (1992) Volume-assured pressure support ventilation (VAPSV). Chest 102:1225–1234
14. Hubmayr RD, Abel MD, Rehder K (1990) Physiologic approach to mechanical ventilation. Crit Care Med 18:103–113
15. Eissa NT, Milic-Emili J (1991) Modern concepts in monitoring and management of respiratory failure. Respiratory mechanics. Anesthesiol Clin N Am 9:199–218
16. Harken AH, Brennan MF, Smith B et al (1974) The hemodynamic response to positive end-expiratory pressure ventilation in hypovolemic patients. Surgery 76:786–793
17. Whittenberg JL, McGregor M, Berglund E et al (1960) Influence of the state of inflation of the lung on pulmonary vascular resistance. J Appl Physiol 15:878–882
18. Petrof BJ, Legaré M, Goldberg P et al (1990) Continuous positive airway pressure reduces work of breathing and dyspnea during weaning from mechanical ventilation in severe chronic obstructive pulmonary disease. Am Rev Respir Dis 141:281–289
19. Kimball WR, Leith DE, Robins AG (1982) Dynamic hyperinflation and ventilator dependence in chronic obstructive pulmonary disease. Am Rev Respir Dis 126:991–995
20. Ranieri VM, Eissa NT, Corbeil C et al (1991) Effects of positive end-expiratory pressure on alveolar recruitment and gas exchange in patients with the adult respiratory distress syndrome. Am Rev Respir Dis 144:544–551
21. Tuxen DV, Lane S (1987) The effects of ventilatory pattern on hyperinflation airway pressures, and circulation in mechanical ventilation of patients with severe airflow obstruction. Am Rev Respir Dis 136:872–879
22. Tobin MJ, Lodato RF (1989) PEEP, auto-PEEP and waterfalls. Chest 96:449
23. Carnevali P, Ferrigno G, Aliverti A et al (1996) A new method for 3D optical analysis of chest wall motion. Technol Health Care 4:43–65

24. Calverley PM, Koulouris NG (2005) Flow limitation and dynamic hyperinflation: key concepts in modern respiratory physiology. Eur Respir J 25:186–199
25. Aliverti A, Dellaca R, Pelosi P et al (2000) Optoelectronic plethysmography in intensive care patients. Am J Respir Crit Care Med 161(5):1546–1552
26. Yan S, Kaminski D, Sliwinski P (1997) Reliability of inspiratory capacity for estimating end-expiratory lung volume changes during exercise in patients with chronic obstructive pulmonary disease. Am J Respir Crit Care Med 156:55–59
27. Aliverti A, Dellaca R, Pelosi P et al (2001) Compartmental analysis of breathing in the supine and prone positions by optoelectronic plethysmography. Ann Biomed Eng 29:60–70
28. Aliverti A, Rodger K, Dellaca RL et al (2005) Effect of salbutamol on lung function and chest wall volumes at rest and during exercise in COPD. Thorax 60(11):916–924
29. Ninane V, Yernault J-C, De Troyer A (1993) Intrinsic PEEP in patients with chronic obstructive pulmonary disease: role of expiratory muscles. Am Rev Respir Dis 148:1037–1042
30. Lessard MR, Lofaso F, Brochard L (1995) Expiratory muscle activity increases intrinsic positive end-expiratory pressure independently of dynamic hyperinflation in mechanically ventilated patients. Am J Respir Crit Care Med 151:562–569
31. Appendini L, Patessio A, Zanaboni S et al (1994) Physiologic effects of positive end-expiratory pressure and mask pressure support during exacerbations of chronic obstructive pulmonary disease. Am J Respir Crit Care Med 149:1069–1076

Interactions Between Pulmonary Circulation and Ventilation

Interactions Between the Pulmonary Circulation and Ventilation: An Overview for Intensivists

A.F. Broccard, F. Feihl

Introduction

The heart and the lungs are coupled both anatomically and physiologically in that the cardiovascular and respiratory systems are functionally linked in the respiratory chain (oxygen and carbon-dioxide exchange). Their close proximity within the thorax and the fact that the lungs serve as a conduit between the right and left heart chambers largely account for the mechanical interactions between these two systems.

Critically ill patients often present with or subsequently develop cardiovascular and/or respiratory dysfunction. Prompt restoration of adequate oxygen delivery is required to avoid anoxic organ injury. Interventions to support the failing cardiovascular system have, however, the potential to worsen lung function and gas exchange (e.g. aggressive fluid resuscitation may lead to pulmonary oedema, hypoxaemia and decreased oxygen delivery). Similarly, ventilatory support with positive airway pressure may reduce blood pressure (e.g. increased thoracic pressure may impede venous return and reduce cardiac output) and impair oxygen delivery and organ perfusion. Interventions that target exclusively one system without taking into account cardiopulmonary interactions thus have the potential to be counterproductive.

In the present review, we focus on the interactions between ventilation and the pulmonary circulation but not on the interaction between ventilation and the systemic circulation (e.g. venous return and cardiac output), as our subject is less well-known we believe, by many intensivists. These interactions are, however, important to consider in critically ill patients for at least three reasons.

Firstly, during mechanical ventilation, alveolar pressure is an important determinant of regional perfusion and ventilation and therefore gas exchange [1]. Secondly, the interplay of ventilation and perfusion generates mechanical stresses that may contribute to ventilator-induced lung injury (VILI) [2–6], which has a significant impact on the outcome of ARDS patients [7]. Thirdly, mechanical ventilation may have significant effects on cardiac function and output through mechanisms distinct [8,9] from the direct effect of positive-pressure

U. Lucangelo, P. Pelosi, W.A. Zin, A. Aliverti (eds.) *Respiratory System and Artificial Ventilation.* © Springer 2008

ventilation on right atrial pressure and venous return, as discussed previously.

Positive airway pressure and lung inflation tend to increase pulmonary vascular resistance (PVR) [10,11]. Because the thin-walled right ventricle has a limited capacity to generate the high systolic pressure needed to maintain cardiac output across an elevated resistance, it is important to consider the possible impact of ventilation on PVR [12,13]. This is especially true in critically ill patients who have pre-existing elevated PVR (e.g. massive pulmonary embolism, ARDS [14]), right ventricular dysfunction (e.g. right ventricular myocardial infarction) or both.

Although lung inflation generally increases total PVR, its effects on the lung haemodynamics are quite complex. For instance, depending on whether a change in lung volume is generated by a reduction in pleural pressure or by an increase in alveolar pressure, it may have markedly different consequences on intrathoracic blood volume, intramural vascular pressures, blood flow across the pulmonary circulation (cardiac output) and PVR (Fig. 1) [15,16]. In other words, the effects of ventilation on vascular resistance are indirectly linked to right and left ventricular functions [17–20].

The effects of airway pressure/lung volume on vascular resistance also depend on the condition of the lungs. PEEP, for instance, has the potential to both recruit and/or distend different regions depending on the specific lung con-

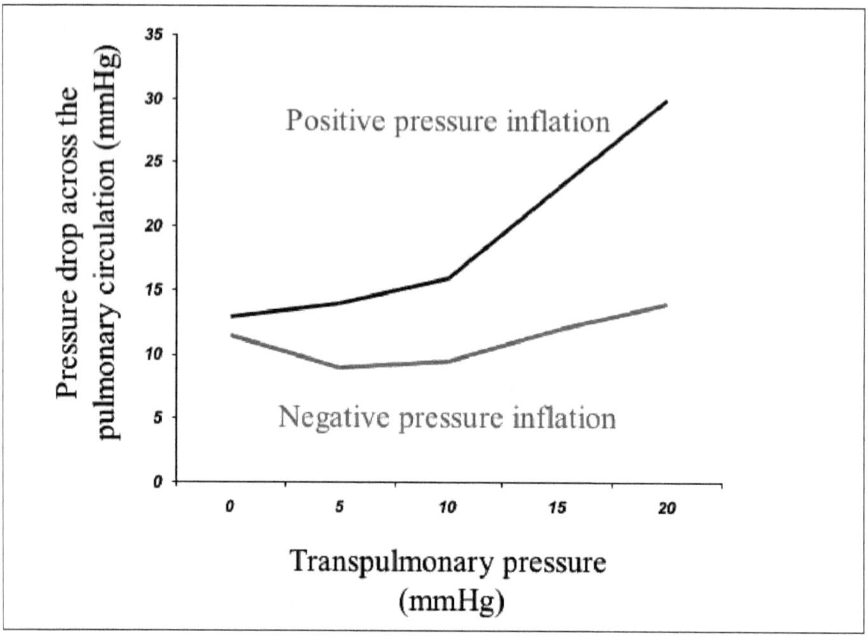

Fig. 1 Effects of rising transpulmonary pressure (inflation) on vascular resistance (pressure drop across the pulmonary circulation: perfusion under constant flow) under positive and negative ventilation conditions. Adapted from [15]

ditions [21–23]. It follows that the effects of positive airway pressure on vascular resistance may vary depending on the type, extent and regional distribution of lung injury, as these factors determine whether a given airway pressure will mainly lead to regional recruitment or distension.

The relationship between airway pressure, lung volume and vascular resistance is not simple, especially in critically ill patients. In subjects at high risk for serious haemodynamic side-effects from positive-pressure ventilation (inadequate preload, right heart dysfunction, high PVR, low chest-wall compliance or high lung compliance), close attention should be paid to the presence of dynamic hyperinflation, high mean airway pressure, acidosis or alveolar hypoxia, since any of these factors has the potential to enhance PVR and right ventricular afterload and thus reduce cardiac output and systemic blood pressure in these patients.

Models of the Pulmonary Circulation: Alveolar and Extra-alveolar Vessels

To understand the interactions between airway pressure, lung volume and the pulmonary circulation, a brief review of the important characteristics of the lung circulation is in order. Two distinct albeit interconnected circulations, namely the pulmonary and bronchial circulations, perfuse the lungs. The former is quantitatively and functionally far more important and will solely be discussed here.

Pulmonary Circulation

Under the physiological conditions of high flow and low pressure (mean PAP$\cong$16 mmHg, mean capillary pressure$\cong$ 10mmHg), low resistance and high compliance characterise the pulmonary circulation. The two major sites of resistance are located upstream and downstream from the capillary vessels, and the vascular resistance distributes approximately equally between the arterial and venous compartments [24,25]. The pulmonary vessels have a lower intramural pressure and are approximately seven times more compliant than the systemic vessels [26]. It follows that the diameters of the pulmonary vessel are largely determined by their transmural pressures (Ptrans)—the pressure difference acting across the vessel wall [intramural pressure (Pi-m) minus extramural pressure (Pe-m)]—and that theses vessels are very sensitive to extramural pressure change. This is especially true for the most compliant vessels, the capillaries [24]. Here, changes in Ptrans may lead to capillary opening/distension or compression/closure, depending on the direction of the Ptrans change.

Other unique characteristics of the pulmonary circulation need to be emphasised. Hypoxia (alveolar PO_2 <70 mmHg) elicits vasoconstriction in the pulmonary vascular bed [27]. This contrasts with the vasodilatation caused by hypoxaemia in the systemic vessels. Respiratory acidosis vasodilates the systemic vessels [28] but does not appear to directly alter pulmonary vessel tone presumably because the vasoconstrictive effects of acidosis are offset by the vasodilatory effect of hypercapnia [29]. If so, the rise in pulmonary artery pressure often associated with permissive hypercapnia [30,31] could be explained by the combination of the increased cardiac output secondary to endogenous catecholamine release [32] and by the implemented low-tidal-volume strategy rather than by a direct effect of respiratory acidosis on vascular tone. In the setting of ARDS, a significant reduction in tidal volume may augment PVR independent of changes in pH and PCO_2, by inducing derecruitment and hypoxic vasoconstriction in the collapsed alveoli [29,31].

Different models have been proposed to describe the relation between the anatomy and the mechanical properties (i.e. compliance and flow resistance) of the pulmonary circulation [24]. The models of West [1] and Hakim [15] have the merit of simplicity and can, we believe, account for most of the clinically relevant interactions between ventilation and perfusion. We shall focus here on these two models. As proposed by Hakim, the pulmonary circulation can be divided in three distinct compartments arranged in series [15]: an arterial, an intermediate and a venous compartment (Fig. 2). These segments can be further characterised as either extra-alveolar (arterial and venous segments) or both alveolar and extra-alveolar (intermediate or middle segment) [15]. Under physiological conditions and at functional residual capacity (FRC), the major sites of resistance to

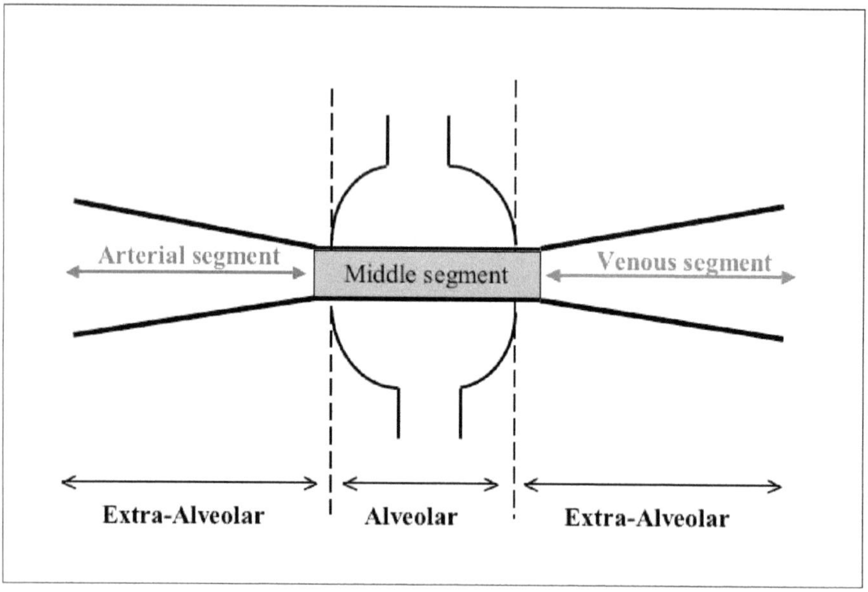

Fig. 2 Pulmonary vascular segments and their relationship to alveolar and extra-alveolar spaces. Adapted from [15]

flow are extra-alveolar (arterial and venous segment) [15,25]. As discussed below, however, the intermediate segment contributes the most to the vascular resistance *change* during ventilation [15]. The latter segment is also the most compliant [24] and is the main site of fluid filtration, as it includes the microcirculation.

Alveolar Vessels

Vessels for which the alveolar pressure is the effective extramural pressure are referred to as alveolar. The definition of alveolar vessels is functional. Anatomically, however, capillaries within alveolar septa constitute the principal alveolar vessels. During lung inflation, the diameters of the alveolar vessels narrow, as they become elongated and compressed (especially during positive-pressure ventilation) by the expanding alveoli. In addition to alveolar size and pressure, other mechanical factors affect vessel transmural pressure, diameter and resistance. Gravity, for instance, accounts for the variation of intramural pressures along the vertical axis, as outlined by West [1].

For the alveolar vessels, West and colleagues have defined different zonal conditions, which are important to consider during positive-pressure ventilation. In brief, conditions are fulfilled for zone III if pulmonary artery pressure (Pap)>pulmonary venous pressure (Pvp)>alveolar pressure (Palv), for zone II if Pap>Palv>Pvp and for zone I if Palv>Pap>Pvp. Under physiological conditions, zone III prevails throughout the lungs and zone I is essentially non-existent. Under zone II conditions (waterfall conditions), the pulmonary circulation has the characteristic of a Starling resistor and flow is independent of the apparent outflow pressure (Ppv) because Palv becomes the effective outflow pressure. Until recently, this gravity-based model (which also includes a Zone IV, not discussed here) was thought to explain regional blood flow differences within the lung. More recent studies have questioned the concept that *under physiological conditions* gravity is a major determinant of regional perfusion [33]. Regional differences in vascular conductance are more important [33]. *During positive-pressure ventilation,* however, both gravity and regional vascular conductance interact and contribute to the distribution of perfusion [34–36], as discussed below.

Extra-alveolar Vessels

Extra-alveolar arterial and venous vessels are not directly influenced by alveolar pressure. The extramural pressure of extra-alveolar vessels (Pe-m) falls relative to pleural pressure when lung volume increases, due to tissue interdependence forces [37,38]. Thus, extra-alveolar vessels expand and their resistance to blood flow may decrease with lung inflation (Fig. 3) up to a point at which the effect of the reduced extramural pressure on the diameter of these vessels is offset by their concomitant elongation as the lungs inflate.

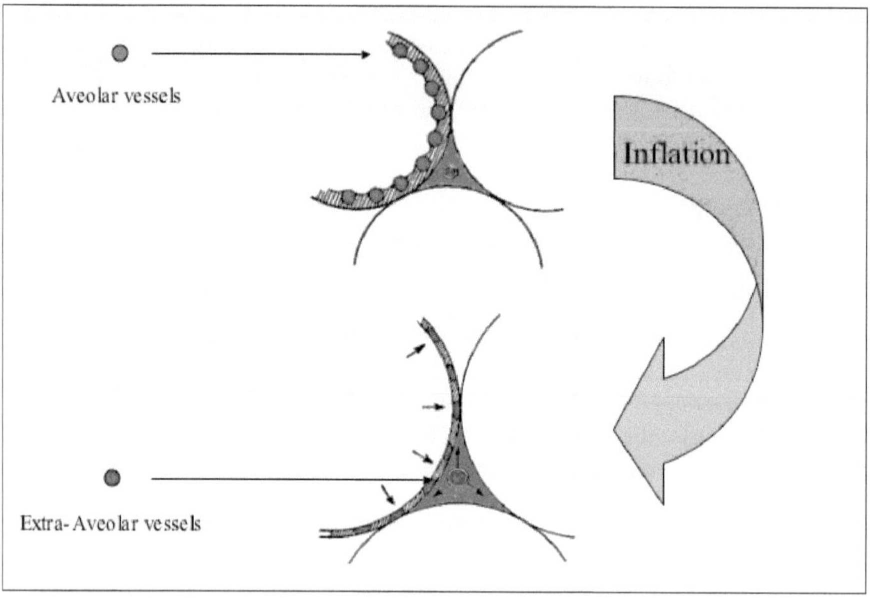

Fig. 3 Effect of lung inflation on alveolar and extra-alveolar vessels. See text for details. Courtesy of Dr Marini, University of Minnesota, St. Paul, USA

If the entire pulmonary circulation is arranged in series, as Hakim's model may suggest, flow should be in essence zero under zone I conditions. This is, however, not the case due to the presence of corner vessels [39]. Despite their close proximity to alveoli, corner vessels remain patent even when Palv is elevated due to their location at the junction of alveolar septa. As the lung inflates, the alveoli expand and tension starts to build up in the septa. The traction on septal–wall junctions reduces the pressure in the spaces adjacent to the corner vessels and their extramural pressures drop below alveolar pressure. Corner vessels thus behave like extra-alveolar vessels kept open by tissue interdependence forces and may act as a central conduit for flow under zone I conditions [40].

Effects of Lung Volume and Airway Pressure on PVR and Regional Blood Flow

Effects on the Longitudinal Distribution of Resistance

The relation between lung volume (from residual volume to total lung capacity) and total PVR is non-linear and differs between negative- and positive-pressure ventilation [15] (Fig. 1). The relation is U-shaped when lung inflation is generated by a decrease in pleural pressure. In contrast, similar changes in transmural pressure and lung volume caused by positive airway pressure are not associated with an initial drop in vascular resistance (PVR rises continuously) [15]. Furthermore, a given increase in lung volume tends to cause a greater rise in PVR when driven by positive airway pressure as opposed to negative pleural pressure [15]. Compared with positive-pressure ventilation, therefore, spontaneous breathing has fewer detrimental effects, not only on cardiac preload but also on right ventricular afterload. This helps explain how ventilatory modes that limit positive pressure and allow spontaneous breathing (e.g. airway pressure release) are less detrimental to cardiac output [41].

The classical U-shape relationship between lung volume and total vascular resistance is best explained by the fact that the latter is a composite measure of extra-alveolar and alveolar vessel resistance [10]. As lung volume increases, traction and compression of alveolar vessels by the expanding alveoli are associated with a progressive increase in alveolar vessel resistance [42]. Simultaneously, traction on the extra-alveolar interstitial compartment leads to its expansion (tissue interdependence) and to a drop in the extramural (Pe-m) pressure of the extra-alveolar vessels [10]. The diameter of those vessels may thus increase more or less depending on the prevailing intramural pressure (Pi-m). The net effect of lung volume on extra-alveolar vessels resistance is mainly due to a balance of opposing forces on vessels: radial traction due to tissue interdependence (decreased extramural pressure relative to intramural pressure) and stretching (reduced vessel diameter). As the lung volume is increased from residual volume (RV) to FRC, the prevailing effect is a drop in extra-alveolar resistance that offsets the concomitant increase in alveolar vessel resistance [10]. Above FRC, vessel stretching tends to offset this effect and extra-alveolar resistance does not change significantly whereas alveolar vessel resistance continues to rise as does total PVR. This largely accounts for the U-shaped relation between lung volume and total vascular resistance.

The effects of positive- and negative-pressure ventilation on PVR need to be considered longitudinally along the different segments defined above, namely the arterial, intermediate and venous segments. Hakim and colleagues demonstrated that only minimal changes in vascular resistance are observed in the arterial and venous segments and that the greatest change in vascular resistance during lung inflation (from RV to total lung capacity) takes place in the intermediate segment (Fig. 4) both during positive- and negative-pressure-generated volume changes [15]. The global vascular resistance increases more with positive airway pressure than with negative pressure generated by transpulmonary changes. This is best explained by the greater compression of alveolar vessels (earlier transition from West's zonal conditions III to II and I) under positive alveolar pressure conditions, everything else being equal. The absence of significant change in resistance in the arterial segment during lung inflation is worth pointing out. It helps to understand the potential interaction between haemodynamics and ventilation in the pathogenesis of VILI, as discussed below. Providing that cardiac output does not concomitantly drop significantly, the

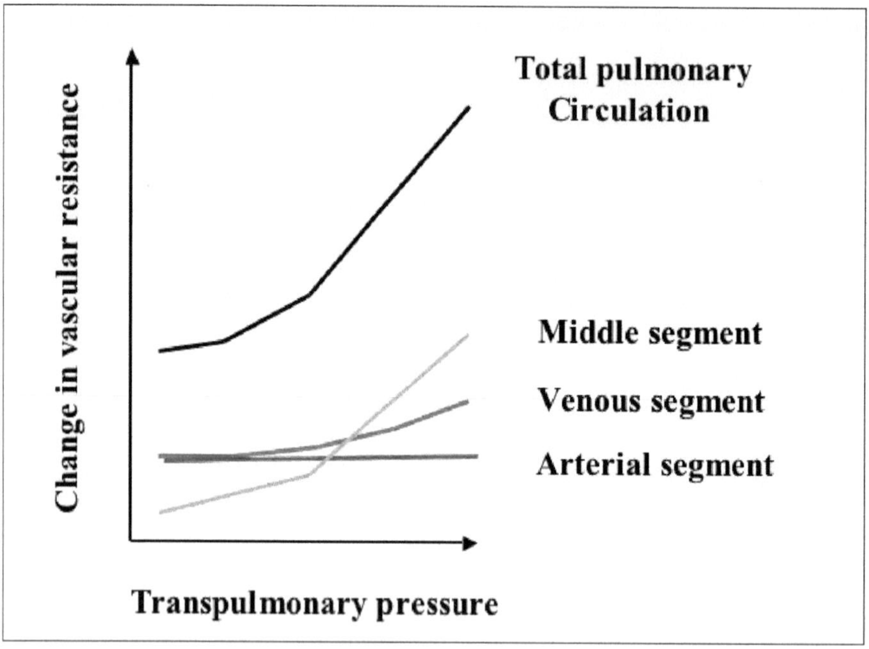

Fig. 4 Effects of inflation on vascular resistance (pressure drop across the pulmonary circulation: perfusion under constant flow) in the vascular segments of the pulmonary circulation. See text for details. Adapted from [15]

intramural pressure in the vessels located upstream rises during positive-pressure ventilation. Since, simultaneously, the extramural pressure of extra-alveolar vessels tends to decrease and that of intra-alveolar pressure to increase [43], the blood volume, vascular resistance and the forces governing fluid filtration and vascular stretch may thus vary in opposite directions in alveolar and extra-alveolar vessels [10,44]. The alveolar vessels tend to collapse and flow redistributes towards extra-alveolar vessels, which experiences a rise in transmural pressure. Such changes enhance fluid filtration [45] and the risk of developing vascular failure, as suggested by the striking distribution of haemorrhage around extra-alveolar vessels in models of VILI [4,46].

Effects of Airway Pressure and Posture on Regional Blood Flow and Gas Exchange

Until recently, gravity was thought to be the main determinant of regional blood flow [1]. It now appears that under physiological conditions regional differences in the anatomy of the pulmonary circulation largely account for the distribution of blood flow within the lung, and the effect of gravity is minor [33,36,47,48].

Given the practical interest in the use of prone positioning to improve gas exchange in patients with ARDS [49,50], we will focus our discussion here on the effects of airway pressure and position on regional perfusion and gas exchange in patients in prone and supine positions.

During spontaneous breathing in the recumbent position, perfusion distributes preferentially in the dorsal lung region in the prone and supine positions (Fig. 5a) both in normal [33] and in oleic-acid-injured lungs [51]. The preferential dorsal distribution of perfusion irrespective of posture cannot be explained by gravity alone and was reported in animals [35] and in humans [47]. Applying positive pressure to the airway (in the form of either PEEP or continuous positive airway pressure) tends, however, to redistribute blood flow away from non-dependent towards dependent regions. In other words, positive airway pressure enhances the contribution of gravity to the distribution of blood flow along the vertical axis. In the supine position, this results in an enhanced vertical flow gradient (Fig. 5b). This is best explained by the fact that positive airway pressure favours the transition from West's zonal condition III to condition II [43]. Under zone III conditions, both the inflow and outflow pressure (venous pressure) are under the influence of gravity and increase along the vertical axis. Under zone II conditions, in contrast, the inflow pressure (pulmonary artery pressure) is highest in the most dependent regions (effect of gravity), whereas the effective outflow pressure (≅alveolar pressure) is gravity-independent. This results in a steep flow gradient along the vertical axis and explains the steeper perfusion pressure gradient along the vertical axis observed in the supine position when airway pressure is supra-atmospheric [1] (Fig. 5).

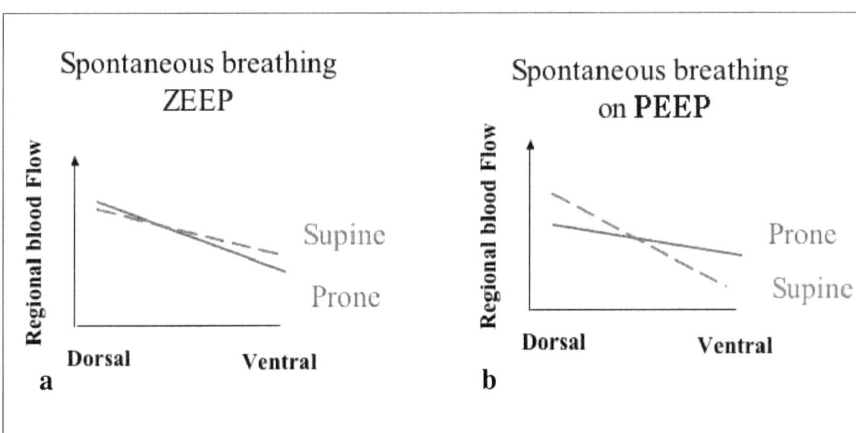

Fig. 5a,b Distribution of perfusion along the vertical axis in the supine and prone positions on ZEEP (**a**) and PEEP (**b**) conditions. Notice how posture alters how the vertical perfusion gradient (flow difference between dependent and non-dependent regions) is affected by positive airway pressure. Adapted from [35,36,47]

Computerised tomography of the chest in animal models of lung injury and in patients with early ARDS not due to pneumonia often demonstrates diffuse and extensive ground-glass opacifications [52] mainly due to increased extravascular water [53,54]. Frank alveolar flooding and/or atelectasis, however, often distribute preferentially in the most dependent lung regions at least in part because this is where the regional pleural pressures are the least negative [55] and because oedematous lungs may, like a sponge, collapse under their own weight [56]. The preferential dependent distribution of lung densities is associated with poor regional tidal ventilation, and the bulk of tidal ventilation is redirected to the non-dependent ventral lung regions [57]. Given the predominantly dorsal (dependent) distribution of perfusion, in the setting of lung injury, VA/Q mismatch and shunting tend to be enhanced in the supine position [58].

In patients with ARDS, the effects of positive airway pressure (e.g. PEEP) on the distribution of perfusion, as discussed above, may theoretically worsen gas exchange in the supine position if ventilation does not concomitantly improve in dependent regions. When positive airway pressure improves ventilation in dependent regions [59] (e.g. in the early phase of non-cardiogenic pulmonary oedema), the concomitant increase in their perfusion is usually associated with improved oxygenation, Theoretically, when consolidated regions cannot be recruited (e.g. pneumonia), modes that allow ventilation at lower positive mean airway pressures or negative-pressure ventilation could be more advantageous by limiting the distribution of blood flow to poorly aerated lung regions. This could explain why PEEP can worsen oxygenation in unilateral pneumonia [60] and why allowing some degree of spontaneous breathing during mechanical ventilation can sometimes help improve gas exchange when dependent regions cannot be recruited and/or ventilated [41,61]. Factors other than minimising positive airway pressure may, however, also be very important: for instance, diaphragmatic contraction may augment the distribution of ventilation to dependent, well-perfused lung regions [41]. It should be emphasised that ARDS is a syndrome. Thus, depending on its cause and its time course (early vs. late ARDS), the effects of airway pressure on regional ventilation and perfusion may vary significantly [62,63].

Gas exchange can also be improved by turning patients with ARDS prone [49]. Although positive airway pressure ventilation tends to redirect blood flow toward the dependent regions regardless of position [35,47] (Fig. 5), the large baseline dorsal *non-dependent* regional blood flow present in the prone position [33] partially offsets the consequence of the emergence of zone II conditions associated with positive airway pressure: non-dependent perfusion is better preserved and overall the perfusion distribution is more uniform along the vertical axis in the prone than in the supine position under positive airway pressure conditions (Fig. 5) [35,47]. Ventilation distributes preferentially away from the consolidated dependent lungs regions both in the prone and the supine positions [57]. The non-dependent well-ventilated lung regions are thus relatively better perfused in the prone than in the supine position and V/Q matching is more favourable in the prone than in the supine position in the setting of lung injury [58,64]. Although other non-mutually exclusive mechanisms have been proposed [65] to explain the improved gas exchange observed in the vast majority (approximately 70%) of patient with ARDS turned prone [49], the difference in blood flow distribution between positions is likely an important factor. Despite a handful of randomised trials [49,66,67], it is still unclear, however, whether prone position can improve these patients' outcome. The results of an ongoing large randomised trial should be available soon.

Lung Volume/Airway Pressure and Oedema Formation

Under physiological conditions, fluid transfer from the microcirculation towards the interstitium mainly takes place between and across endothelial cells and involves specific water channels (aquaporines) [68]. The largest bulk of filtration occurs in the capillaries (50%) and the rest in the arterioles (25%) and venules (25%). The key factors governing the filtration rate are interdependent, as described by the Starling equation: Filtration = K_f [(Pc - Pt) - σ (Πp - Πt)], where K_f is the ultrafiltration coefficient (a measure of permeability to water), σ the reflection coefficient for protein (a measure of permeability to protein), Pc and Pt, the hydrostatic intramural and extramural pressures across the walls of the microcirculation, respectively, and Πp and Πt represent the plasma and tissue oncotic pressures [69]. Although this equation is clearly an oversimplification, it remains clinically useful.

The ultrafiltration coefficient (K_f) is a composite measure of the vascular permeability to water and of the effective exchange surface [69,70]. The latter varies with the lung volume and the prevailing West zone conditions. In other words, K_f and filtration are altered by lung volume and positive pressure. For instance, positive airway pressure promotes the transition from the predominant zone III to zone II or I, which reduces the vascular filtration surface and rate in normal lungs [71]. Other factors to consider regarding the effects of airway pressure and lung volume on filtration include their magnitudes respective to the prevailing haemodynamics (e.g. intramural pressure and flow conditions) and their distinct effects on the transmural hydrostatic pressures of alveolar and extra-alveolar vessels, as previously discussed.

The complex interactions between these variables explain why filtration may differ under different experimental conditions. For example, in an isolated lung study, Bo et al. found that: (1) increasing Palv at constant lung volume reduced filtration, (2) lung inflation at constant Palv enhanced filtration, and (3) lung inflation due to increasing Palv tended to reduce filtration when pulmonary artery pressure was kept constant [72]. In isolated perfused rabbit lungs, PEEP increased filtration [73].

Effects of PEEP on Fluid Filtration

In vivo, the effects of a given airway pressure/volume change on the transmural pressures of pulmonary vessels and filtration are rendered more complex by heart-lung interactions and may vary with myocardial preload, contractility and lung and chest-wall compliances. Although in high-surface-tension pulmonary oedema, PEEP may accelerate the accumulation of water in the lung [74], positive airway pressure seems, however, to have generally little effect on filtration. In intact animals, for instance, PEEP does not protect against hydrostatic pulmonary oedema [75,76]. Similarly, in non-cardiogenic pulmonary oedema (oleic-acid-induced lung injury), PEEP does not reduce fluid filtration but merely redistributes oedema from the alveolar to the extra-alveolar space, which helps to recruit alveolar surface for gas exchange [59].

Haemodynamic Effect of PEEP and Lung Injury

Although the early administration of PEEP has experimentally been found to limit oleic-acid-induced lung injury and oedema formation [77,78], its prophylactic use in patients was not beneficial [79]. However, the protective effects of PEEP against permeability pulmonary oedema have been well-documented in experimental ventilator-induced lung injury [80,81]. The mechanism that best accounts for the lung protective effect of PEEP is still uncertain [82], but may be explained partially by a reduction in cardiac output from the resulting increased intrathoracic pressure [3,4]. Although clinical studies consistent with a lung protective effect of PEEP have been published [83,84], definitive proof regarding the protective effects of PEEP against lung injury are still lacking in patients. While a recent large trial found that PEEP was not protective [85], the study lacked a solid physiological basis and only demonstrated that PEEP titration has no merit and fails to take into account that the response to PEEP (recruiter and non-recruiter) may vary between patients [86].

Effect of the Ventilatory Pattern on Fluid Filtration

In isolated lungs, increasing minute ventilation either by raising tidal volume (V_T) at constant respiratory rate or by increasing respiratory rate at constant V_T equally promoted oedema formation [87]. These data indicate that breathing pattern impacts fluid filtration by mechanisms partially independent of peak tidal lung volume/airway pressure.

Haemodynamics and VILI

Mechanical ventilation is frequently needed to restore adequate gas exchange and alleviate the increased work of breathing that is often associated with respiratory failure. Numerous animal studies have demonstrated that mechanical ventilation can cause lung injury, as reviewed elsewhere [82]. More recently, a multi-centre NIH-sponsored trial confirmed the concept that excessive tidal breathing adversely affects outcome in ARDS patients [7]. Excessive end-inspiratory stretch (overdistension/volutrauma) and cyclic opening and collapse of the airways (atelectrauma) are thought to be instrumental in the development of VILI, which is characterised by diffuse structural and functional alterations of the epithelium and endothelium barrier and by inflammation [88].

Pulmonary haemodynamics may, however, also play an important role in the pathogenesis of VILI. In the setting of increased vascular permeability in general and of VILI in particular, the prevailing haemodynamic conditions have important consequences on oedema formation [89] and so may indirectly contribute to injury [90]. For instance, the exudation of protein-rich fluid may inactivate surfactant and further alter membrane permeability by increasing surface tension and radial traction on the microcirculation [91]. In addition, there are now solid experimental data to support a more direct role of haemodynamics in the pathogenesis of VILI. One of the first studies along this line was carried out in rats by Dreyfuss et al., who found that the protective effect of PEEP against VILI was partly due to a reduced pulmonary perfusion [3]. Later on, we demonstrated in the isolated rabbit lung perfused with constant flow that the same injurious pattern of ventilation caused the greatest structural damage when blood flow was highest (Fig. 6a) [4]. In addition, the magnitude of the rise in vascular pressure caused by the change in vascular resistance imposed by a given mechanical breath (tidal vascular pressure change) tightly correlated with the degree of VILI (Fig. 6b) [4]. This suggested that the effects of flow on VILI were mediated by changes in vascular pressure. A similar correlation of tidal vascular pressure changes with intensity of lung injury was also found in this experimental model, when the animals were exposed to different ventilatory patterns while lung perfusion was kept constant [5]. Although direct extrapolation from this isolated perfused model to the intact organism is not warranted, these findings point to the importance of haemodynamic factors as modulators of VILI. Later, we discuss the potential mechanistic basis for these observations, notwithstanding the very limited amount of presently available knowledge.

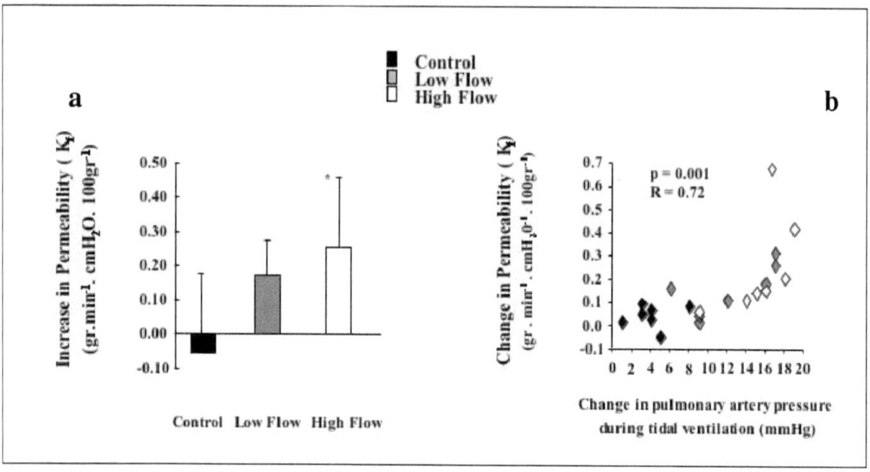

Fig. 6a,b Effect of perfusion level (flow) on VILI in an isolated perfused rabbit lung. The highest perfusion is associated with the largest degree of lung injury, everything else being equal (**a**). This finding is best explained by the greater tidal change in vascular pressure with high perfusion rate (**a,b**: high-flow group). Adapted from [4]

VILI and Extra-alveolar Vessel Haemodynamics

As previously discussed, lung inflation decreases the pressure in the space surrounding the extra-alveolar vessels relative to pleural pressure. Simultaneously, it raises the resistance of the intermediate segment, which comprises alveolar capillaries and small extra-alveolar vessels [15]. Thus, the tidal increase in pulmonary arterial pressure must propagate to at least some of the latter, namely those near the arterial end of the intermediate segment. In short, lung inflation must raise the transmural pressure in at least part of the extra-alveolar vessels by an amount obviously dependent on pulmonary blood flow. Dilatation of extra-alveolar vessels in the course of lung inflation has been substantiated [10].

The tidal increase in transmural pressure has two distinct consequences in these vessels. First, it shifts the balance of hydrostatic forces toward filtration [45,92]. Second, if large enough, the strain generated by the transmural pressure change may inflict structural damage on the vascular wall. As a result, vascular permeability increases and ultimately full-blown vascular failure with protein-rich oedema and red blood cell extravasation may ensue [93]. This scenario could explain the presence of haemorrhages around extra-alveolar vessels in isolated lungs ventilated with high peak alveolar pressure and perfused with constant flow [5]. Such perivascular haemorrhages were found to be most prominent when blood flow was the highest [5].

VILI and Alveolar Vessel Haemodynamics

West et al. introduced the concept of stress failure incurred by pulmonary capillaries subjected to excessive mechanical stress [93–100]. According to the analysis developed by these authors, the total mechanical stress incurred by alveolar capillaries has three components: (1) hoop stress, which depends on the transmural pressure and vessel radius (Laplace's law); (2) alveolar surface tension, which acts as a support to those capillaries that bulge into the alveolar space and (3) longitudinal traction exerted by the alveolar wall as it expands (Fig. 7). With overdistension, the extramural pressure of the alveolar vessels tends to decrease, as previously seen. Furthermore, alveolar surface tension increases. These two changes would appear to counteract the concomitant increase in longitudinal traction, such that the net effect of overdistension on capillary stress is not easily predicted. In isolated lungs, VILI is manifested by the extravasation of red blood cells (Fig. 8), not only around extra-alveolar vessels but also in alveoli, indicating concomitant damage to lung capillaries [4]. For the same injurious ventilatory pattern, the intensity of this abnormality was found to increase in direct proportion to lung perfusion [4], suggesting that haemodynamic factors modulate the capillary injury associated with VILI. At present, the mechanistic pathways of such modulation may only be speculated upon. One possibility is suggested by the aforementioned increase in the resistance of the middle segment with lung inflation [15]: the resulting pulmonary artery pressure and pressure gradient across the pulmonary microcirculation might be such that in some alveolar vessels (i.e.

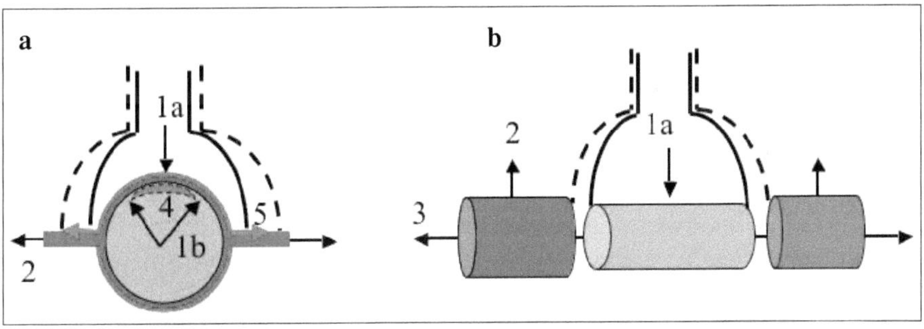

Fig. 7a,b a Alveolar vessels are subjected to a complex set of forces. Wall tension is determined by wall thickness, transmural pressure (difference between *1a* and *1b*) and vessel radius (*4*). Intraluminal pressure (*1b*) opposes alveolar vessels compression and collapse during inflation. Surface tension (*5*) may be protective by limiting the tendency of alveolar capillaries to bulge into the airspace, which increases vessel radius and wall tension. Lung inflation tends to elongate pulmonary vessels and to alter transmural pressure. **b** During positive -pressure ventilation, the alveolar /extramural pressure increases and tends to compress alveolar vessels (*1a*). In contrast, extramural pressure (*2*) of extra-alveolar vessels tends to be reduced, which increases extra-alveolar vessel size

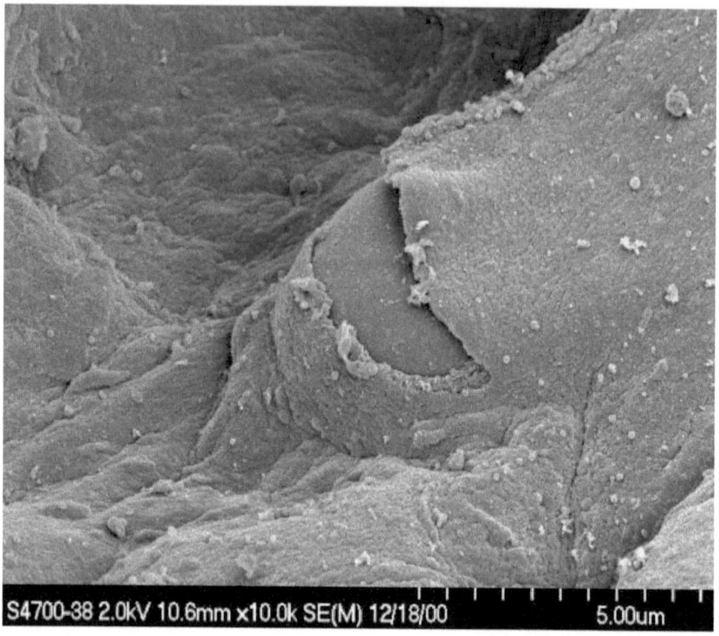

Fig. 8 Excessive forces applied to alveolar capillaries may lead to capillary failure. In this electronic microscopy illustration, complete endothelial and epithelial rupture has occurred and a red blood cell on the verge of entering the alveolar space can be seen. Courtesy of Dr Dries and Dr Marini, University of Minnesota, St. Paul, and Dr Hotchkiss, University of Pittsburgh, Pittsburgh, USA

those closest to the arterial side) intramural pressure would increase more than alveolar pressure. In these particular vessels, hoop stress would be larger rather than smaller with lung inflation, a phenomenon that would be amplified by an increase in lung perfusion. Along another line, incipient alveolar edema—the development rate and intensity of which are highly dependent on haemodynamic factors—might abolish the protection afforded by alveolar surface tension to bulging capillaries. In support of this hypothesis, suppression of the gas-liquid surface-tension by filling alveoli with normal saline may result in augmented damage to some parts of the alveolar-capillary barrier, when the latter is subjected to high transmural pressures [101].

VILI and Outflow Pressure of the Pulmonary Circulation

In rabbit lungs, Fu et al. reported that the number of alveolar epithelial and endothelial breaks varied directly with both lung volume and vascular pressure [2]. These observations were made in the absence of ventilation and perfusion (i.e. airway and vascular pressures were kept constant in any given experiment).

Nevertheless, the possibility is thereby suggested that VILI is aggravated by excessive repletion of the pulmonary vascular bed with blood in perfused and ventilated conditions. The latter is directly related to outflow pressure, namely, left atrial pressure (LAP).

Interestingly, an abnormally *low* LAP may also potentiate VILI, as we recently found in the isolated perfused rabbit lung [102] (Fig. 9). The possible contribution of a low LAP to VILI can be explained as follows: tidal ventilation with high positive pressure tends to promote transition from West zone III to zone II or I conditions (depending on the magnitude of perfusion and how flow is generated: e.g. constant flow or pressure [71]). Furthermore, tidal inflation has opposite effects on vascular resistance and the volume of the alveolar and extra-alveolar vessels [10,44], such that the alveolar vessels collapse and the extra-alveolar vessels expand, as previously discussed. Due to the upstream propagation of LAP, the accompanying reduction in pressure enhances the compressibility of the alveolar vessels, so that a transition from a zone III to a zone II or I condition occurs earlier in the course of tidal inflation. This may lead to vascular failure by promoting the repeated collapse of the alveolar vessels during inflation followed by reopening as intramural pressure builds upstream from the closed vessels and the airway pressure decreases at the beginning of expiration. In addition, the earlier zone III to zone II transition during tidal inflation with

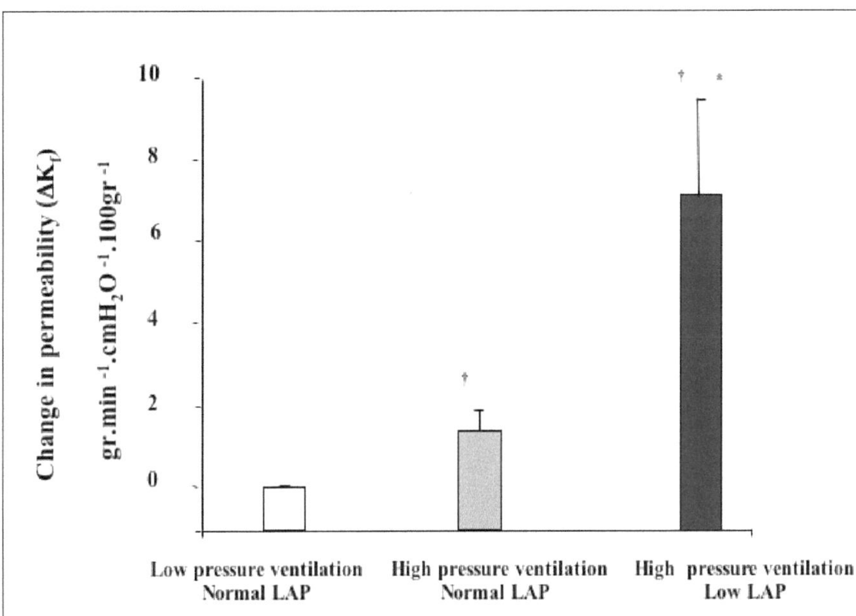

Fig. 9 Atrial pressure may modulate the degree of VILI. Low atrial pressure enhances the permeability alteration associated with VILI and the risk of vascular failure. See text for details. Adapted from [102]

low rather than normal LAP may increase blood volume in the extra-alveolar vessels. The combination of augmented blood volume and reduced extramural pressure results in a rise in both transmural pressure and lumen radius, thereby enhancing the amount of stress incurred by these vessels. Further studies are needed to determine which of these possible mechanisms predominate.

Conclusions

In conclusion, pulmonary haemodynamics have the potential to contribute not only to edema but also to injury in non-cardiogenic pulmonary oedema caused by MV. Here we have limited the discussion regarding the possible contribution of haemodynamics to VILI to mechanical stress and material failure. It should be outlined, however, that mechanical-force-induced signal transduction in lung cells is also very important as recently reviewed [103,104].

The burden of evidence regarding the role of haemodynamics to VILI comes from animal models, which preclude direct extrapolation to patients. These results thus need to be confirmed in intact animals. In the mean time, in patients with pulmonary oedema who require MV it may be prudent to avoid potentially harmful therapeutic interventions, such as increasing cardiac output to supra-physiological levels, altering pulmonary vascular resistance with vaso-active drugs [105] or shifting the left-heart filling pressure towards high or extremely low values. A conservative approach to fluid balance (keeping the patient on the 'dry side') appears, however, to be helpful in reducing the duration of mechanical ventilation [106].

References

1. West JB (1966) Distribution of blood and gas in lungs. Phys Med Biol 11(3):357–370
2. Fu Z, Costello ML, Tsukimoto K et al (1992) High lung volume increases stress failure in pulmonary capillaries. J Appl Physiol 73(1):123–133
3. Dreyfuss D, Saumon G (1993) Role of tidal volume, FRC, and end-inspiratory volume in the development of pulmonary edema following mechanical ventilation. Am Rev Respir Dis 148(5):1194–1203
4. Broccard AF, Hotchkiss JR, Kuwayama N et al (1998) Consequences of vascular flow on lung injury induced by mechanical ventilation. Am J Respir Crit Care Med 157(6 Pt 1):1935–1942
5. Broccard AF, Hotchkiss JR, Suzuki S et al (1999) Effects of mean airway pressure and tidal excursion on lung injury induced by mechanical ventilation in an isolated perfused rabbit lung model. Crit Care Med 27(8):1533–1541
6. Hotchkiss JR Jr, Blanch L, Naveira A et al (2001) Relative roles of vascular and airspace pressures in ventilator-induced lung injury. Crit Care Med 29(8):1593–1598
7. The Acute Respiratory Distress Syndrome Network (2000) Ventilation with lower tidal volumes as compared with traditional tidal volumes for acute lung injury and the acute respiratory distress syndrome. N Engl J Med 342(18):1301–1308

8. Robotham JL, Lixfeld W, Holland L et al (1980) The effects of positive end-expiratory pressure on right and left ventricular performance. Am Rev Respir Dis 121(4):677–683
9. Cheifetz IM, Craig DM, Quick G et al (1998) Increasing tidal volumes and pulmonary overdistention adversely affect pulmonary vascular mechanics and cardiac output in a pediatric swine model. Crit Care Med 1998 26(4):710–716
10. Howell J, Permutt D, Proctor, Riley R (1961) Effect of inflation of the lung on different parts of the pulmonary vascular bed. Journal of Applied Physiology 16:71–76
11. Sun RY, Nieman GF, Hakim TS, Chang HK (1987) Effects of lung volume and alveolar surface tension on pulmonary vascular resistance. J Appl Physiol 62(4):1622–1626
12. Henning RJ (1986) Effects of positive end-expiratory pressure on the right ventricle. J Appl Physiol 61(3):819–826
13. Romand JA, Donald FA, Suter PM (1995) Acute right ventricular failure, pathophysiology and treatment. Monaldi Arch Chest Dis 50(2):129–133
14. Monchi M, Bellenfant F, Cariou A et al (1998) Early predictive factors of survival in the acute respiratory distress syndrome. A multivariate analysis. Am J Respir Crit Care Med 158(4):1076–1081
15. Hakim TS, Michel RP, Chang HK (1982) Effect of lung inflation on pulmonary vascular resistance by arterial and venous occlusion. J Appl Physiol 53(5):1110–1115
16. Ducas J, Schick U, Girling L, Prewitt RM (1988) Effects of altered left atrial pressure on pulmonary vascular pressure-flow relationships. Am J Physiol 255(1 Pt 2):H19-H25
17. Graham R, Skoog C, Oppenheimer L et al (1982) Critical closure in the canine pulmonary vasculature. Circ Res 1982 50(4):566–572
18. Warrell DA, Evans JW, Clarke RO et al 1972) Pattern of filling in the pulmonary capillary bed. J Appl Physiol 32(3):346–356
19. Glazier JB, Hughes JM, Maloney JE, West JB (1969) Measurements of capillary dimensions and blood volume in rapidly frozen lungs. J Appl Physiol 26(1):65–76
20. Borst HG, McGregor M, Whittenberger JL, Berglund E (1956) Influence of pulmonary arterial and left atrial pressure on pulmonary vascular resistance. Circ Res 4:393–399
21. Malbouisson LM, Muller JC, Constantin JM et al (2001) Computed tomography assessment of positive end-expiratory pressure-induced alveolar recruitment in patients with acute respiratory distress syndrome. Am J Respir Crit Care Med 163(6):1444–1450
22. Crotti S, Mascheroni D, Caironi P et al (2001) Recruitment and derecruitment during acute respiratory failure: a clinical study. Am J Respir Crit Care Med 164(1):131–140
23. Kloot TE, Blanch L, Melynne YA et al (2000) Recruitment maneuvers in three experimental models of acute lung injury. Effect on lung volume and gas exchange. Am J Respir Crit Care Med 161(5):1485–1494
24. Presson RG Jr, Audi SH, Hanger CC et al (1998) Anatomic distribution of pulmonary vascular compliance. J Appl Physiol 84(1):303–310
25. Hakim TS, Michel RP, Chang HK (1982) Partitioning of pulmonary vascular resistance in dogs by arterial and venous occlusion. J Appl Physiol 52(3):710–715
26. Shoukas AA (1975) Pressure-flow and pressure–volume relations in the entire pulmonary vascular bed of the dog determined by two-port analysis. Circ Res 37(6):809–818
27. Dawson CA (1984) Role of pulmonary vasomotion in physiology of the lung. Physiol Rev 64(2):544–616
28. Feihl F, Perret C (1994) Permissive hypercapnia. How permissive should we be? Am J Respir Crit Care Med 150(6 Pt 1):1722–1737
29. Brimioulle S, Lejeune P, Vachiery JL et al (1990) Effects of acidosis and alkalosis on hypoxic pulmonary vasoconstriction in dogs. Am J Physiol 258(2 Pt 2):H347-H353
30. Puybasset L, Stewart T, Rouby JJ et al (1994) Inhaled nitric oxide reverses the increase in pulmonary vascular resistance induced by permissive hypercapnia in patients with acute respiratory distress syndrome. Anesthesiology 80(6):1254–1267
31. Feihl F, Eckert P, Brimioulle S et al (2000) Permissive hypercapnia impairs pulmonary gas exchange in the acute respiratory distress syndrome. Am J Respir Crit Care Med 162(1):209–215

32. Hickling KG, Walsh J, Henderson S, Jackson R (1994) Low mortality rate in adult respiratory distress syndrome using low-volume, pressure-limited ventilation with permissive hypercapnia: a prospective study. Crit Care Med 22(10):1568–1578
33. Glenny RW, Lamm WJ, Albert RK, Robertson HT (1991) Gravity is a minor determinant of pulmonary blood flow distribution. J Appl Physiol 71(2):620–629
34. Mure M, Domino KB, Lindahl SG et al (2000) Regional ventilation-perfusion distribution is more uniform in the prone position. J Appl Physiol 88(3):1076–1083
35. Walther SM, Domino KB, Glenny RW, Hlastala MP (1999) Positive end-expiratory pressure redistributes perfusion to dependent lung regions in supine but not in prone lambs. Crit Care Med 27(1):37–45
36. Glenny RW, Bernard S, Robertson HT, Hlastala MP (1999) Gravity is an important but secondary determinant of regional pulmonary blood flow in upright primates. J Appl Physiol 86(2):623–632
37. Smith JC, Mitzner W (1980) Analysis of pulmonary vascular interdependence in excised dog lobes. J Appl Physiol 1980 48(3):450–467
38. Albert RK, Lamm WJ, Rickaby DA et al (1993) Lung inflation distends small arteries (<1 mm) in excised dog lungs. J Appl Physiol 75(6):2595–2601
39. Koyama S, Lamm WJ, Hildebrandt J, Albert RK (1989) Flow characteristics of open vessels in zone 1 rabbit lungs. J Appl Physiol 66(4):1817–1823
40. Lamm WJ, Kirk KR, Hanson WL et al (1991) Flow through zone 1 lungs utilizes alveolar corner vessels. J Appl Physiol 70(4):1518–1523
41. Putensen C, Mutz NJ, Putensen-Himmer G, Zinserling J (1999) Spontaneous breathing during ventilatory support improves ventilation–perfusion distributions in patients with acute respiratory distress syndrome. Am J Respir Crit Care Med 159(4 Pt 1):1241–1248
42. Gil J (1980) Organization of microcirculation in the lung. Annu Rev Physiol 42:177–186
43. Brower R, Wise RA, Hassapoyannes C et al (1985) Effect of lung inflation on lung blood volume and pulmonary venous flow. J Appl Physiol 58(3):954–963
44. Permutt S, Howell J, Proctor, Riley R (1961) Effect of lung inflation on static pressure–volume characteristics of pulmonary vessels. J Appl Physiol 16:64–70
45. Albert RK, Lakshminarayan S, Kirk W, Butler J (1980) Lung inflation can cause pulmonary edema in zone I of in situ dog lungs. J Appl Physiol 49(5):815–819
46. Broccard A, Shapiro RS, Schmitz LL et al (2000) Prone positioning attenuates and redistributes ventilator-induced lung injury in dogs. Crit Care Med 28(2):295–303
47. Nyren S, Mure M, Jacobsson H et al (1999) Pulmonary perfusion is more uniform in the prone than in the supine position: scintigraphy in healthy humans. J Appl Physiol 86:1135–1141
48. Kallas HJ, Domino KB, Glenny RW et al (1998) Pulmonary blood flow redistribution with low levels of positive end-expiratory pressure. Anesthesiology 88(5):1291–1299
49. Gattinoni L, Tognoni G, Pesenti A et al (2001) Effect of prone positioning on the survival of patients with acute respiratory failure. N Engl J Med 345(8):568–573
50. Chatte G, Sab JM, Dubois JM et al (1997) Prone position in mechanically ventilated patients with severe acute respiratory failure. Am J Respir Crit Care Med 155(2):473–478
51. Wiener CM, Kirk W, Albert RK (1990) Prone position reverses gravitational distribution of perfusion in dog lungs with oleic acid-induced injury. J Appl Physiol 68(4):1386–1392
52. Puybasset L, Cluzel P, Chao N et al (1998) A computed tomography scan assessment of regional lung volume in acute lung injury. The CT Scan ARDS Study Group. Am J Respir Crit Care Med 158(5 Pt 1):1644–1655
53. Scillia P, Kafi SA, Melot C et al (2001) Oleic acid-induced lung injury: thin-section CT evaluation in dogs. Radiology 219(3):724–731
54. Sandiford P, Province MA, Schuster DP (1995) Distribution of regional density and vascular permeability in the adult respiratory distress syndrome. Am J Respir Crit Care Med 151(3 Pt 1):737–742
55. Mutoh T, Lamm WJ, Embree LJ et al (1992) Volume infusion produces abdominal distension, lung compression, and chest wall stiffening in pigs. J Appl Physiol 72(2):575–582

56. Gattinoni L, D'Andrea L, Pelosi P et al (1993) Regional effects and mechanism of positive end-expiratory pressure in early adult respiratory distress syndrome. JAMA 269(16):2122–2127
57. Martynowicz MA, Minor TA, Walters BJ, Hubmayr RD (1999) Regional expansion of oleic acid-injured lungs. Am J Respir Crit Care Med 160(1):250–258
58. Lamm WJ, Graham MM, Albert RK (1994) Mechanism by which the prone position improves oxygenation in acute lung injury. Am J Respir Crit Care Med 150(1):184–193
59. Malo J, Ali J, Wood LD (1984) How does positive end-expiratory pressure reduce intrapulmonary shunt in canine pulmonary edema? J Appl Physiol 57(4):1002–1010
60. Hasan FM, Beller TA, Sobonya RE et al (1982) Effect of positive end-expiratory pressure and body position in unilateral lung injury. J Appl Physiol 52(1):147–154
61. Hormann C, Baum M, Putensen C et al (1997) Effects of spontaneous breathing with BIPAP on pulmonary gas exchange in patients with ARDS. Acta Anaesthesiol Scand Suppl 111:152–155
62. Gattinoni L, Pelosi P, Suter PM et al (1998) Acute respiratory distress syndrome caused by pulmonary and extrapulmonary disease. Different syndromes? Am J Respir Crit Care Med 158(1):3–11
63. Gattinoni L, Caironi P, Pelosi P, Goodman LR (2001) What has computed tomography taught us about the acute respiratory distress syndrome? Am J Respir Crit Care Med 164(9):1701–1711
64. Pappert D, Rossaint R, Slama K et al (1994) Influence of positioning on ventilation-perfusion relationships in severe adult respiratory distress syndrome. Chest 106(5):1511–1516
65. Pelosi P, Tubiolo D, Mascheroni D et al (1998) Effects of the prone position on respiratory mechanics and gas exchange during acute lung injury. Am J Respir Crit Care Med 157(2):387–393
66. Guerin C (2006) Ventilation in the prone position in patients with acute lung injury/acute respiratory distress syndrome. Curr Opin Crit Care 12(1):50–54
67. Mancebo J, Fernandez R, Blanch L et al (2006) A multicenter trial of prolonged prone ventilation in severe acute respiratory distress syndrome. Am J Respir Crit Care Med 173(11):1233–1239
68. Verkman AS, Matthay MA, Song Y (2000) Aquaporin water channels and lung physiology. Am J Physiol Lung Cell Mol Physiol 278(5):L867-L879
69. Drake RE, Laine GA (1988) Pulmonary microvascular permeability to fluid and macromolecules. J Appl Physiol 64(2):487–501
70. Taylor AE (1981) Capillary fluid filtration. Starling forces and lymph flow. Circ Res 49(3):557–575
71. Goldberg HS, Mitzner W, Batra G (1977) Effect of transpulmonary and vascular pressures on rate of pulmonary edema formation. J Appl Physiol 43(1):14–19
72. Bo G, Hauge A, Nicolaysen G (1977) Alveolar pressure and lung volume as determinants of net transvascular fluid filtration. J Appl Physiol 42(4):476–482
73. Zabner J, Angeli LS, Martinez RR, Sanchez dL (1990) The effects of graded administration of positive end expiratory pressure on the fluid filtration rate in isolated rabbit lungs, using normal lungs, hydrostatic oedema lungs and oleic acid induced oedema. Intensive Care Med 16(2):89–94
74. Nieman GF, Bredenberg CE, Paskanik AM (1990) Positive end-expiratory pressure accelerates lung water accumulation in high surface tension edema. Surgery 107(2):156–162
75. Wickerts CJ, Berg B, Blomqvist H (1992) Influence of positive end-expiratory pressure on extravascular lung water during the formation of experimental hydrostatic pulmonary oedema. Acta Anaesthesiol Scand 36(4):309–317
76. Hirakawa A, Sakamoto H, Shimizu R (1996) Effect of positive end-expiratory pressure on extravascular lung water and cardiopulmonary function in dogs with experimental severe hydrostatic pulmonary edema. J Vet Med Sci 58(4):349–354
77. Ruiz-Bailen M, Fernandez-Mondejar E, Hurtado-Ruiz B et al (1999) Immediate application of positive-end expiratory pressure is more effective than delayed positive-end expiratory

pressure to reduce extravascular lung water. Crit Care Med 27(2):380–384
78. Colmenero-Ruiz M, Fernandez-Mondejar E, Fernandez-Sacristan MA et al (1997) PEEP and low tidal volume ventilation reduce lung water in porcine pulmonary edema. Am J Respir Crit Care Med 155(3):964–970
79. Pepe PE, Hudson LD, Carrico CJ (1984) Early application of positive end-expiratory pressure in patients at risk for the adult respiratory-distress syndrome. N Engl J Med 311(5):281–286
80. Corbridge TC, Wood LD, Crawford GP et al (1990) Adverse effects of large tidal volume and low PEEP in canine acid aspiration. Am Rev Respir Dis 142(2):311–315
81. Muscedere JG, Mullen JB, Gan K, Slutsky AS (1994) Tidal ventilation at low airway pressures can augment lung injury. Am J Respir Crit Care Med 149(5):1327–1334
82. Dreyfuss D, Saumon G (1998) Ventilator-induced lung injury: lessons from experimental studies. Am J Respir Crit Care Med 157(1):294–323
83. Amato MB, Barbas CS, Medeiros DM et al (1998) Effect of a protective-ventilation strategy on mortality in the acute respiratory distress syndrome. N Engl J Med 338(6):347–354
84. Ranieri VM, Suter PM, Tortorella C et al (1999) Effect of mechanical ventilation on inflammatory mediators in patients with acute respiratory distress syndrome: a randomized controlled trial. JAMA 282(1):54–61
85. Brower RG, Lanken PN, MacIntyre N et al (2004) Higher versus lower positive end-expiratory pressures in patients with the acute respiratory distress syndrome. N Engl J Med 351(4):327–336
86. Grasso S, Fanelli V, Cafarelli A et al (2005) Effects of high versus low positive end-expiratory pressures in acute respiratory distress syndrome. Am J Respir Crit Care Med 171(9):1002–1008
87. Bshouty Z, Ali J, Younes M (1988) Effect of tidal volume and PEEP on rate of edema formation in in situ perfused canine lobes. J Appl Physiol 64(5):1900–1907
88. Slutsky AS (1999) Lung injury caused by mechanical ventilation. Chest 116(1 Suppl):9S-15S
89. Taylor AE, Khimenko PL, Moore TM, Adkins WK (1997) Fluid Balance. In: Crystal RG, West JB, Weibel ER, Barnes PJ (eds) The lung scientific foundations. Lippincott-Raven. Philadelphia, pp 1549–1566
90. Dreyfuss D, Saumon G (1996) Synergistic interaction between alveolar flooding and distension during mechanical ventilation. Am J Respir Crit Care Med 153(Suppl):A12
91. Albert RK, Lakshminarayan S, Hildebrandt J et al (1979) Increased surface tension favors pulmonary edema formation in anesthetized dogs' lungs. J Clin Invest 63(5):1015–1018
92. Albert RK, Lakshminarayan S, Charan NB et al (1983) Extra-alveolar vessel contribution to hydrostatic pulmonary edema in in situ dog lungs. J Appl Physiol 54(4):1010–1017
93. West JB, Mathieu-Costello O (1992) Stress failure of pulmonary capillaries in the intensive care setting. Schweiz Med Wochenschr 122(20):751–757
94. West JB, Mathieu-Costello O (1995) Vulnerability of pulmonary capillaries in heart disease. Circulation 92(3):622–631
95. West JB, Mathieu-Costello O, Jones JH et al (1993) Stress failure of pulmonary capillaries in racehorses with exercise- induced pulmonary hemorrhage. J Appl Physiol 75(3):1097–1109
96. West JB, Mathieu-Costello O (1992) High altitude pulmonary edema is caused by stress failure of pulmonary capillaries. Int J Sports Med 13(Suppl 1):S54-S58
97. West JB, Mathieu-Costello O (1992) Stress failure of pulmonary capillaries: role in lung and heart disease. Lancet 340(8822):762–767
98. West JB, Mathieu-Costello O (1992) Strength of the pulmonary blood-gas barrier. Respir Physiol 88(1–2):141–148
99. Tsukimoto K, Mathieu-Costello O, Prediletto R et al (1991) Ultrastructural appearances of pulmonary capillaries at high transmural pressures. J Appl Physiol 71(2):573–582
100. West JB, Tsukimoto K, Mathieu-Costello O, Prediletto R (1991) Stress failure in pulmonary capillaries. J Appl Physiol 70(4):1731–1742

101. Namba Y, Kurdak SS, Fu Z et al (1995) Effect of reducing alveolar surface tension on stress failure in pulmonary capillaries. J Appl Physiol 79(6):2114–2121
102. Broccard AF, Vannay C, Feihl F, Schaller MD (2002) Impact of low pulmonary vascular pressure on ventilator-induced lung injury. Crit Care Med 30(10):2183–2190
103. Han B, Lodyga M, Liu M (2005) Ventilator-induced lung injury: role of protein-protein interaction in mechanosensation. Proc Am Thorac Soc 2(3):181–187
104. Lionetti V, Recchia FA, Ranieri VM (2005) Overview of ventilator-induced lung injury mechanisms. Curr Opin Crit Care 11(1):82–86
105. Adhikari NK, Burns KE, Friedrich JO et al (2007) Effect of nitric oxide on oxygenation and mortality in acute lung injury: systematic review and meta-analysis. BMJ 334(7597):779
106. Wiedemann HP, Wheeler AP, Bernard GR et al (2006) Comparison of two fluid-management strategies in acute lung injury. N Engl J Med 354(24):2564–2575

Monitoring of the Respiratory Mechanics

Monitoring of Respiratory Mechanics in the Intensive Care Unit: Models, Techniques and Measurement Methods

A. Aliverti

Introduction

Any assessment of respiratory-system mechanics from measured data is strongly dependent on the model adopted to describe the structure of the respiratory system and its components: airways, lung and chest wall. Sometime, the model may be very complex, with multiple alveolar compartments and airway branches representing the tracheo-bronchial tree, or many chest-wall structures representing the rib cage, the respiratory muscles and the abdomen. This modelling approach is used mainly for research purposes, when an analytical description is required to study the respiratory system in detail and data that cannot be obtained in humans are available.

In most clinical applications, the model adopted is instead very simple, typically involving only a single compartment. The model of respiratory or pulmonary mechanics most frequently employed as the basis for lung-function measurements is that of a single elastic compartment served by a single flow-resistive airway (Fig. 1). This model assumes that the lungs are homogeneously ventilated and that all alveolar pressures are equal to each other at all times.

Resistance and Elastance

The single-compartment model of respiratory mechanics is described by a simple and extremely useful mathematical equation, if the model is linear. If the resistive pressure drop between one end of the airway and the other is considered to be proportional to the flow of gas (V') through it, then the constant of proportionality (R) is termed 'resistance'. Similarly, the elastic recoil pressure inside the compartment is defined as being proportional to the volume of the compartment above some elastic equilibrium volume, with its constant of proportionality (E) termed 'elastance'. Also, the model takes into account the possibility that the pressure (P) applied across the model (from the entrance to the airway through to

U. Lucangelo, P. Pelosi, W.A. Zin, A. Aliverti (eds.) *Respiratory System and Artificial Ventilation*. © Springer 2008

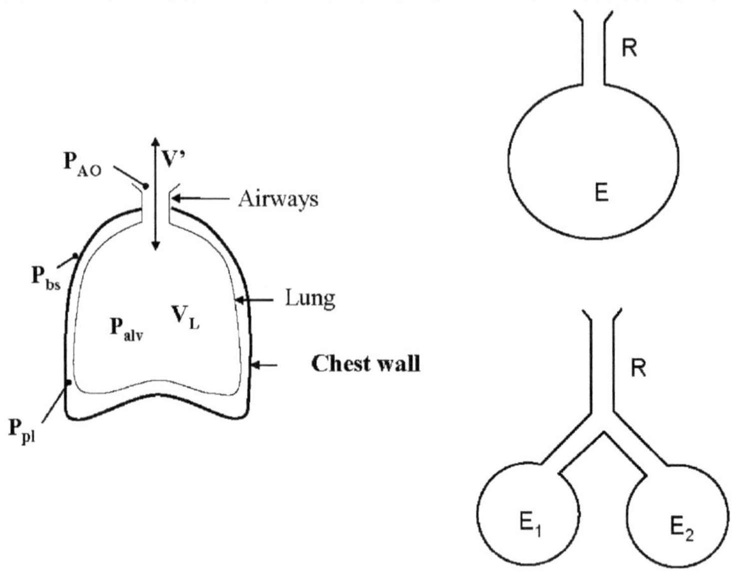

Fig. 1 The respiratory system, comprising the airways, the lung and the chest wall. V', airflow; V_L, lung volume; P_{AO}, pressure at airway opening; P_{alv}, alveolar pressure; P_{pl}, pleural pressure; Pbs, pressure at the body surface (*left*). *Right*, the single-compartment model of the respiratory system, where R is resistance and E is elastance (top); a double-compartment model, where two elastances E_1 and E_2 account for regional differences in mechanical function throughout the lung

the outside of the elastic compartment) has some finite value P_0 when V' and V are both zero. P is the sum of the resistive and elastic pressures:

$$P(t)=RV'(t)+EV(t)+P_0 \quad \text{(Eq. 1)}$$

where the variables P, V and V' are written as functions of time (t) as they all vary during breathing. Equation 1 is used to estimate R, E and P_0 by multiple linear regression. This statistical approach provides those values that give the closest approximation to the measured P, in the least squares sense, which means that the sum of the squared differences between the measured value of P and the model values is minimal. R and E are measures of the resistance and elastance of the lung or respiratory system, respectively, if P is the pressure across the total respiratory system (i.e. the pressure at the airway opening, P_{ao}) or the pressure across the lung (i.e. the trans-pulmonary pressure, equal to P_{ao}-P_{pl}, where P_{pl} is pleural pressure). In this approach, R and E are the parameters of the model that has been designed to match the measured signals (pressure, flow and volume) as well as possible.

The usefulness of R and E depends on how much the single-compartment linear model accurately describes the behaviour of the system under study. When this linear model is accurate, then the meaning of R is not just the flow resistance of the airway tree, as studies with the alveolar capsule in animal models have allowed total resistance (R) to be partitioned into airway resistance and tissue resistance [1,2]. The latter has been shown to depend greatly on the frequency at which the lungs are oscillated and, at normal breathing frequencies, may constitute the great majority of R [3]. Only at frequencies well above the range of normal breathing (above about 2 Hz) is a good estimate of airway resistance alone [4–6]. R also contains a significant contribution from the chest wall [7].

Non-linear Single-Compartment Models

When the single-compartment linear model does not describe a set of respiratory data with acceptable accuracy (e.g. when the volume excursions of the lungs are large or when the stiffness of the lung tissue increases, as in certain diseases), a more realistic (and more complex) model must be considered. In this case, the elastic properties of the tissues are described by a curvilinear function of volume rather than a straight line as in the linear model.

It has been shown in humans [8] and in animals [9] that the equation

$$P(t) = RV'(t) + E_1V(t) + E_2V^2(t) + P_0 \qquad \text{(Eq. 2)}$$

sometimes fits the data significantly better than the linear model described by Eq. 1.

The non-linear model described by Eq. 2 is structurally the same as the linear model described by Eq. 1 as both have a single compartment that is ventilated through a single airway. The difference is that the elastic properties of the tissues surrounding the compartment are non-linear. Similarly, the linear resistance R in Eq. 1 can be replaced by two terms representing a flow-dependent resistance, as originally proposed by Rohrer [9]:

$$R = K_1 + K_2 \times |V'(t)| \qquad \text{(Eq. 3)}$$

An important use of the single-compartment model of respiratory mechanics is the assessment of the stiffness of the lung or respiratory system from the quasi-static pressure–volume (PV) curve. The PV curve is obtained by inflating the compartment slowly enough such that the resistive pressure drop across the airways can be neglected. The result is a relationship that embodies the elastic properties of the pulmonary tissues, viewed as a single compartment. The model invoked to account for the PV curve is thus again a single compartment model, but now it is non-linear because the elastic recoil pressure inside the compartment increases disproportionately as volume approaches total lung capacity.

Several parameters derived from the PV curve have been considered to be of potential clinical interest, such as the lower and upper inflection points. Initially, these parameters were manually identified. In an attempt to standardise their definitions, the lower and upper inflection points were computed as the point of intersection of the 'inflation' compliance (or chord compliance) and, respectively, the starting and 'final compliance'. Roupie et al. [10] defined 'final compliance' as the portion of PV curve in which compliance is decreased at least 20%, whereas Nunes et al. [11] suggested a threshold of 10%.

A commonly used equation for describing the descending limb of the PV curve is the exponential expression originally proposed by Salazar et al. [12]:

$$V = A - B \times e^{-KP} \qquad \text{(Eq. 4)}$$

where A, B and K are constants chosen to make the right side of the equation match the left side as closely as possible.

The ascending limb of the PV curve lies to the right of the descending limb, thus showing a phenomenon known as *hysteresis*. The amount of hysteresis depends on the volume range over which V is cycled and is caused by a number of factors. One of the most important is recruitment of closed airspaces during inspiration that remain open during expiration. Hysteresis may become markedly enhanced in acute lung injury [13].

The Super-Syringe Technique

The super-syringe static method consists of inflating the lungs in steps of 50–100 ml up to 1.5 or 3.0 l starting from the functional residual capacity (FRC) [14]. The volume of gas administered is determined by the displacement of the piston. The airway pressure is measured by a pressure transducer, with zero referred to the atmospheric pressure. The patients are sedated, paralysed and ventilated at a fractional inspired oxygen of 1.0 without any positive end-expiratory pressure (PEEP) for 15 min before the measurement, and the syringe is filled beforehand with humidified oxygen. The patient must be disconnected from the ventilator for a few seconds to empty the lungs completely. The syringe is then connected to the endotracheal tube and the inflation manoeuvre is started from the FRC. The interval between two successive inflations should be 3 s in order to ensure a stable plateau pressure. The same manoeuvre can be performed during deflation in successive steps of 50–100 ml (Fig.2). The pressures and the volumes are recorded simultaneously and the pressure–volume curve is constructed from the obtained data. The entire procedure takes about 60 s. The super-syringe technique was largely used during the 1980s to describe the different stages of acute respiratory distress syndrome (ARDS) [14,15]. This method has some disadvantages, however; the patient has to be disconnected from the ventilator and there is a loss of lung volume during the inflation procedure due to consumption of the oxygen contained in the syringe. The errors in measurement that occur with the use of the super-syringe technique were evaluated by Dall'Ava-Santucci et al. [16] and Gattinoni et al. [17]. Those investigators compared the variations in lung volumes obtained using the syringe technique with those measured by respiratory inductance plethysmography (RIP). The PV curves obtained with RIP exhibited lesser

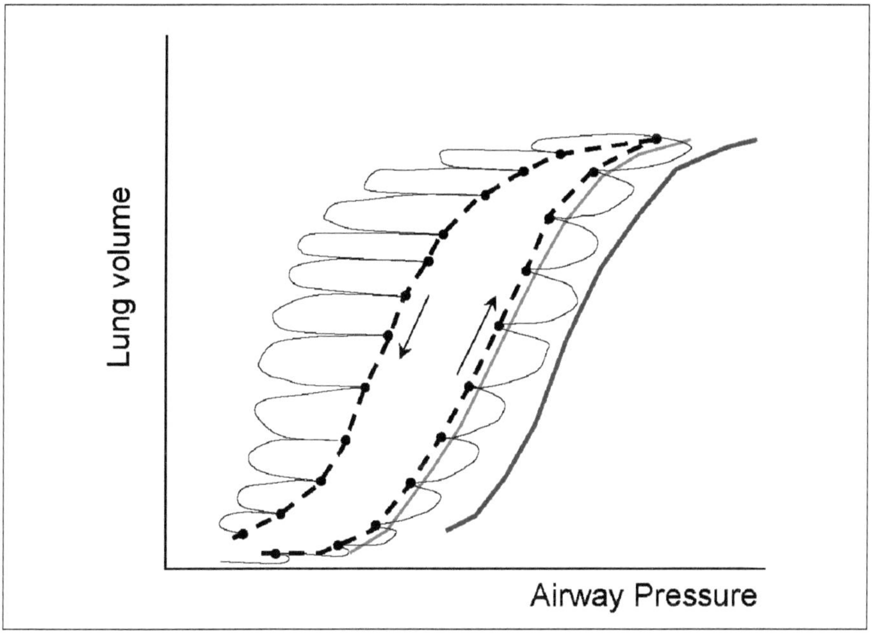

Fig. 2 *Dashed line*, pressure–volume curve obtained with the super-syringe method, showing the inspiratory and expiratory limbs of the curve. Each point (pressure and volume) is obtained during stepwise inflation and deflation of the lungs. *Red solid line*, pressure–volume curve obtained by a quasi-static technique, i.e. inflating the respiratory system by a constant flow delivered by the ventilator, with a low inspiratory flow (10 l/min). *Blu solid line*, pressure–volume curve obtained with an high inspiratory constant flow (between 20 and 60 l/min)

degrees of hysteresis (difference between the lung volumes during inflation and deflation for the same level of pressure), and the compliance during deflation was higher (73 vs. 67 ml/cmH_2O). This difference was observed only if the duration of the inflation was prolonged (>45 s) and was related to the gas exchange that occurred in the lung during the manoeuvre. The loss of lung volume due to oxygen uptake was only partially compensated for by the production of CO_2 [17]. A rapid inflation of <40 s helps to minimise this error [16]. The temperature and the humidity of the gas in the syringe may also influence the measurement of the PV curve. Administration of unwarmed and unhumidified gas causes a displacement of the curve to the left [17,18].

More recently, Chiumello et al. [19] used optoelectronic plethysmography (see below) during the super-syringe method in patients with acute lung injury (ALI) and ARDS in order to measure the difference between total chest-wall and gas volume changes (ΔV_{cw}-ΔV_{gas}). This, corrected for thermodynamic and gas exchange, is an index of blood volume shifts (V_{bs}) from the thorax to the periphery. They found that hysteresis, i.e. the difference between the inspired and expired volumes, was significantly affected by V_{bs}. As this was partially attributed to recruitment [20,21], i.e. alveolar opening during inspiration and persistent opening during expiration, these findings partly smoothed the concept. In fact, these differences may be due not only to recruitment, but also to the shift of blood from the thorax to the periphery and vice versa. At the same airway pressure on the inspiratory and expiratory limbs (20 cmH_2O), the difference in volume possibly due to the blood shift averaged 0.099±0.058 l, ranging from -0.014 to 0.164 l, the same order of magnitude as the 'recruitment' in some ALI/ARDS patients [22] (Fig. 3). All these studies demonstrate that the relation between modifications of chest-wall volume, lung volume, and blood shift during PV curve assessment need further investigation, especially when the curve is used to estimate pulmonary recruitment.

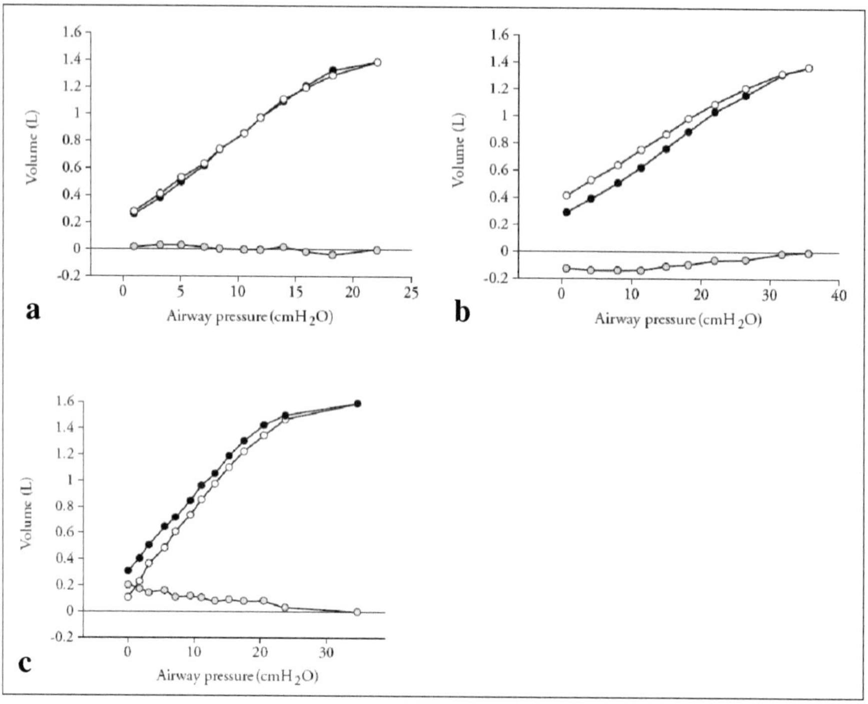

Fig. 3a-c Possible patterns of deflation limbs of the pressure–volume (PV) curve. *Black circles,* PV curves of the entire chest wall as obtained by optoelectronic plethysmography (OEP); *white circles,* gas volume (corrected by thermodynamics and gas exchange); *grey circles,* discrepancy between the two curves. **a** The volume decrease of the chest wall is equal to the volume of gas withdrawn from the system, suggesting that the net shift of blood volume is zero. **b** The chest-wall volume decreases more than the gas volume withdrawn from the lung, suggesting a further volume shift out of the chest wall. **c** The chest-wall volume decreases less than the gas volume withdrawn, suggesting a net entry of blood volume in the chest wall. From [19], with permission

The Quasi-static Method Using Continuous Inflation at Constant Flow

Another relatively simple technique to obtain a PV curve from a critically ill patient without having to disconnect the patient from the ventilator is to inflate the respiratory system by a constant flow delivered by the ventilator (Fig. 2) [23,24]. This quasi-static technique can be performed on any intensive-care ventilator that is equipped with a constant-flow generator and has software and a display screen for plotting and analysing the PV curve. Several studies have been performed to compare the quasi-static technique at constant flow with the static technique [25–27]; the results showed that the compliances obtained by the two methods are very similar. An important parameter to be defined is the value of delivered constant flow. High constant flows (between 20 and 60 l/min) reliably estimate only the slope of the PV curve, while upper and lower inflection points are overestimated because of the resistive effect (Fig. 2) [23,24]. While very low flow allows accurate estimates, long measurement periods are required to inflate the lungs, which may result in a loss of lung volume during the manoeuvre because of oxygen uptake by the lungs.

Two solutions have been proposed to decrease the resistive component when quasi-static methods are used: (a) subtraction of the resistive pressure in the connecting tubes and in the airways from the measured total pressure [23,28]; (b) reduction of the constant flow. Recent studies [24,29] showed that the influence of the resistive factor on the PV curves obtained using the quasi-static method is not clinically relevant if the flow is administered at a rate less than 9 l/min (Fig. 2).

The continuous-flow technique presents a number of advantages over the super-syringe and the inspiratory occlusion techniques: it does not require disconnection of the patient from the ventilator; it does not modify the lung volume before the manoeuvre is performed; construction of the PV curve on the ventilator screen takes only 10 s and the entire procedure, including the analysis of the characteristics of the PV curves, takes around 2 min; the loss of volume due to oxygen uptake by the lungs is negligible; and the technique is simple to carry out at the bedside, without the need for any special equipment other than a respirator. However, the software for freezing and analysing the PV curve is not available on most intensive-care ventilators. Systems are being developed that deliver constant flows between 0 and 10 l/min and which include software that allows analysis of the PV curves. These ventilators should facilitate routine measurement of the PV curves at the bedside.

Methods Based on Multi-compartment Models

The single-compartment linear model generally reliably describes respiratory pressure-flow data when volume excursions are modest and the volume oscillations are concentrated around a single frequency, such as, for example, during normal breathing or mechanical ventilation. Nonetheless, the values of R and E obtained using this model vary with frequency. In particular, R decreases markedly as frequency is increased over the range of normal breathing, whereas E correspondingly increases. The main reason for this frequency dependence of R and E in normal lungs is the fact that the respiratory tissues are viscoelastic; that is, they exert a recoil pressure that is a function not only of volume but also of volume history [30]. In diseased lungs, additional variation of R and E with frequency may be caused by regional variations in mechanical function throughout the lung, leading to transient redistribution of gas as the lungs are dynamically inflated and deflated [31,32]. In any case, the single-compartment linear model is no longer valid as a description of pulmonary or respiratory mechanics when multiple frequencies are involved. Instead, it is necessary to consider models featuring two or more compartments to account for regional differences in mechanical function throughout the lung (Fig. 1) [33].

Interrupter Technique

A technique for assessing lung function that was first introduced nearly a century ago involves the rapid interruption of airflow at the airway opening, while pressure just behind the point of interruption is measured. This technique is performed using a mechanical ventilator equipped with facilities for end-inspiratory and end-expiratory occlusions. It is not necessary to disconnect the patient from the ventilator, and the loss of volume due to lung oxygen uptake is negligible because each measurement lasts only 3 s. The patient is ventilated in a volume-controlled mode with a constant flow. Between two measurements, ventilation is normalised by using the same ventilatory parameters. The different tidal volumes are administered in a randomised sequence. These tidal volumes are obtained by changing the respiratory rate while maintaining the inspiratory flow constant (lengthening or shortening the duration of inflation). The intrinsic PEEP is determined before each inflation to ensure that the lung volume and the end-expiratory pressure are stable. The occlusion manoeuvre is performed at end-inspiration and the plateau pressure is measured after a few seconds of occlusion (Fig. 4). The PV curve is constructed from the different plateau pressures that correspond to the administered volumes.

The inspiratory occlusion technique offers the advantage of avoiding disconnection of the patient from the ventilator and it allows measurements from any level of PEEP. Since the beginning of the 1990s, this technique has been extensively used to determine the lower and upper inflection points on the PV curve [34,36] and to quantify the effect of PEEP on alveolar recruitment in patients with ARDS [27,37]. Initially, it was thought that this manoeuvre would simply obliterate any resistive pressure drop across the airways, so that the observed sudden change in pressure would reflect Raw. However, work over the past two decades has shown that the sudden change in pressure occurring with interruption of flow is accompanied by rapid damped oscillations and a subsequent fur-

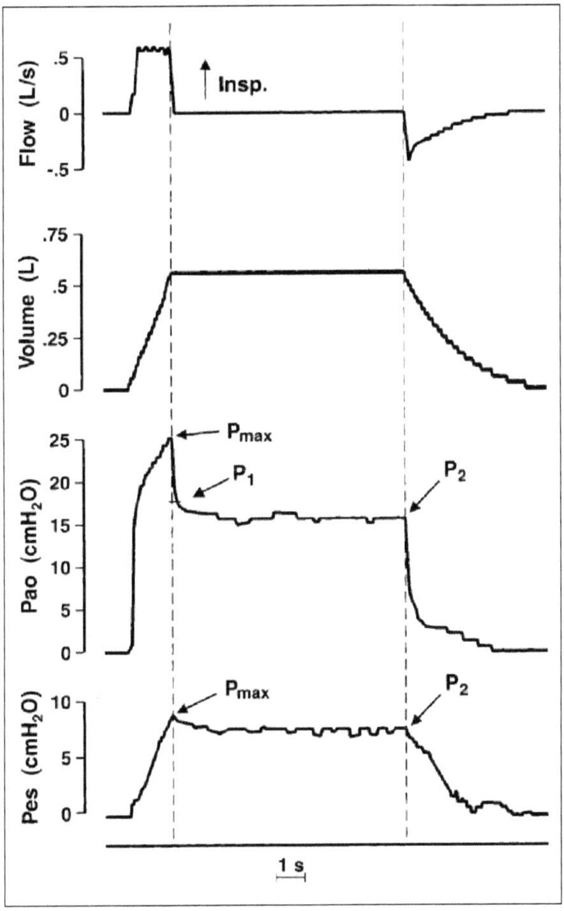

Fig. 4 Interrupter technique. Tracings (top to bottom) of flow, volume, airway pressure (P_{ao}) and oesophageal pressure (P_{oes}). After an end-expiratory occlusion, there is an immediate drop in P_{ao} from a maximum pressure (P_{max}) to a lower value (P_1), followed by a slow decay to a plateau (P_2) that represents the end-inspiratory recoil pressure of the respiratory system ($P_{st,rs}$)

ther transient change in pressure to a stable plateau. The oscillations are mainly due to ringing of the gas in the central airways [37], whereas the secondary slow pressure change is due to the viscoelastic properties of the respiratory tissues when the lung is normal [38] and may be accentuated by gas redistribution in pathologic situations [39]. The initially rapid and subsequently slower pressure changes have been interpreted on the basis of two-compartment models of respiratory mechanics [33,40,41].

The interrupter technique is currently gaining interest among paediatricians [42], who face a particular challenge in trying to assess lung function in young children and infants unable to perform the voluntary manoeuvres necessary to generate forced expired flows. However, the interruption of flow is merely a specialised kind of flow perturbation. The information obtained by applying general flow perturbations to the lungs is best understood in the context of the forced oscillation technique and impedance.

Input Impedance

The frequency dependence of R and E has led researchers to move to a more general assessment of respiratory mechanics based on a quantity known as input impedance (Zin). Zin can be determined over a range of frequencies by imposing an oscillatory flow signal that contains multiple frequencies to the lung. Zin is then determined by taking the ratio of the Fourier transform of P to the Fourier transform of'. This yields a complex function of frequency

$$Zin(f)=R(f)+iX(f) \qquad \text{(Eq. 5)}$$

where R(f) is the real part and X(f) is the imaginary part.

The value of R at each value of f is equal to the resistance of an equivalent single-compartment linear model, such that the R(f) is called the resistance. X(f) is the reactance and at each f it is related to the elastance of the equivalent single-compartment model by

$$X(f)=\frac{-E(f)}{2\pi f} \qquad \text{(Eq. 6)}$$

Zin is thus nothing more than a description of how R and E vary over a range of frequencies. Zin still requires that the system under study be linear. This assumes that whatever values of R and E are obtained at a particular frequency, their values do not depend on the amplitudes of the P, and V signals used to measure them.

Forced Oscillation Technique

The measurement of Zin is achieved by the so-called forced oscillation technique, originally proposed by Dubois et al. [43], in which a flow generator (such as a loudspeaker or piston pump) is used to drive an oscillatory flow into the lungs via the airway opening (see [44] for a comprehensive review). The frequency range over which the signal oscillates determines the kind of information that will be obtained about respiratory mechanical function. At frequencies below about 2 Hz, much of Zin is determined by the rheologic properties of the tissues, as well as regional mechanical heterogeneities throughout the lung, should they exist. Regional heterogeneities can affect the shape of Zin above 2 Hz as well [31,32]. At frequencies of hundreds of Hz, information is obtained about the acoustic characteristics of the airways. Whatever the frequency range, the interpretation of Zin in physiologic terms requires some kind of model of the system under investigation. For example, normal respiratory or pulmonary Zin is described very accurately below about 20 Hz by a model consisting of a uniformly ventilated compartment surrounded by viscoelastic tissue. The compartment is served by a single airway having a Newtonian resistance R_N, whereas the viscoelastic tissue has an impedance with real and imaginary parts that both decrease hyperbolically with f. This construct is frequently referred to as the constant-phase model [45]. It is described by four parameters that allow Zin to be partitioned into a component pertaining to the airways and a component pertaining to the lung periphery.

The input impedance measured by the forced oscillation technique (FOT) reflects the mechanical properties of the entire respiratory system under most conditions. Recently, Dellacà et al. [46] showed that in the presence of expiratory flow limitation (EFL), a condition frequently occurring in patients with chronic obstructive pulmonary disease (COPD) even during spontaneous breathing, the impedance measured by the FOT is only a measure of the mechanical properties of airways downstream from the choke points. This is because a change in pressure cannot be transmitted upstream through the choke points and thus only the downstream airways are oscillated [47]. It was found that the threshold is independent of subject size and the severity of the disease [46]. This suggests that the differences in the mechanical properties of the airways downstream of choke points (measured by total respiratory-system Zin during expiration if the patient is flow limited) versus the mechanical properties of the entire respiratory system (measured by Zin during inspiration) must be much greater than any possible inter-subject variability of airway wall mechanics and location of choke points. Therefore, the measurement of expiratory reactance during tidal breathing can reliably detect breaths that are flow-limited and potentially the time at which flow limitation begins.

A possible application of this approach is the identification of minimum constant positive airway pressure (CPAP) or PEEP values required to minimise the development of EFL in mechanically ventilated COPD patients [48]. This information may guide the clinician's choice of CPAP, eliminating unnecessary effects on haemodynamics and impairment of inspiratory muscle function by increasing operating volumes. Moreover, as FOT has already been proved to be very well-tolerated by patients when combined with non-invasive mechanical ventilation [48–50], it may be useful to incorporate this measurement into mechanical ventilators able to continuously optimise the PEEP level to changes in patient posture, conditions, lung volumes and breathing pattern.

Measurement of Respiratory Variables

As expressed by Eq. 1, the basic variables that allow the assessment of respiratory mechanics are pressure, flow and volume. In the following sections, the main devices, their principles of measurement, and the most important problems associated with the different techniques are reviewed.

Pressure

Pressure Transducers

Pressure transduction is based on the deformation of a mechanical element whose altered configuration is read by some electronic means. Until about 20 years ago, the most frequently used device for pressure measurement in the respiratory physiology laboratory was the *variable reluctance transducer*, in which a thin metal disk is placed between the primary and secondary coils of a transformer excited by several kHz of alternating electric current. A pressure difference on either side of the disk causes it to deform in a way that alters the magnetic-flux linkage between the transformer coils, thereby changing the induced voltage in the secondary coil. The change in voltage is then transformed into a DC voltage that is proportional to the pressure difference. These transducers are sensitive and accurate. They also typically have a frequency response that is flat to 20 Hz or more, depending on the length of the tubing connecting its ports to the sites of pressure measurement. However, they are somewhat cumbersome and can be damaged by over-pressurisation. In more recent years, respiratory pressure measurement has been taken over by the piezoresistive transducer, in which the pressure-sensitive element changes its electrical resistance as it deforms. If a constant voltage (or current) is passed through the piezoresistive element when it is configured to be one of the four arms of a suitably balanced Wheatstone bridge, the voltage across the bridge is then proportional to the change in the element's resistance. A medium-gain amplifier and an anti-aliasing filter are the only remaining elements required to produce an electrical signal that is proportional to pressure and ready for digitisation. When piezoresistive pressure transducers were first used in respiratory physiology in the 1980s, they tended to suffer from baseline drift, were affected by orientation and temperature and were not very sensitive. These problems have now been essentially overcome, allowing piezoresistive transducers to be exploited for their several advantages. These include an extremely high-frequency response (typically flat to several hundred Hz), robustness (they can be pressurised to many times their nominal full-scale range without damage), and the fact that they can be manufactured using solid-state technology to be very small and light. Piezoresistive transducers are also much cheaper than their variable reluctance counterparts and require simpler electronic signal conditioning circuitry.

Measuring Pressure at the Airway Opening

The assessment of pulmonary function frequently requires that the pressure in a flowing stream of gas be measured, such as at the entrance to the endotracheal tube in a mechanically ventilated patient. The easiest way is to insert a perpendicular tap into the tube and connect it to a pressure transducer. However, this approach provides what is known as lateral pressure (P_{lat}), which corresponds to the pressure exerted perpendicular to the direction of flow as the gas moves past the point of measurement. It turns out, however, that P_{lat} is less than the pressure driving the gas along the tube (P_{stat}) because of a phenomenon known as the Bernoulli effect, which occurs because of the principle of conservation of energy: the faster gas moves along the tube, and consequently the larger its kinetic energy, the more it loses in potential energy, manifest as a drop in P_{lat}. Thus, P_{lat} underestimates true driving pressure, e.g. in a tube of cross-sectional area of a value

$$\Delta P = P_{stat} - P_{lat} = \frac{\beta \rho V'}{2A^2} \qquad \text{(Eq. 7)}$$

where ρ is the density of the gas and β is a factor determined by the flow velocity profile.

The problem of the Bernoulli effect on the measurement of respiratory pressure is apparent from Eq. 7, which shows that the difference between P_{stat} and P_{lat} depends on the square of flow divided by the cross-sectional area. When the area is large enough, this difference is negligible; however, as the area decreases there comes a point at which the difference starts to become important. Indeed, Eq. 7 shows that for small tube areas P_{lat} may even become negative. Thus, it is important in any application in which lateral pressures are measured to be sure that the Bernoulli effect is not significantly disturbing the measurement of the desired quantity, namely driving pressure [51]. The Bernoulli effect may also be an important factor influencing the measurement of pressures at the distal end of an endotracheal tube in an intubated patient [52].

Oesophageal Pressure Measurements

Oesophageal pressure (P_{oes}) is used to estimate P_{pl}. It can be measured using a thin catheter with a 10-cm-long balloon at the tip. The balloon is filled with 0.5 ml of air (a volume sufficient to prevent the walls of the balloon from occluding all the multiple holes in the end of the catheter, but not so much that there is tension in the balloon walls) and usually positioned in the middle third of the oesophagus. It is crucial to confirm correct positioning by the occlusion test [53]. When inspiratory efforts are made against an occluded airway, the deflections in P_{oes} should match P_{ao}. Thus, a regression of P_{oes} vs. P_{ao} should yield a slope of unity. In practice, slopes that differ from 1.0 by up to 10% are common. Although the occlusion test requires that the subject be able to breathe spontaneously, it has been shown that the oesophageal balloon also works well during paralysis [54].

The method has not reached widespread acceptance as it is difficult to introduce the relatively soft balloon catheter into the oesophagus of an unconscious patient, particularly if the patient already has a gastric tube in place. Karason and colleagues [55] suggested the use of a double-lumen gastric tube, the narrow lumen being connected to a standard pressure transducer and filled with fluid. Correct positioning was checked by compression of the rib cage during an expiratory hold, i.e. an occlusion-compression test, which can be carried out in paralysed patients. When this is done, the changes in oesophageal and airway pressures should be equal. The advantage of this method is the easy introduction of the device, but it is difficult to position the transducer at the appropriate level for correct absolute oesophageal pressure measurements. However, the absolute value is less important than the difference between the end-inspiratory and end-expiratory oesophageal pressures, which is used to estimate the compliance of the chest wall.

The frequency response of the oesophageal balloon is obviously somewhat compromised by the fact that pressure changes in the oesophageal lumen must be transmitted through the air inside a long thin catheter to a pressure transducer some distance away. However, a reasonably good response to 30 Hz has been observed [56]. Oesophageal pressure has also been measured using catheter-tip piezoresistive transducers, which have been shown to perform well [57] and have a much better frequency response than balloon catheter systems.

Gastric Pressure

Similar methods can be used for gastric pressure (P_{ga}) measurements, which will reflect intra-abdominal pressure (P_{ab}). When a fluid-filled measurement system is used, the mid-axillary line can be set as a zero reference for the transducer. In most patients with secondary ARDS, the elastance of the abdomen is greater than that of the chest wall, indicated by intra-abdominal and oesophageal pressure measurements, respectively. For gastric-pressure monitoring, positioning of the pressure line is easy and the pressure is probably measured more reliably than from the oesophagus.

Bladder Pressure

Abdominal pressure can also be measured via a urinary catheter. The bladder is drained of its content after which 50±100 ml of saline is instilled and the catheter is clamped distal to the pressure measurement position [58]. Collee and colleagues [59] compared measurements of intra-abdominal pressure using a gastric tube and using bladder pressure, and found that the two pressures were within 2.5 cmH_2O. Variations in bladder and central venous pressure correlated well with oesophageal and gastric pressures, respectively [60].

As for most pressure measurements of respiratory events, a frequency response that is flat up to 10–15 Hz is adequate to measure both dynamic and static pressures related to contractions of respiratory muscles, unless particular testing must be performed (e.g. application of the FOT). The frequency response of a transducer can be greatly altered by the characteristics of the systems attached to it, including balloons, tubing, and interconnecting fittings [61]. Thus, testing the response characteristics of any transducer with the specific connectors and fittings that are to be used to make the pressure measurements is highly recommended [61]. When differential pressure transducers are used, care must be taken that their two sides have identical frequency responses. Calibration is best made with water manometers. The required range and sensitivity of the transducers depend on the test in question.

Flow

Pneumotachographs

The basis of flow measurement in respiratory physiology is the pneumotachograph, which is a calibrated resistance (R) across which a differential pressure is measured (Fig. 5). When gas flows through the pneumotachograph, there is a pressure drop (ΔP) from the upstream side of the resistance to the downstream side that increases as flow (V') increases:

$$\Delta P = RV' \qquad \text{(Eq. 8)}$$

If R is independent of V' over the range of flows of interest, then the pneumotachograph is said to be linear. Linearity is generally achieved only within a range of flow values, and therefore it is necessary to invert Eq. 8 to calculate flow from a measurement of ΔP. The frequency response of a pneumotachograph depends on the construction of its resistive element, which may have a honeycomb arrangement of conduits or consist of a wire screen. The honeycomb type is less likely to become partially blocked by secretions but has a poorer frequency response than the screen type, as ΔP become dependent on a second term proportional to the derivative of the flow time through the inertia of the gas (which in turn is proportional to gas density and to the volume of the resistive element). Either type should be heated to above body temperature during prolonged use to avoid breath condensate from settling on the resistive element and changing its resistance (and hence altering the calibration of the device). Pneumotachographs can have a good frequency response above 20 Hz with a resonance occurring at

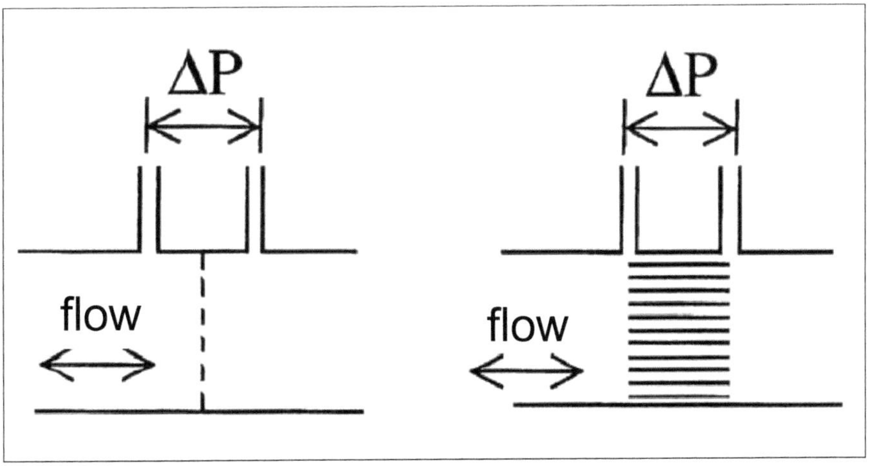

Fig. 5 The pneumotachograph (longitudinal view). Flow-resistive elements can consist of either wire screen (*left*) or a honeycomb arrangement of conduits (*right*)

around 70 Hz, provided that the associated differential transducer has a response at least that good and is connected with the shortest possible lengths of tubing [61]. The frequency response of a pneumotachograph degrades rapidly as the tubing connecting the transducer to the lateral taps either side of the resistance element increases in length. Although the resistive pneumotachograph is the principal device used to measure flow in respiratory applications, other devices have been proposed. Ultrasonic transducers based on differences in time-of-flight of sound propagating into the direction of flow versus away from it have an excellent frequency response and avoid the problems of a resistive element becoming clogged with secretions [62]. Devices based on the rate of cooling of a heated wire are also used [63].

Volume

Integration of Flow

Before the advent of the modern laboratory digital computer, integration was typically achieved in real time using an electronic circuit based on the charging of a capacitor. Nowadays, integration is performed digitally on a computer. The digitised flow signal consists of a series of data points separated by equal time intervals. A simple method for numerical integration is to calculate the area under the curve defined by the series of measured data (Fig. 6). The key problem is that the sampling frequency should be high enough so that the errors involved in approximating the true curve between points are negligible.

Another important problem is integration drift. When flow is integrated to yield volume, an upward or downward drift in the volume baseline is invariably seen. Some degree of drift is expected for purely physiological reasons. For example, the respiratory exchange ratio (i.e. carbon dioxide production/oxygen consumption) is usually ~0.8, i.e. the volume of O_2 absorbed by the lungs is 20% greater than the volume of CO_2 excreted. This is reflected in a slightly greater volume of gas being inspired than expired with each breath. Also, if the inspired air is not warmed to body temperature and pre-humidified, the volume of gas expired with each breath can be increased by up to 5%, relative to that inspired, by a gain in water-vapour content. These physiological effects contribute to a gradually increasing or decreasing volume measured at the mouth, but not to a real change in baseline lung volume. In addition to the physiological factors discussed above, the following methodological factors also contribute to volume drift [64].

1. *Temperature changes between inspired and expired gas.* If the inspired air is not warmed to body temperature before passing through the pneumotachograph, it has a different viscosity and density than expired air, which causes the pneumotachograph to register the transit of an equal number of molecules differently between inspiration and expiration. Variations in temperature may also affect the physical dimensions of the pneumotachograph due to the coefficients of thermal expansion of its components.

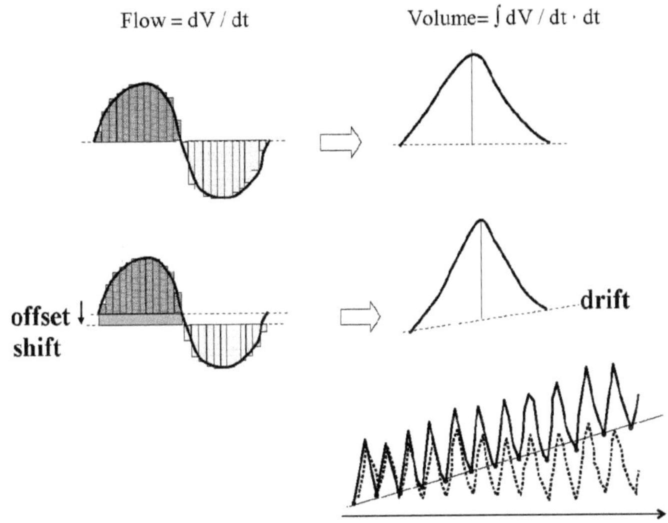

Fig. 6 *Top panel*, volume is obtained by numeric integration of flow signal. *Middle panel*, different physiological and methodological factors (see text) contribute to an offset shift in the flow signal, which determines a drift in its numeric integration. *Bottom panel*, example of volume drift correction. The oscillating volume signal drifting upwards (*solid line*) has a straight line that characterises its drift. Subtracting this line from the volume yields a drift-corrected signal that oscillates about a stable baseline (*dotted line*)

2. *Changes in gas composition between inspiration and expiration.* Inspired and expired gases differ in their partial pressures of O_2 and CO_2. This leads to slight differences in the viscosities of the gas mixtures, with concomitant effects on the flows registered during inspiration and expiration by the pneumotachograph.
3. *Leaks.* Any leaks between the airway opening and the pneumotachograph, whether through the mask seal or around a tracheal tube, cause a discrepancy between the volume registered by the apparatus and that entering or leaving the lungs, and hence a drift in volume. This problem is most likely to occur immediately after mask displacement, such as if an infant patient moves, or in a pressurised system (e.g. during artificial ventilation).
4. *Zero offset in flow calibration.* If the true zero flow is registered as some finite value, then integration of this offset over time results in a linear drift in volume with a slope equal to the offset. Accurate delineation of the zero flow point is more difficult as the sensitivity of the pneumotachograph decreases, which generally occurs as the linear range increases. The resolution of the A/D converter used to sample the flow also sets a limit on how accurately the

zero flow point can be identified. Therefore, perfect offset compensation is never possible. To prevent this volume drift, a dead band around the zero flow, in which all values are set to zero, is used in some devices. However, a dead band can hamper breath detection, especially when flow is very low; thus its use and the flow thresholds of the dead band should be described by the manufacturer of the equipment [65].

5. *Imperfections in the pneumotachometer response*. If the transducer for measuring flow does not function as a perfect measuring instrument (which is always the case to some degree and may be significantly so under dynamic conditions), it is unlikely that the inspiratory and expiratory flows are measured equally. This produces asymmetries in the recorded flow. Such asymmetry can often be seen in measurements from infants intubated with small endotracheal tubes, due to the geometric differences on either side of the pneumotachograph.

Correcting Volume Drift

The analysis of tidal breathing data requires the examination of data records containing a substantial number of breaths (typically about 20) obtained during regular breathing (Fig. 6). In principle, it might be possible to avoid drift in volume in this type of data record by pre-conditioning the inspired gas to body temperature pressure saturated (BTPS) conditions, continuously monitoring gas partial pressures in both the alveoli and the pulmonary arterial and venous blood to correct for respiratory-exchange ratios not equal to unity and eliminating all the methodological factors discussed above. However, this is extremely difficult, if not impossible, in practice. Consequently, it is never known how much of the baseline drift in volume is due to drift and how much represents a true change in absolute lung volume. Also, because the subject is assumed to be in the physiological steady state when data are recorded, the assumption is generally made that Functional Residual Capacity (FRC) remains more or less constant throughout the study period. Such a situation is thus forced on the measured volume signal by some kind of drift correction algorithm that first assesses the drift and then removes it. This does not, of course, mean that FRC must be identical from one breath to the next, but merely that there is no net upward or downward trend in FRC over a period containing many breaths.

Direct Measurement of Volume

The volume of gas entering the lungs can be measured directly with a spirometer attached to the mouth or from the pressure or flows emanating from a whole-body plethysmograph when the subject breathes through a conduit connected outside the plethysmograph. A more convenient but less accurate plethysmographic method is provided by the changes in trunk volume assessed with an inductance plethysmograph [66]. Recently, a more accurate optical device, optoelectronic plethysmography (OEP), has been developed that allows detailed measurement of thoracic movement during breathing [67–69].

Optoelectronic Plethysmography

As shown in Fig. 7, OEP is based on an automatic motion analyser that detects passive markers composed of a thin film of retro-reflective paper on plastic hemispheres (5–10 mm diameter). The markers are placed on the skin by bio-adhesive hypo-allergenic tape. Special TV cameras (solid-state CCDs) operate up to 120 frames per second synchronised with coaxial infrared flashing LEDs. A dedicated software processes in real time the images coming from the different cameras (six in the typical configuration,) to compute their 3D co-ordinates by stereo-photogrammetric techniques. From the 3D co-ordinates of the points belonging to the chest-wall surface, the volume enclosed by any surface described by proper geometrical models can be computed at each frame. Different geometrical descriptions of the chest wall can be achieved in order to obtain the volume enclosed by the whole chest wall surface or those of its different compartments. In the first studies based on OEP measurements, the chest wall was modelled as being composed of three different compartments: the pulmonary rib cage (RCp), i.e. the part of the rib cage apposed to the lung; the abdominal rib cage (RCa), i.e. the part of the rib cage apposed to the diaphragm, and the abdomen (Ab). Thus, the total chest-wall volume is the sum of V_{RCp}, V_{RCa} and V_{Ab}.

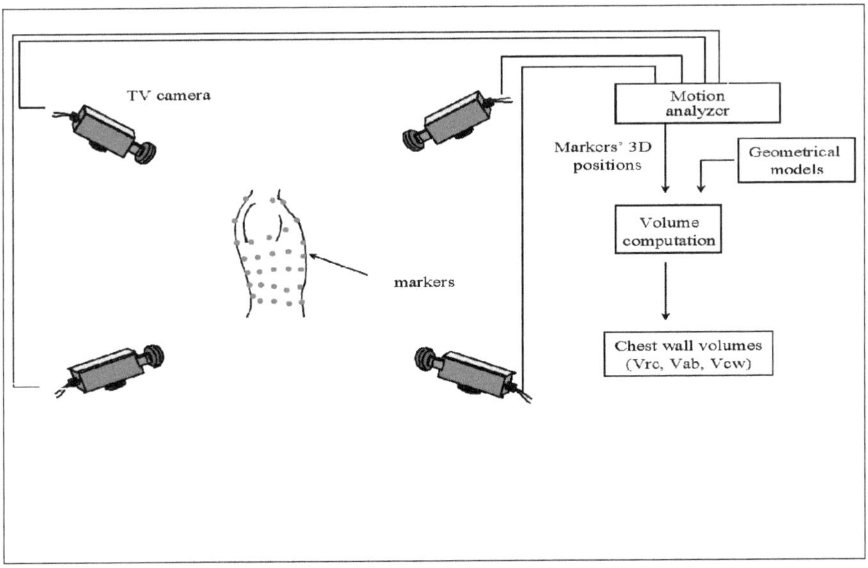

Fig. 7 Optoelectronic plethysmography: principle of measurement (see text for details)

One of the most useful characteristics of OEP is that the subdivision of the chest-wall volume into different compartments is totally free and, in this context, the ability of the OEP to measure the subdivision between right and left chest-wall expansion is particularly useful when asymmetries of respiratory-muscle action and chest-wall compliance are being considered.

OEP has been used following various measurement protocols specifically developed for different applications and different experimental and clinical situations. In the arrangement designed for the analysis of subjects in sitting and standing positions [67], 89 markers are arranged at different levels on the anterior and posterior surfaces of the chest wall. OEP has been successfully used also in constrained postures, such as supine and prone position [68,69]. In these situations, the analysis is performed by placing the markers only on the visible part of the trunk surface, while the inferior part should be fixed to the support (e.g. the bed).

OEP was validated by comparing the lung volume changes obtained by spirometry or pneumotachography with chest-wall total volumes measured by OEP during different manoeuvres, firstly in healthy subjects [67,68] and subsequently in the ICU setting in patients receiving pressure-support ventilation and continuous positive pressure ventilation, both in prone and supine positions [69]. In the ICU setting, the method was reliable and reproducible with a difference of 1.7±5.9% compared to spirometry and -1.6±5.4% compared to pneumotachography.

However, in the last validation study [69], there was a slight but systematic underestimation of chest-wall volume when the total inspired volume in patients treated with positive pressure was increased. The small but systematic discrepancy between gas volume and chest-wall volume during normal mechanical or spontaneous breathing was hypothesised to be due to the shift of blood out of the thorax as the intrathoracic pressure rose, or into the thorax (chest-wall volume changes greater than gas volume changes) when the subjects were in spontaneous breathing with negative intrathoracic pressures. This phenomenon is greater and clinically relevant during a long and sustained rise of intrathoracic pressure, as occurs when the PV curve is constructed with the super-syringe method [19].

The introduction of OEP solves the difficult problem of tracking absolute lung-volume changes on a breath-to-breath basis during almost any activity in which the chest wall can be visualised. In another recent study [70], it was shown that the OEP method can be adopted in the ICU in all situations in which end-expiratory lung volume (EELV) measurements are required, both on a breath-by-breath and on a long-term basis. A typical example of a breath-by-breath study is the measurement of dynamic pulmonary hyperinflation during mechanical ventilation in COPD patients. An important application of long-term monitoring of ΔEELV is the assessment of lung recruitment and derecruitment during different ventilatory settings and inspired oxygen concentrations (F_IO_2) [71]. The monitoring of ΔEELV should allow limitation of volutrauma and alveolar overdistension. In patients with assisted mechanical ventilation, for example, assist-controlled or pressure-support ventilation, the presence of dynamic hyperinflation and the resulting intrinsic PEEP may explain why patients sometimes fight the respirator and why they fail the weaning process and remain ventilator dependent [72]. Of interest, and unique to this method of measurement, are the data obtained during the non-steady and steady states after sudden PEEP changes. In fact, as shown by continuous OEP monitoring of EELV, when PEEP is increased several breaths are required to reach the new end-expiratory volume as a result of two 'compartments' moving with different time constants—slow and fast. The study determined that the 'slow' time constant is mainly related to axial rather than radial expansion of the lung, because the 'slow' EELV change was confined to the abdominal compartment of the chest wall. In fact, the rib-cage compartments reached the new equilibrium immediately, whereas the abdominal compartment required several breaths. In contrast, when PEEP was decreased, all three compartments immediately reached the new steady state, suggesting that end-expiratory 'collapse' is governed by a different time constant.

OEP has been also combined with oesophageal and gastric pressure measurements (performed with standard balloon-catheter-transducer systems) to accurately quantify respiratory muscle dynamics and energetics [73]. This approach to the assessment of respiratory-muscle activity was originally proposed by Rahn et al. [74], who showed that compartmental volume change is the result of the elastic recoil of the compartment and the pressure generated by the different groups of muscles acting on each compartment. By compartmental volume analysis obtained with OEP and oesophageal and gastric pressure measurements, the pressures developed by the abdominal muscles and by the inspiratory and expiratory rib-cage muscles can be estimated as the difference between the dynamic compartmental pressure–volume loops and the corresponding relaxation curves of the abdomen and the rib cage, respectively. Integrating the area under the curves of these PV diagrams gives the work and power of various muscle groups. Since the pressure is known, power can be partitioned into the relative contributions of force and velocity of shortening [73,75].

This approach was recently applied to evaluate patient-ventilator interactions during pressure-support ventilation in a group of patients with moderate to severe ALI/ARDS, excluding those patients with known chronic obstructive lung disease. It was shown that the degree to which pressure-support ventilation leads to synchronised (that is, natural) chest and abdominal mechanics during respiration depends on the level of pressure support used [76]. Respiratory parameters, thoraco-abdominal muscle synchrony and respiratory-muscle action were measured at three levels of pressure support (3, 15 and 25 cmH_2O). The breathing pattern was significantly modified by changes in the level of pressure support, with large variations in the frequency/tidal volume ratio while minute ventilation remained constant. Specifically, when the pressure-support level was less than 10 cmH_2O there was recruitment of both the inspiratory and expiratory muscles during early expiration, leading to asynchrony in thoraco-abdominal expansion and an alteration in the distribution of the tidal volume. Therefore, during pressure-support ventilation the ventilatory pattern is very different depending on the level of pressure support; furthermore, in patients with ALI, pressure support greater than 10 cmH_2O permits homogeneous recruitment of respiratory muscles, with resulting synchronous thoraco-abdominal expansion. The results suggest that when pressure-support ventilation is used in patients with ALI/ARDS, support levels higher than 10 cmH_2O may reduce the work of breathing and potentially improve the distribution of the delivered breath. Clinicians should thus be vigilant to evaluate such patients for thoraco-abdominal asynchrony and other indicators of increased respiratory workload.

Conclusions

The assessment of respiratory mechanics involves three levels: (1) measurement of the basic variables (pressure, flow and volume), (2) estimation of key physiologic parameters (such as resistance and compliance) by using a given procedure to be performed either in the research or in the clinical setting and (3) a definition of a suitable mathematical model of respiratory mechanics. At any level, there is no universally correct decision to be made because the appropriate action to be taken (e.g. the choice of the transducer to perform the measurement, the method to assess respiratory mechanics or the mathematical model) depends on the physiologic questions being addressed. It is therefore crucially important to understand the basics of measurement theory as it applies to both the collection of physiologic signals and their interpretation through mathematical models.

References

1. Fredberg JJ, Keefe DH, Glass GM et al (1984) Alveolar pressure nonhomogeneity during small-amplitude high-frequency oscillation. J Appl Physiol 57:788–800
2. Fredberg JJ, Ingram RH Jr, Castile RG et al (1985) Nonhomogeneity of lung response to inhaled histamine assessed with alveolar capsules. J Appl Physiol 58:1914–1922
3. Ludwig MS, Dreshaj I, Solway J et al (1987) Partitioning of pulmonary resistance during constriction in the dog: effects of volume history. J Appl Physiol 62:807–815
4. Sato J, Davey BL, Shardonofsky F, Bates JH (1991) Low-frequency respiratory system resistance in the normal dog during mechanical ventilation. J Appl Physiol 70:1536–1543
5. Hantos Z, Daroczy B, Suki B, Nagy S (1987) Low-frequency respiratory mechanical impedance in the rat. J Appl Physiol 63:36–43
6. Hantos Z, Daroczy B, Suki B et al (1992) Input impedance and peripheral inhomogeneity of dog lungs. J Appl Physiol 72:168–178
7. Bates JH, Abe T, Romero PV, Sato J (1989) Measurement of alveolar pressure in closed-chest dogs during flow interruption. J Appl Physiol 67:488–492
8. Bersten AD (1998) Measurement of overinflation by multiple linear regression analysis in patients with acute lung injury. Eur Respir J 12:526–532
9. Wagers S, Lundblad L, Moriya HT et al (2002) Nonlinearity of respiratory mechanics during bronchoconstriction in mice with airway inflammation. J Appl Physiol 92:1802–1807

10. Roupie E, Dambrosio M, Servillo G et al (1995) Titration of tidal volume and induced hypercapnia in acute respiratory distress syndrome. Am J Respir Crit Care Med 152:121–128
11. Nunes S, Uusaro A, Takala J (2004) Pressure–volume relationships in acute lung injury: methodological and clinical implications. Acta Anaesthesiol Scand 48:278–286
12. Salazar E, Knowles JH (1964) An analysis of pressure–volume characteristics of the lungs. J Appl Physiol 19:97–104
13. Hickling KG (1998) The pressure–volume curve is greatly modified by recruitment. A mathematical model of ARDS lungs. Am J Respir Crit Care Med 158:194–202
14. Matamis D, Lemaire F, Harf A et al (1984) Total respiratory pressure–volume curves in the adult respiratory distress syndrome. Chest 86:58–66
15. Gattinoni L, Pesenti A, Avalli L et al (1987) Pressure–volume curve of total respiratory system in acute respiratory failure. Computed tomographic scan study. Am Rev Respir Dis 136:730–736
16. Dall'Ava-Santucci J, Armaganidis A, Brunet F (1988) Causes of error of respiratory pressure–volume curves in paralyzed subjects. J Appl Physiol 64:42–49
17. Gattinoni L, Mascheroni D, Basilico E et al (1987) Volume/pressure curve of total respiratory system in paralyzed patients: artifacts and correction factors. Intensive Care Med 13:19–25
18. Sydow M, Burchardi H, Zinserling J et al (1991) Improved determination of static compliance by automated single volume steps in ventilated patients. Intensive Care Med 17:108–114
19. Chiumello D, Carlesso E, Aliverti A et al (2007) Effects of volume shift on the pressure–volume curve of the respiratory system in ALI/ARDS patients. Minerva Anestesiol 73:109–118
20. Benito S, Lemaire F, Mankikian B, Harf A (1985) Total respiratory compliance as a function of lung volume in patients with mechanical ventilation. Intensive Care Med 11:76–79
21. Lachmann B (1992) Open up the lung and keep the lung open. Intensive Care Med 18:319–321
22. Ranieri VM, Eissa NT, Corbeil C et al (1991) Effects of positive end-expiratory pressure on alveolar recruitment and gas exchange in patients with the adult respiratory distress syndrome. Am Rev Respir Dis 144:544–551
23. Servillo G, Svantesson C, Beydon L et al (1997) Pressure–volume curves in acute respiratory failure. Automated low flow inflation versus occlusion. Am J Respir Crit Care Med 155:1629–1636
24. Lu Q, Vieira S, Richecoeur J et al (1999) A simple automated method for measuring pressure–volume curve during mechanical ventilation. Am J Respir Crit Care Med 159:275–282
25. Suratt PM, Owens DH, Kilgore WT et al (1980) A pulse method of measuring respiratory system compliance. J Appl Physiol 49:1116–1121
26. Suratt PM, Owens DH (1981) A pulse method of measuring respiratory system compliance in ventilated patients. Chest 80:34–38
27. Ranieri VM, Giuliani R, Flore T et al (1994) Volume–pressure curve of the respiratory system predicts effects of PEEP in ARDS: 'occlusion' versus 'constant flow' technique. Am J Respir Crit Care Med 149:19–27
28. Jonson B, Richard JC, Straus C et al (1999) Pressure–volume curves and compliance in acute lung injury. Am J Respir Crit Care Med 159:1172–1178
29. Rodriguez L, Marquer B, Mardrus P et al (1999) A new simple method to perform pressure–volume curves obtained under quasi-static conditions during mechanical ventilation. Intensive Care Med 25:173–179
30. Bates JH, Brown KA, Kochi T (1989) Respiratory mechanics in the normal dog determined by expiratory flow interruption. J Appl Physiol 67:2276–2285
31. Kaczka DW, Ingenito EP, Israel E, Lutchen KR (1999) Airway and lung tissue mechanics in asthma. Effects of albuterol. Am J Respir Crit Care Med 159:169–178
32. Lutchen KR, Greenstein JL, Suki B (1996) How inhomogeneities and airway walls affect frequency dependence and separation of airway and tissue properties. J Appl Physiol 80:1696–1707

33. Similowski T, Bates JHT (1991) Two compartment modelling of respiratory system mechanics at low frequencies: gas redistribution or tissue rheology? Eur Respir J 4:353–358
34. Roupie E, Dambrosio M, Servillo G et al (1995) Titration of tidal volume and induced hypercapnia in acute respiratory distress syndrome. Am J Respir Crit Care Med 152:121–128
35. Amato MBP, Barbas CSV, Mediros DM et al (1998) Effect of a protective ventilation strategy on mortality in the acute respiratory distress syndrome. N Engl J Med 338:347–354
36. Ranieri VM, Mascia LM, Fiore T et al (1995) Cardiorespiratory effects of positive end-expiratory pressure during progressive tidal volume reduction (permissive hypercapnia) in patients with acute respiratory distress syndrome. Anesthesiology 83:710–720
37. Romero PV, Sato J, Shardonofsky F, Bates JH (1990) High-frequency characteristics of respiratory mechanics determined by flow interruption. J Appl Physiol 69:1682–1688
38. Bates JH, Ludwig MS, Sly PD et al (1988) Interrupter resistance elucidated by alveolar pressure measurement in open chest normal dogs. J Appl Physiol 65:408–414
39. Ludwig MS, Romero PV, Sly PD et al (1990) Interpretation of interrupter resistance after histamine-induced constriction in the dog. J Appl Physiol 68:1651–1656
40. Bates JH, Baconnier P, Milic-Emili J (1988) A theoretical analysis of interrupter technique for measuring respiratory mechanics. J Appl Physiol 64:2204–2214
41. Bates JH, Rossi A, Milic-Emili J (1985) Analysis of the behavior of the respiratory system with constant inspiratory flow. J Appl Physiol 58:1840–1848
42. Frey U, Silverman M, Kraemer R, Jackson AC (1998) High-frequency respiratory input impedance measurements in infants assessed by the high speed interrupter technique. Eur Respir J 12:148–158
43. DuBois AB, Brody AW, Lewis DH, Burgess BF (1956) Oscillation mechanics of lungs and chest in man. J Appl Physiol 8:587–594
44. Oostven E, Macleod D, Lorino H et al (2003) The forced oscillation technique in clinical practice: methodology, recommendations and future developments. Eur Respir J 22:1026–1041
45. Hantos Z, Daroczy B, Suki B et al (1992) Input impedance and peripheral inhomogeneity of dog lungs. J Appl Physiol 72:168–178
46. Dellaca RL, Santus P, Aliverti A et al (2004) Detection of expiratory flow limitation in COPD using the forced oscillation technique. Eur Respir J 23:232–240
47. Peslin R, Farre R, Rotger M, Navajas D (1996) Effect of expiratory flow limitation on respiratory mechanical impedance: a model study. J Appl Physiol 81:2399–2406
48. Dellaca RL, Rotger M, Aliverti A et al (2006) Noninvasive detection of expiratory flow limitation in COPD patients during nasal CPAP. Eur Respir J 27:983–991
49. Randerath WJ, Schraeder O, Galetke W et al (2001) Autoadjusting CPAP therapy based on impedance efficacy, compliance and acceptance. Am J Respir Crit Care Med 163:652–657
50. Badia JR, Farre R, Rigau J et al (2001) Forced oscillation measurements do not affect upper airway muscle tone or sleep in clinical studies. Eur Respir J 18:335–339
51. Bates JHT, Sly PD, Sato J et al (1992) Correcting for the Bernoulli effect in lateral pressure measurements. Pediatr Pulmonol 12:251–256
52. Navalesi P, Hernandez P, Laporta D et al (1994) Influence of site of tracheal pressure measurement on in situ estimation of endotracheal tube resistance. J Appl Physiol 77:2899–2906
53. Baydur A, Behrakis PK, Zin WA et al (1982) A simple method for assessing the validity of the esophageal balloon technique. Am Rev Respir Dis 126:788–791
54. Dechman G, Sato J, Bates JHT (1992) Factors affecting the accuracy of esophageal balloon measurement of pleural pressure in dogs. J Appl Physiol 72:383–388
55. Kárason S, Karlsen KL, Lundin S, Stenqvist O (1999) A simplified method for separate measurements of lung and chest wall mechanics in ventilator-treated patients. Acta Anaesthesiol Scand 43(3):308–315
56. Peslin R, Navajas D, Rotger M, Farre R (1993) Validity of the esophageal balloon technique at high frequencies. J Appl Physiol 74:1039–1044

57. Panizza JA (1992) Comparison of balloon and transducer catheters for estimating lung elasticity. J Appl Physiol 72:231–235
58. Iberti TJ, Kelly KM, Gentili DR, Hirsch S (1987) A simple technique to accurately determine intra-abdominal pressure. Crit Care Med 15:1140–1142
59. Collee GG, Lomax DM, Ferguson C, Hanson GC (1993) Bedside measurement of intra-abdominal pressure (IAP) via an indwelling naso-gastric tube: clinical validation of the technique. Intensive Care Med 19(8):478–480
60. Chieveley-Williams S, Dinner L, Puddicombe A et al (2002) Central venous and bladder pressure reflect transdiaphragmatic pressure during pressure support ventilation. Chest 121:533–538
61. Jackson AC, Vinegar A (1979) A technique for measuring frequency response of pressure, volume, and flow transducers. J Appl Physiol 47:462–467
62. Schibler A, Hall GL, Businger F et al (2002) Measurement of lung volume and ventilation distribution with an ultrasonic flow meter in healthy infants. Eur Respir J 20:912–918
63. Clary AL, Fouke JM (1991) Fast-responding automated airway temperature probe. Med Biol Eng Comput 29:501–504
64. Bates JH, Schmalisch G, Filbrun D, Stocks J (2000) Tidal breath analysis for infant pulmonary function testing. Eur Respir J 16:1180–1192
65. Schmalisch G, Foitzik B, Wauer RR, Stocks J (2001) In vitro assessment of equipment and software used to assess tidal breathing parameters in infants. Eur Respir J 17(1):100–107
66. Cohen KP, Ladd WM, Beams DM et al (1997) Comparison of impedance and inductance ventilation sensors on adults during breathing, motion, and simulated airway obstruction. IEEE Trans Biomed Eng 44:555–566
67. Cala SJ, Kenyon C, Ferrigno G et al (1996) Chest wall and lung volume estimation by optical reflectance motion analysis. J Appl Physiol 81:2680–2689
68. Aliverti A, Dellacà R, Pelosi P et al (2001) Compartmental analysis of breathing in the supine and prone positions by Opto-Electronic Plethysmography. Ann Biomed Eng 29:60–70
69. Aliverti A, Dellacà R, Pelosi P et al (2000) Opto-electronic plethysmography in intensive care patients. Am J Respir Crit Care Med 161:1546–1552
70. Dellacà RL, Aliverti A, Pelosi P et al (2001) Estimation of end-expiratory lung volume variations by opto-electronic plethysmography (OEP). Crit Care Med 29:1807–1811
71. Gattinoni L, Pelosi P, Crotti S et al (1995) Effects of positive end-expiratory pressure on regional distribution of tidal volume and recruitment in adult respiratory distress syndrome. Am J Respir Crit Care Med 151:1807–1814
72. Guerin C, Tantucci C (1999) Respiratory mechanics in intensive care unit. Eur Respir Mon 12:255–278
73. Aliverti A, Cala SJ, Duranti R et al (1997) Human respiratory muscle actions and control during exercise. J Appl Physiol 83:1256–1269
74. Rahn H, Otis AB, Chadwick LE, Fenn WO (1946) The pressure–volume diagram of the thorax and lung. Am J Physiol 146:161–178
75. Aliverti A, Iandelli I, Duranti R et al (2002) Respiratory muscle dynamics and control during exercise with externally imposed expiratory flow-limitation. J Appl Physiol 92:1953–1963
76. Aliverti A, Carlesso E, Dellacà RL et al (2006) Chest wall mechanics during pressure support ventilation. Crit Care 10:R54

Acute Lung Injury–ARDS, Controlled Mechanical Ventilation in ARDS and the Open Lung Concept

Pathophysiology of ARDS

D. Chiumello, C.S. Valente Barbas, P. Pelosi

Introduction

Acute respiratory distress syndrome (ARDS) is a quite common disease, with an annual incidence ranging from 1.5 to 8.3 cases for every 100000 patients and a mortality of 30–50% [1]. In 1994, the American European Consensus Conference defined ARDS as: 'an acute and persistent lung disease characterized by an arterial hypoxemia (PaO_2/FiO_2<200 mmHg), resistant to oxygen therapy and bilateral infiltrates on chest X ray' [2]. In general, ARDS has two different pathogeneses: a direct 'pulmonary' insult to the lung cell or an indirect "extrapulmonary' insult resulting in a systemic inflammatory response. ARDS is a progressive disease, with different stages, different mediators, and both inflammatory and anti-inflammatory activity (cellular and humoural). At the beginning of the inflammatory response, changes occur in the alveolar capillary barrier, including the formation of a protein-rich fluid, alteration of surfactant and migration into the lung of neutrophils, lymphocytes and macrophages. Plasma factors, such as complement, and mediators generated by the cells, such as cytokines, oxidants and leucotrienes, are secreted inappropriately and at high levels. Resolution of the disease starts with a decrease in the levels of inflammatory mediators, the migration of fibroblasts into the lung, collagen deposition and the re-absorption of oedema fluid.

In this chapter, we discuss the different cellular and humoural mediators involved in the pathogenesis of ARDS, and the microscopic and submicroscopic aspects of pulmonary and extrapulmonary ARDS.

The Alveolar Capillary Barrier and Surfactant

The recent literature suggests that mutations or polymorphisms in surfactant protein genes can impart a phenotype consisting of a propensity to develop ARDS [3,4]. An individual's genetic background may explain why, with similar

U. Lucangelo, P. Pelosi, W.A. Zin, A. Aliverti (eds.) *Respiratory System and Artificial Ventilation*. © Springer 2008

comorbidities, and similar stimuli for ARDS, one patient progresses to ARDS, multiple organ failure and death while another patient of the same age either does not develop ARDS or presents with ARDS that differs in the degrees of severity and without multiple organ failure [5].

The alveolar capillary barrier consists of type I and type II alveolar epithelial cells and capillaries. The alveolar wall serves as a minimal tissue barrier to alveolar air, and normal type II and type I epithelial cells to endothelial cells. The alveolar capillary barrier consists of cytoplasmic leaflets of epithelium and endothelium that are joined by fused basement membranes. The epithelial and endothelial leaflets are bounded by plasma membranes, as is the erythrocyte. A substantial interstitial space, with collagen fibres and fibroblasts, is present only on the endothelial side, whereas a minimal air/blood barrier is formed on the epithelial side by the fusion of basement membrane. The capillaries usually show a regular pattern of nuclear chromatin.

In the acute phase of ARDS, damage to the alveolar capillary barrier, including an increase in its permeability, causes the accumulation of a protein-rich fluid. The degree of injury to the epithelium and endothelium influences both the severity of lung injury and the clinical outcome [6]. The protein-rich fluid may gradually become organised, producing the characteristic hyaline membrane that further destroys the alveolar structure. Matthay et al. measured the protein concentration in sequential samples of pulmonary oedema fluid and found that the protein concentration remained unchanged in patients whose clinical status did not improve but it rose in patients who eventually improved [7]. These data suggest that active ion-transport across the alveolar capillary barriers is important for the clearance of oedematous fluid from the airspaces of the lung.

In the presence of lung injury, alveolar type I epithelial cells, which are the majority, are destroyed and replaced by the more resistant type II cells. Under normal conditions, type II cells cover only 10% of the total alveolar surface. Among the different functions of type II cells, such as ion transport and proliferation, they are able to release surfactant, which is a complex mixture of phospholipids and surfactant proteins (SP-A, SP-B, SP-C, SP-D) [8]. The main function of SP-A, SP-B, and SP-C is to reduce the surface tension at the alveolar air–liquid interface, while SP-D has a primary role in host pulmonary defences.

Gregory et al. reported that endogenous surfactant was lower in ARDS patients and in patients at risk of developing ARDS than in normal subjects [9]. Similarly, Pison et al. found a decrease in the surfactant concentration in ARDS in multiple-trauma patients. The levels remained low in the most severely injured patients but returned to normal in patients with less severe injuries [10]. In contrast to the low levels of SP-A and SP-B, the concentration of SP-D in bronchoalveolar lavage (BAL) fluid of ARDS patients was found to be normal [11]. This was confirmed by the inverse correlation between blood oxygenation and static respiratory system compliance and the plasma level of SP-A and SP-B in patients with ARDS [12].

Recently, Cheng et al. showed that, at the onset of acute lung injury, reduced

SP-D and elevated plasma SP-A concentrations in pulmonary oedema fluid may be associated with more severe disease and worse clinical outcome. Thus, these proteins may serve as valuable biochemical markers of prognosis [13]. Rasaiah et al. showed that the administration of exogenous surfactant at the time of a systemic insult (cecal ligation and perforation surgery) protect the lung from the damaging effects of mechanical ventilation 18 h later [14].

Macrophages and Neutrophils

In the early phases of ARDS, there is an intense alveolar inflammatory process that is characterised by the local accumulation and activation of neutrophils and macrophages. These cells, in turn, release oxidants and inflammatory mediators.

The lung per se has a large reservoir of alveolar and interstitial macrophages, both of which come from blood monocytes. Alveolar macrophages release oxygen metabolites, cytokines, hormones, proteases and anti-proteases, all of which are fundamental for normal lung homeostasis and have the ability to eliminate microorganisms.

According to an animal model of lung injury, there is an initial accumulation of neutrophils and then macrophages, which is followed by resolution of the inflammatory process [15].

During phagocytosis, macrophages produce oxygen radicals and proteases, which eliminate most particulate matter and microorganism from the distal airways, thus keeping the alveoli 'clean'.

Steinger et al. evaluated the BAL composition in ARDS patients, those who survived and those who later died, on days 3, 7 and 14 after disease onset [16]. The percentage of macrophages and their concentration in BAL fluid were lowest on day 3, intermediate on day 7 and highest at day 14, but, more importantly, were low in patients who died. These findings support the theory that, in humans, macrophages are essential both for the normal resolution of alveolar inflammation and for a favourable outcome.

Several experimental and clinical studies confirmed the prompt accumulation of neutrophils in the BAL and in histological specimens from the ARDS lung [15]. Weiland et al. evaluated the number of neutrophils in the BAL of ARDS patients within 24 h of admission [17]. Neutrophils made up 68% of the lavage cells in ARDS patients compared with only 4% in mechanically ventilated non-ARDS subjects. The percentage was directly correlated with the degree of hypoxaemia and total protein concentration. In addition, the neutrophil concentration in the BAL was higher on days 7 and 14 in surviving ARDS patients than in those who died, whereas in ARDS patients the neutrophil concentration in the BAL fluid after trauma did not differ between survivors and non-survivors.

In normal subjects, neutrophils are intravascular and only a few are present within the alveoli. To migrate into the alveolar lumen, neutrophils must adhere to the endothelium. Several substances, such as tumour necrosis factor-α, platelet-derived products, leucotrienes, and complement fragment facilitate neutrophil adhesion to the endothelium [18]. Similar to macrophages, neutrophils secrete several enzymes, such as hydrolases, myeloperoxidate, lysozyme and neutral proteases, which can cause further damage to the injured lung. Among the proteases the most representative are elastase and collagenase. Elastase degrades elastin and activates/inactivates complement components. There is a direct correlation between the degree of lung injury and the level of neutrophil elastase [19]. Collagenase destroys collagen types I, II and III. Like elastase, there is a high level of collagenase in ARDS patients [20].

Although there is evidence, at least in ARDS patients, of a relationship between neutrophil accumulation and induced lung injury, the accumulation of neutrophil on its own is not always dangerous and may in fact be useful, as is the case in primary pneumonia. Neutrophils that accumulate in the lungs in models of acute lung injury (ALI) express several properties: (1) increased activation of the kinases AKt and p38, (2) increased nuclear accumulation of the transcriptional regulatory factor NFκB, (3) increased production of pro-inflammatory cytokines, particularly those whose transcription is dependent on NFκB and (4) decreased apoptosis. Inhibition of the activation of p38, AKt, or NFκB reduces the severity of endotoxin- or haemorrhage-induced ALI [21]. Martin et al. identified soluble Fas ligand in the BAL of patients before and after the onset of ALI, and this apoptotic protein was shown to be biologically active in human epithelial cells, as demonstrated using specific inhibitors of sFasL. Patients with a higher concentration of sFasL in BAL fluid were more likely to die [22]. Human sFasL caused concentration-dependent apoptosis of human lung epithelial cells. Distal airway and alveolar epithelial cells were much more sensitive than proximal epithelial cells, suggesting that the effect of sFasL in the airspace is focused on the distal airways and alveolar units–the major site of injury in ALI. In addition, sFasL induces inflammation, as evidenced by the finding that human alveolar macrophages produce pro-inflammatory cytokines following Fas-dependent activation and do not undergo apoptosis.

In animal models, direct instillation of human sFasL into rabbit lungs caused areas of haemorrhage, with evidence of apoptosis in the alveolar walls and the induction of pro-inflammatory cytokines in alveolar macrophages. In mice, direct activation of membrane Fas using a specific activating antibody caused alveolar-wall apoptosis and acute neutrophilic inflammation in the airspaces within 4–6 h. This was associated with an increase in the concentration of alveolar proteins, the induction of mRNAs of pro-inflammatory cytokines and caspase activation in the alveolar walls. Thus, Fas-dependent pathways in the lungs initiate apoptosis of the distal lung epithelium and stimulate macrophage-dependent inflammatory responses [23].

Complement

In the presence of lung injury there is also breakdown of alveolar cells, with the subsequent release of nuclear debris and membrane damage and thus activation of the complement pathway. In this pathway, generation of the biologically active fragments C3 and C5 further accentuates the inflammatory response and vascular endothelial injury [1,23]. In vitro, C3 and C5 have been shown to activate neutrophils, causing chemotaxis and the production of superoxide anion [24]. A prospective study in patients at risk for ARDS found a strong correlation between the aggregating activity of plasma neutrophils (i.e. the activity of the complement fragments) and the development of ARDS [25]. Another prospective study, in which 50 patients, 36 of whom developed ARDS, were examined, found lower haemolytic activity, but higher C3 levels than in normal subjects [26].

The infusion of C5 fragments into healthy animals caused neutrophil sequestration in lung capillaries without any migration of the cells into the alveolar space or any change in arterial oxygenation [27]. These findings suggest that C5 is a chemotactic factor and does not per se cause lung injury; instead, additional factors are required to injure the lung.

Oxygen Radicals

Toxic oxygen metabolites released by neutrophils, macrophages and monocytes in response to a variety of mediators cause tissue damage. The most common oxygen metabolites are hydrogen peroxide (H_2O_2), superoxide ion (O_2-) and hydroxyl radical (OH). Of these, H_2O_2 is not only the most stable but it also enhances the toxicity of neutrophil elastase, increasing the amount of cell damage. H_2O_2 levels were higher in the expired gases of ARDS patients than in mechanically ventilated patients without pulmonary infiltrates. Patient with ALI plus pulmonary infiltrates but without ARDS had higher concentrations of H_2O_2 than patients without pulmonary infiltrates.

Measuring H_2O_2 in expired breath is cumbersome and can only be done in intubated patients. To avoid these problems, Mathru et al. measured H_2O_2 in the urine of ARDS patients with and without sepsis [28]. During the first 48 h of enrolment, urinary H_2O_2 of ARDS patients was significantly lower than that of ARDS patients with sepsis, although the lung injury scores were not different. Furthermore, in ARDS patients who did not survive, urinary H_2O_2 was higher in those with sepsis than in those without sepsis. Thus, there may be an additional source of H_2O_2 in patients with sepsis and the urinary H_2O_2 concentration could be useful to stratify disease severity.

To antagonise the effect of toxic oxygen metabolites, human beings have several antioxidant systems. Of these, glutathione, which reduces the oxygen metabolites to less toxic substances, is one of the most important [29]. However, the concentration of glutathione is significantly lower and the percentage of total glutathione in oxidised form higher in ARDS patients than in healthy subjects [30]. Presumably, therefore, the ARDS lung, with its deficit of glutathione, is more susceptible to injury by oxygen metabolites.

Cytokines

These soluble proteins are released by specific cells and affect the behaviour of adjacent cells. In the lung, cytokines are produced by local cells, such as macrophages, pneumocytes and fibroblasts or by the neutrophils, lymphocytes and platelets that arrive in the lung in response to a stimulus [31]. Although cytokines are essential for an adequate inflammatory response, their overproduction or protracted release, by promoting neutrophil-endothelial adhesion and microvascular leakage, can have deleterious effects.

Among the various cytokines, three in particular, tumour necrosis factor-α (TNF-α), interleukin-1β (IL-1β) and the interleukin-8 (IL-8) play the largest role in the inflammatory response during ALI [24]. TNF-α and IL-1β levels in BAL fluid were significantly higher in ARDS patients than in healthy subjects [19,32].

TNF-α increases pulmonary permeability, IL-1β secretions and the accumulation of neutrophils in the lung. In an animal model of septic shock, pre-treatment with monoclonal antibody to TNF-α reduced both the sequestration of neutrophils in the lung and damage of the alveolar capillary membrane [33].

Several studies investigated a correlation between the level of TNF-α and the development of ARDS in patients at risk of this syndrome [34]. However, the results were contradictory, probably because of the rapid clearance of TNF-α from the blood or its neutralisation by endogenous inhibitors that may alter its final effects [34].

It is also worth recalling that the cytokine concentration may not be related to the biological effect, and when cytokines are released there is sudden secretion of specific cytokine inhibitors or antagonist receptors. Consequently, the final effect will depend on the balance between pro-inflammatory and inflammatory agents. Pugin et al. measured pro-inflammatory activity in the BAL of ARDS patients and found that it was maximal during the first 3 days after ARDS onset and higher in patients at risk. Furthermore, the prevalence of pro-inflammatory activity was due more to IL-1β than to TNF-α [35].

IL-8, which is a potent chemotactic agent, was elevated in the BAL fluid of ARDS patients and correlated with the neutrophil concentration in the lavage fluid but not with the outcome [36]. The presence of IL-8 is associated with the release of anti-IL-8 autoantibody. The anti IL-8/IL-8 complex is higher in ARDS patients than in patients at risk. In fact, ARDS patients with a higher anti IL-8/IL-8 complex concentration were approximately three times more likely to die than patients with lower concentrations. Thus, the presence of the complex in the BAL of ARDS patients may be an important prognostic indicator of outcome. Although cytokines are necessary for an adequate immune response, their persistent and exaggerated production seems to be associated with a poor outcome. ARDS patients with persistently high levels of TNF-α, IL-1β and IL-8 had a poorer outcome than patients with lower values and a rapid reduction of these cytokines [37].

Leucotrienes

Leucotrienes (LTs) are derived from arachidonic acid through the action of the enzyme 5-lipooxygenase. It has been suggested that these compounds play a role in cellular damage in the lungs of ARDS patients by increasing lung permeability and inducing pulmonary and vessel constriction [24]. In the serum and BAL of ARDS patients, LT levels were higher than in normal subjects [38,39]. In addition, LTs are chemotactic for lung neutrophils. In an animal model of hyperoxia during ALI, the increase of LTs in BAL fluid was significantly correlated with the number of neutrophils [40]. When the animals were pre-treated with an inhibitor of 5-lipooxygenase, exposure to hyperoxia did not increase LTs or neutrophils in the BAL. Thus, the importance of LTs may be due to their ability to induce several damaging effects and to perpetuate lung injury.

Coagulation, Fibrinolysis and Fibrin Deposition in Acute Lung Injury

Fibrin deposition in the alveolar compartment is a characteristic of ALI, indicating that pathways regulating regulate fibrin turnover are altered under these circumstances. Local pro-coagulant activity in the alveolar compartment is increased and coagulation is initiated mainly through the extrinsic coagulation pathway—specifically, tissue factor associated with factor VIIa. Resident lung cells can contribute to the overexpression of tissue factor in ALI. Increased pro-coagulant activity in ALI overwhelms the capacity of endogenous inhibitors to prevent alveolar coagulation. The formation of a fibrin-rich neo-matrix in ALI promotes the local inflammatory response as well as associated lung dysfunction. Impairment of the alveolar fibrinolytic capacity and overexpression of extravascular pro-coagulant activity are concurrent events in ALI. These derangements favour persistent alveolar fibrin deposition in the alveolar compartment. The fibrinolytic defect largely relates to the inhibition of urokinase plasminogen activator by plasminogen activators, and downstream inhibition of locally produced plasmin by anti-plasmins. The overexpression of plasminogen activator inhibitor-1 (PAI-1) makes an important contribution to the defective alveolar fibrinolytic activity in ALI [41]. Recently, Prabbakaran et al. showed that, in patients with ALI, elevated levels of PAI-1 in pulmonary oedema fluid and in plasma are associated with a higher mortality rate and fewer days of assisted ventilation [42]. Recently, Ware LB et al. showed that protein C levels were lower in ALI/ARDS patients than in normal subjects and were associated with worse clinical outcomes, including death, fewer ventilator-free days, and more non-pulmonary organ failures, even when only those patients without sepsis were analysed. Levels of thrombomodulin in the pulmonary oedema fluid of patients with ALI/ARDS were more than ten-fold higher than in normal plasma and two-fold higher than in ALI/ARDS plasma. Higher thrombomodulin levels in oedema fluid were associated with worse clinical outcomes. Decreasing circulating protein C and increased circulating thrombomodulin are markers of the pro-thrombotic, anti-fibrinolytic state [43].

Mediators of Pulmonary Hypertension

Pulmonary hypertension is frequently seen in patients with ARDS and is related to prognosis. Studies with knockout mice have shown that nitric oxide plays a pivotal role in the normal modulation of pulmonary vascular tone. The mechanisms by which this is lost in lung injury are not clear, but it is known that endotoxin induces the expression of COX-2 and inducible nitric oxide synthase (iNOS) in the pulmonary vasculature. The situation is complicated, however, as endotoxin contributes to early, marked pulmonary hypertension despite the induction of iNOS and irrespective of pulmonary-artery occlusion pressure or cardiac output.

Increased expression of the powerful vasoconstrictor endothelin-1 is associated with pulmonary hypertension in sepsis and ARDS. Thromboxane B2, another pulmonary vasoconstrictor, may also be an important mediator of pulmonary hypertension in ARDS since COX inhibitors reduce the early pulmonary hypertension induced by endotoxin. Other pulmonary vasoconstrictors may also be released in ARDS and additional mechanisms of pulmonary hypertension, such as microthromboembolism, probably contribute. Inflammation leads to a pro-coagulant state and to disseminated intravascular coagulation, which is a well-recognised component of ARDS and sepsis. Thrombin can also potentiate inflammation and cause endothelial barrier dysfunction, in addition to its pro-fibrotic effects [8].

Microscopic, Submicroscopic and Biochemical Alterations in Primary and Secondary ARDS

Although, as noted above, the American-European Consensus Conference has recognised two pathogenetic pathways leading to ARDS: a direct (primary or pulmonary) form and an indirect (secondary or extrapulmonary) form, there have been only a few investigations into the differences between them.

Experimental Data

A direct insult was studied in experimental models by using intra-tracheal instillation of endotoxin [44], complement [45], TNF [46] or bacteria [47]. An increase in the number of apoptotic neutrophils and altered type I and type II cells was reported as was an increase in interleukins 6, 8 and 10 in the BAL after direct injury compared to indirect injury [48]. The prevalence of epithelial damage leads to a localization of the pathologic abnormality in the intra-alveolar space, with alveolar filling by oedema, fibrinous exudate, collagen, neutrophil aggregates and/or blood, with a minimum interstitial oedema. This pattern has often been described as pulmonary ARDS (ARDSp) and consists of pulmonary consolidation and probably represents a combination of alveolar collapse, prevalent fibrinous exudates and alveolar-wall oedema.

Rocco et al., in a pulmonary experimental model of ARDS, used electron microscopy to show degenerative changes in type I pneumocytes, especially over the thinnest part of the membrane, exposing a bare basement membrane. The changes included cytoplasmic swelling and membrane fragmentation. Some type I cells showed a prominent fragmented endoplasmic reticulum with fibrin in some of them. Type II pneumocytes proliferated inside the alveolar lumina. Hyaline membranes, comprising a mixture of plasma proteins, fibrin strands and cell debris, and degenerative changes in elastic fibres were also noted. In the extracellular matrix of the alveolar barrier, collagen and elastic fibres were modified by increased synthesis, resulting in fibroelastosis and a thickened basement membrane. In the exudative phase of ARDS, the afflux of neutrophils likely causes destruction of the elastic fibre system [48].

Indirect insult has been studied in experimental models by intravenous or intra-peritoneal toxic injection. In these models, lung injury originates from the action of inflammatory mediators released from extrapulmonary foci into the systemic circulation. The first target of damage is the pulmonary vascular endothelium, with an increase in vascular permeability and interstitial oedema. The number of apoptotic cells was reported to be reduced in an experimental model of extrapulmonary ARDS (ARDSexp) and there was a decrease in the amount of interleukins in the BAL [48]. Thus, the pathological alterations resulting from an indirect insult are primarily microvascular congestion and interstitial oedema, with relative sparing of the intra-alveolar spaces. The electron microscopy findings of Rocco et al., in an extrapulmonary experimental model of ARDS, showed alveolar collapse and interstitial oedema, most marked in the thick regions of the alveolar septa. Hyaline membranes and neutrophil exudates were also observed. There was evidence of endothelial injury in the form of apoptosis and degenerative changes in type II pneumocytes. The rich lysosomal content of neutrophils and their relationship with the elastic fibres was evident.

Hyaline membranes, interstitial oedema and endothelial apoptosis tend to characterise the exudative phase of ARDS. Margination of neutrophils in the alveolar barrier has been also observed [48].

Human Data

In a recent study, Hoelz et al. described the morphological differences between pulmonary lesions in patients with ARDSp and ARDSexp [49]. They found a predominance of alveolar collapse, fibrinous exudate and alveolar-wall oedema in the pulmonary form. However, the acute inflammatory phase of lung injury is also associated with a fibroproliferative response that leads to alveoli obliteration and derangements in the spatial distribution of the extracellular matrix.

Negri et al. found that the collagen content was higher in ARDSp than in ARDSexp in the early phase of the disease, but there were no differences in the content of elastic fibres [50]. The authors concluded that remodelling of the extracellular matrix occurs early in ARDS and depends on the site of the initial insult, being prevalent in ARDSp.

Chollet-Martin et al. measured elevated levels of IL-8 in BAL fluid and serum in extrapulmonary ARDS [51] as did Bauer et al. [52], who also noted a higher level of serum TNF-α in patients with ARDSexp than in those with ARDSp. Shutte et al. found high levels of IL-6 and IL-8 in the BAL regardless of the aetiology in the first ten days of mechanical ventilation [53]. However, as expected, with time the BAL levels of IL-6 and IL-8 decreased in ARDSexp but not in ARDSp.

These experimental and in vivo findings suggest that damage in the early stage of direct insult primarily involves the alveolar epithelium, whereas it is the vascular endothelium that is affected by indirect injury. Inflammatory agents increase to a greater extent in serum in ARDSexp, and in the BAL in ARDSp.

Thoracic tomography can help to establish the diagnosis of ARDS. The typical pattern is a heterogeneous infiltrate with gravitationally dependent densities. In patients with clinical and functional deterioration despite standard treatment and in those with atypical tomographic findings (associated interstitial infiltrates), a pulmonary biopsy can help in establishing the diagnosis. We evaluated 12 patients by open lung biopsy after clinical deterioration despite optimised medical treatment and mechanical ventilation. Diffuse alveolar damage due to viral infections in six patients (cytomegalovirus, herpes and influenza viruses) and to unsuspected diseases, such as leukaemic infiltrates and malaria, were diagnosed [54].

Respiratory Mechanics

The mechanical alterations of the respiratory system observed in ARDS have always been attributed to the lung because chest-wall elastance was believed to be nearly normal [55]. Studies in which the mechanics of the respiratory system, lung, and chest wall were partitioned showed that this assumption was wrong. We found that the elastance of the respiratory system was similar in ARDSp and ARDSexp, but the elastance of the lung was higher in ARDSp, i.e. the lung was stiffer. Conversely, the elastance of the chest wall was more than two-fold higher in ARDSexp than in ARDSp, i.e. the chest wall was stiffer in the former. The increase in the elastance of the chest wall was related to an increase in intra-abdominal pressure, which was three times greater in ARDSexp.

Data on intra-abdominal pressure in critically ill patients are surprisingly scarce. In most of our patients, the high values could be explained by primary abdominal disease or oedema of the gastrointestinal tract. We analysed the sonographic findings of the abdomen in normal spontaneously breathing subjects, in patients with ARDSexp due to abdominal sepsis, and in patients with ARDSp due to community-acquired pneumonia. In normal subjects, it was difficult to identify the abdominal wall and the anatomical structures of the gut. In patients with ARDSexp and related abdominal problems, the increased dimension and thickness of the gut, due to intra-luminal debris, fluid and reduced peristaltic movements, were visible. In patients with ARDSp, the gut was slightly enlarged but its wall was not thickened and there was no consistent debris or fluid present. Thus, it is evident that patients with abdominal problems present with important anatomical alterations of the gut, which may explain the increased intra-abdominal pressure. These findings suggest that in ARDS the increased elastance of the respiratory system is produced by two different mechanisms: in ARDSp, the high elastance of the lung is the major component; in ARDSexp, the increased elastance of the lung and of the chest wall contribute equally to the high elastance of the respiratory system.

However, it should be noted that most of the patients in the extrapulmonary group had ARDS caused by intra-abdominal pathologies, and some of the changes in chest-wall elastance were very likely related to the intra-abdominal mechanics and its effects on diaphragmatic movements. Altered lung elastance with relatively normal chest-wall elastance was also reported in patients with severe *Pneumocystis carinii* pneumonia [56]. Similarly, Ranieri et al. reported a marked alteration in chest-wall mechanics in patients with ARDSexp, but not in those with ARDSp [57]. Rouby et al., however, found significantly lower respiratory-system compliance (higher elastance) and worse oxygenation in the pulmonary group [58]. All these data suggest the importance of respiratory partitioning for better characterisation of the pathology underlying ARDS and thus improved clinical management.

Ventilator-Induced Lung Injury

Mechanical ventilation is frequently used in the symptomatic treatment of ARDS patients. However, there is ample evidence that mechanical ventilation itself, using high volume or high pressure, can induce alveolar and airway damage (barotrauma–volutrauma). The first seminal study was done by Webb and Tierney, who ventilated intact animals with different peak pressures. Microscopic examinations showed moderate interstitial oedema in animals ventilated with moderate peak pressure, but profuse oedema and alveolar flooding in animals ventilated with high peak pressures [59].

Further studies confirmed these data and showed that mechanical ventilation with high pressure and volume (i.e. using high transpulmonary pressure, which is the true distending force of the lung) may cause lung injury by increasing endothelial and epithelial permeability, alveolar haemorrhage and hyaline membrane formation.

A second type of injury is due to the increased shear stress in bronchioles and alveoli due to the repeated opening and closing of alveolar units. Several studies that evaluated the effects of mechanical ventilation on injured lungs with and without PEEP showed that PEEP had a beneficial effect on the lung. However, in more recent studies, mechanical ventilation increased the amounts of several inflammatory cells and mediators [60]. This type of injury is called biotrauma. Mechanical ventilation, by applying stress and strain on alveolar cells, may induce mechanotransduction (i.e. the conversion of physical forces on the cell membrane/receptors into activation of intracellular signal and transduction pathways), with subsequent release of cytokines. The cytokines, in turn, pass into the systemic circulation, thus playing a role in the pathophysiology of systemic multiple organ failure and shock. Consequently, to limit the negative effects of mechanical ventilation, the less traumatic techniques of mechanical ventilation should always be administered to ARDS patients.

Resolution and Fibrosing Alveolitis

Although the mortality from ARDS has dropped in the last decade, it is still too high. The course of disease ranges from a sudden full recovery of lung function to late recovery, but in some patients there is progression to a fibrotic lung with persistently altered lung function. In a prospective analysis of lung function in ARDS patients, total lung capacity and diffusing capacity were substantially improved at 3 months, with further slight improvement at 6 months [61]. In the most severe cases of ARDS, i.e. patients who had the greatest impairment of total lung capacity, and diffusing capacity, evidence of the disease was still present after one year. Chest radiographs revealed changes such as bullous cysts and linear fibrosis in up to 20% of these patients [62] and only 49% were able to return to their original jobs.

During recovery from ARDS, the increased endothelial and epithelial permeability is resolved by fluid clearance from the lung and elimination of soluble and insoluble materials from the interstitium and alveolar spaces. Resolution of pulmonary oedema is mediated by active transepithelial sodium transport. When severe lung injury occurs, the decreased clearance of alveolar fluid may be related to changes in either alveolar permeability or the activity or expression of sodium and chloride transport molecules. Multiple pharmacological tools, such as β-adrenergic agonists, vasoactive drugs, and gene therapy, may prove effective in stimulating the resolution of alveolar oedema in the injured lung [63]. However, at the same time, fibrosing alveolitis may develop, with deposition and accumulation of collagen in the lung. In a series of consecutive ARDS patients who had undergone transbronchial lung biopsy, 64% presented with fibrosing alveolitis and the mortality rate was 57% higher than in patients without signs of pulmonary fibrosis. In that study, the severity of pulmonary fibrosis did not influence outcome [64]. Lung collagen is composed of fibrillar collagen, mainly types I and III (CI and CIII), and intracellular galactosyl-hydroxylysylglucosyltransferase (GGT) catalyses intracellular collagen synthesis. In a post-mortem series of lung biopsies obtained from patients with pulmonary fibrosis, an increase of CI and CIII fibres were found. Farianel et al. evaluated the products of collagen metabolism (CI, CIII and GGT) in BAL and serum of ARDS patients, patients with pneumonia and healthy subjects. ARDS patients had higher levels of collagen metabolism and GGT in BAL than patients with pneumonia or healthy subjects [65]. In addition, when the amount of procollagen type III peptide, which derives from the amino-terminal of procollagen type III fibre, was measured in ARDS patients, a relationship with the degree of arterial hypoxaemia was noted [66]. Chesnutt et al. reported that, as early as 1 h after disease onset, the concentration of procollagen type III peptide in the BAL of mechanically ventilated ARDS patients was higher than in patients with hydrostatic pulmonary oedema [67]. Moreover, the median procollagen III peptide level was significantly higher in non-survivors than in survivors, with positive and negative predictive values for non-survival of 71 and 83%, respectively.

These results suggest that fibrosing alveolitis may develop even in the early phase and that procollagen III peptide could be used to identify patients at risk of death.

Conclusions

Since ARDS was first described, in 1967, substantial advance have been made in our understanding of its pathogenesis. It is also now clear that outcome depends not only on the elimination of the initial event, but also on the balance between the inflammatory and anti-inflammatory responses. How we ventilate an ARDS lung may play a major role in amplifying the inflammatory response. Increased dead-space fraction is a feature of early-phase ARDS and elevated values are associated with an increased risk of death. Nevertheless, whether directing the initial ventilatory support at decreasing the dead space and the shunt fraction can alter the evolution and the mortality of ARDS remains to be determined.

Several trials that have attempted to modify the inflammatory/anti-inflammatory response have yielded discouraging results. Thus, further studies are needed to better explain the complex relationship between the cellular and humoural factors involved in the pathogenesis of ARDS.

References

1. Ware LB, Matthay MA (2000) The acute respiratory distress syndrome. N Engl J Med 342:1334–1349
2. Bernard GR, Artigas A, Brigham KL et al (1994) Report of the American-European consensus conference on ARDS: definitions, mechanisms, relevant outcomes and clinical trial coordination. The Consensus Committee. Intensive Care Med 20:225–232
3. Haataja R, Ramet M, Marttila R et al (2000) Surfactant proteins A and B as interactive genetic determinants of neonatal respiratory distress syndrome. Hum Mol Genet 9:2751–2760
4. Lin Z, Pearson C, Chinchilli V et al (2000) Polymorphisms of human SP-A, SP-B, and SP-D genes: association of SP-B Thr131Ile with ARDS. Clin Genet 58:181–191
5. Wong HR (2002) ARDS. The future. Crit Care Clin 18:177–196
6. Atabai K, Matthay MA (2002) The pulmonary physician in critical care. 5: Acute lung injury and the acute respiratory distress syndrome: definitions and epidemiology. Thorax 57:452–458
7. Matthay MA, Wiener-Kronish JP (1990) Intact epithelial barrier function is critical for the resolution of alveolar edema in humans. Am Rev Respir Dis 142:1250–1257
8. Bellingan GJ (2002) The pulmonary physician in critical care 6: The pathogenesis of ALI/ARDS. Thorax 57:540–546
9. Gregory TJ, Longmore WJ, Moxley MA et al (1991) Surfactant chemical composition and biophysical activity in acute respiratory distress syndrome. J Clin Invest 88:1976–1981
10. Pison U, Obertacke U, Seeger W et al (1992) Surfactant protein A (SP-A) is decreased in acute parenchymal lung injury associated with polytrauma. Eur J Clin Invest 22:712–718
11. Greene KE, Wright JR, Steinberg KP et al (1999) Serial changes in surfactant-associated proteins in lung and serum before and after onset of ARDS. Am J Respir Crit Care Med 160:1843–1850
12. Doyle IR, Bersten AD, Nicholas TE (1997) Surfactant proteins-A and -B are elevated in plasma of patients with acute respiratory failure. Am J Respir Crit Care Med 156:1217–1229
13. Cheng IW, Ware LB, Greene KE et al (2003) Prognostic value of surfactant proteins A and D in patients with acute lung injury. Crit Care Med 31:20–27
14. Rasaiah VP, Malloy JL, Lewis JF et al (2003) Early surfactant administration protects against lung dysfunction in a mouse model of ARDS. Am J Physiol Lung Cell Mol Physiol 284:L783-L790
15. Larsen GL, McCarthy K, Webster RO et al (1980) A differential effect of C5a and C5a des Arg in the induction of pulmonary inflammation. Am J Pathol 100:179–192
16. Steinberg KP, Milberg JA, Martin TR et al (1994) Evolution of bronchoalveolar cell populations in the adult respiratory distress syndrome. Am J Respir Crit Care Med 150:113–122
17. Weiland JE, Davis WB, Holter JF et al (1986) Lung neutrophils in the adult respiratory distress syndrome. Clinical and pathophysiologic significance. Am Rev Respir Dis 133:218–225
18. Sibille Y, Reynolds HY (1990) Macrophages and polymorphonuclear neutrophils in lung defense and injury. Am Rev Respir Dis 141:471–501
19. Suter PM, Suter S, Girardin E et al (1992) High bronchoalveolar levels of tumor necrosis factor and its inhibitors, interleukin-1, interferon, and elastase, in patients with adult respiratory distress syndrome after trauma, shock, or sepsis. Am Rev Respir Dis 145:1016–1022

20. Christner P, Fein A, Goldberg S et al (1985) Collagenase in the lower respiratory tract of patients with adult respiratory distress syndrome. Am Rev Respir Dis 131:690–695
21. Abraham E. (2003) Neutrophils and acute lung injury. Crit Care Med 31:S195-S199
22. Martin TR, Nakamura M, Matute-Bello G (2003) The role of apoptosis in acute lung injury. Crit Care Med 31:S184-S188
23. Martin TR, Pistorese BP, Hudson LD et al (1991) The function of lung and blood neutrophils in patients with the adult respiratory distress syndrome. Implications for the pathogenesis of lung infections. Am Rev Respir Dis 144:254–262
24. Pittet JF, Mackersie RC, Martin TR et al (1997) Biological markers of acute lung injury: prognostic and pathogenetic significance. Am J Respir Crit Care Med 155:1187–1205
25. Hammerschmidt DE, Weaver LJ, Hudson LD et al (1980) Association of complement activation and elevated plasma-C5a with adult respiratory distress syndrome. Pathophysiological relevance and possible prognostic value. Lancet 1:947–949
26. Duchateau J, Haas M, Schreyen H et al (1984) Complement activation in patients at risk of developing the adult respiratory distress syndrome. Am Rev Respir Dis 130:1058–1064
27. Webster RO, Larsen GL, Mitchell BC et al (1982) Absence of inflammatory lung injury in rabbits challenged intravascularly with complement-derived chemotactic factors. Am Rev Respir Dis 125:335–340
28. Mathru M, Rooney MW, Dries DJ et al (1994) Urine hydrogen peroxide during adult respiratory distress syndrome in patients with and without sepsis. Chest 105:232–236
29. Cochrane CG, Spragg R, Revak SD (1983) Pathogenesis of the adult respiratory distress syndrome. Evidence of oxidant activity in bronchoalveolar lavage fluid. J Clin Invest 71:754–761
30. Bunnell E, Pacht ER (1993) Oxidized glutathione is increased in the alveolar fluid of patients with the adult respiratory distress syndrome. Am Rev Respir Dis 148:1174–1178
31. Meduri GU, Kohler G, Headley S et al (1995) Inflammatory cytokines in the BAL of patients with ARDS. Persistent elevation over time predicts poor outcome. Chest 108:1303–1314
32. Hyers TM, Tricomi SM, Dettenmeier PA et al (1991) Tumor necrosis factor levels in serum and bronchoalveolar lavage fluid of patients with the adult respiratory distress syndrome. Am Rev Respir Dis 144:268–271
33. Windsor AC, Walsh CJ, Mullen PG et al (1993) Tumor necrosis factor-alpha blockade prevents neutrophil CD18 receptor upregulation and attenuates acute lung injury in porcine sepsis without inhibition of neutrophil oxygen radical generation. J Clin Invest 91:1459–1468
34. Berthiaume Y, Albertine KH, Grady M et al (1989) Protein clearance from the air spaces and lungs of unanesthetized sheep over 144 h. J Appl Physiol 67:1887–1897
35. Pugin J, Ricou B, Steinberg KP et al (1996) Proinflammatory activity in bronchoalveolar lavage fluids from patients with ARDS, a prominent role for interleukin-1. Am J Respir Crit Care Med 153:1850–1856
36. Folkesson HG, Matthay MA, Westrom BR et al (1996) Alveolar epithelial clearance of protein. J Appl Physiol 80:1431–1445
37. Meduri GU, Headley S, Kohler G et al (1995) Persistent elevation of inflammatory cytokines predicts a poor outcome in ARDS. Plasma IL-1 beta and IL-6 levels are consistent and efficient predictors of outcome over time. Chest 107:1062–1073
38. Antonelli M, Bufi M, De Blasi RA et al (1989) Detection of leukotrienes B4, C4 and of their isomers in arterial, mixed venous blood and bronchoalveolar lavage fluid from ARDS patients. Intensive Care Med 15:296–301
39. Stephenson AH, Lonigro AJ, Hyers TM et al (1988) Increased concentrations of leukotrienes in bronchoalveolar lavage fluid of patients with ARDS or at risk for ARDS. Am Rev Respir Dis 138:714–719
40. Taniguchi H, Taki F, Takagi K et al (1986) The role of leukotriene B4 in the genesis of oxygen toxicity in the lung. Am Rev Respir Dis 133:805–808
41. Idell S (2003) Coagulation, fibrinolysis, and fibrin deposition in acute lung injury. Crit Care Med 31:S213-S220

42. Prabhakaran P, Ware LB, White KE et al (2003) Elevated levels of plasminogen activator inhibitor-1 in pulmonary edema fluid are associated with mortality in acute lung injury. Am J Physiol Lung Cell Mol Physiol 285:L20-L28
43. Ware LB, Fang X, Matthay MA (2003) Protein C and thrombomodulin in human acute lung injury. Am J Physiol Lung Cell Mol Physiol 285:L514-L521
44. Muller-Leisse C, Klosterhalfen B, Hauptmann S et al (1993) Computed tomography and histologic results in the early stages of endotoxin-injured pig lungs as a model for adult respiratory distress syndrome. Invest Radiol 28:39–45
45. Harris JA, Hyde DM, Wang QJ et al (1991) Repeated episodes of C5a-induced neutrophil influx do not result in pulmonary fibrosis. Inflammation 15:233–250
46. Ryan AJ, McCoy DM, McGowan SE et al (2003) Alveolar sphingolipids generated in response to TNF-alpha modifies surfactant biophysical activity. J Appl Physiol 94:253–258
47. Suntres ZE, Omri A, Shek PN (2002) Pseudomonas aeruginosa-induced lung injury: role of oxidative stress. Microb Pathog 32:27–34
48. Rocco PRM, Leite-Junior JHP, Souza AB et al (2002) Acute respiratory distress sindrome caused by pulmonary and extrapulmonary disease: effects of corticosteroid. Eur Respir J 20:P343
49. Hoelz C, Negri EM, Lichtenfels AJ et al (2001) Morphometric differences in pulmonary lesions in primary and secondary ARDS. A preliminary study in autopsies. Pathol Res Pract 197:521–530
50. Negri EM, Hoelz C, Barbas CS et al (2002) Acute remodeling of parenchyma in pulmonary and extrapulmonary ARDS. An autopsy study of collagen-elastic system fibers. Pathol Res Pract 198:355–361
51. Chollet-Martin S, Montravers P, Gibert C et al (1993) High levels of interleukin-8 in the blood and alveolar spaces of patients with pneumonia and adult respiratory distress syndrome. Infect Immun 61:4553–4559
52. Bauer TT, Monton C, Torres A et al (2000) Comparison of systemic cytokine levels in patients with acute respiratory distress syndrome, severe pneumonia, and controls. Thorax 55:46–52
53. Schutte H, Lohmeyer J, Rosseau S et al (1996) Bronchoalveolar and systemic cytokine profiles in patients with ARDS, severe pneumonia and cardiogenic pulmonary edema. Eur Respir J 9:1858–1867
54. Barbas CS, Capellozzi VL, Hoelz C (2002) Impact of lung biopsy in acute respiratory distress syndrome. Am J Respir Crit Care Med 165:A218
55. Pesenti A, Pelosi P, Rossi N et al (1991) The effects of positive end-expiratory pressure on respiratory resistance in patients with the adult respiratory distress syndrome and in normal anesthetized subjects. Am Rev Respir Dis 144:101–107
56. D'Angelo E, Calderini E, Robatto FM et al (1997) Lung and chest wall mechanics in patients with acquired immunodeficiency syndrome and severe Pneumocystis carinii pneumonia. Eur Respir J 10:2343–2350
57. Ranieri VM, Brienza N, Santostasi S et al (1997) Impairment of lung and chest wall mechanics in patients with acute respiratory distress syndrome: role of abdominal distension. Am J Respir Crit Care Med 156:1082–1091
58. Puybasset L, Gusman P, Muller JC et al (2000) Regional distribution of gas and tissue in acute respiratory distress syndrome. III. Consequences for the effects of positive end-expiratory pressure. CT Scan ARDS Study Group. Adult Respiratory Distress Syndrome. Intensive Care Med 26:1215–1227
59. Webb HH, Tierney DF (1974) Experimental pulmonary edema due to intermittent positive pressure ventilation with high inflation pressures. Protection by positive end-expiratory pressure. Am Rev Respir Dis 110:556–565
60. Slutsky AS, Tremblay LN (1998) Multiple system organ failure. Is mechanical ventilation a contributing factor? Am J Respir Crit Care Med 157:1721–1725
61. McHugh LG, Milberg JA, Whitcomb ME et al (1994) Recovery of function in survivors of the acute respiratory distress syndrome. Am J Respir Crit Care Med 150:90–94

62. Herridge MS, Cheung AM, Tansey CM et al (2003) One-year outcomes in survivors of the acute respiratory distress syndrome. N Engl J Med 348:683–693
63. Berthiaume Y, Folkesson HG, Matthay MA (2002) Lung edema clearance: 20 years of progress: invited review: alveolar edema fluid clearance in the injured lung. J Appl Physiol 93:2207–2213
64. Martin C, Papazian L, Payan MJ et al (1995) Pulmonary fibrosis correlates with outcome in adult respiratory distress syndrome. A study in mechanically ventilated patients. Chest 107:196–200
65. Farjanel J, Hartmann DJ, Guidet B et al (1993) Four markers of collagen metabolism as possible indicators of disease in the adult respiratory distress syndrome. Am Rev Respir Dis 147:1091–1099
66. Waydhas C, Nast-Kolb D, Trupka A et al (1993) Increased serum concentrations of procollagen type III peptide in severely injured patients: an indicator of fibrosing activity? Crit Care Med 21:240–247
67. Chesnutt AN, Matthay MA, Tibayan FA et al (1997) Early detection of type III procollagen peptide in acute lung injury. Pathogenetic and prognostic significance. Am J Respir Crit Care Med 156:840–845

Ventilator-Associated Lung Injury

E. Crimi, L. Del Sorbo, V.M. Ranieri

Types of Lung Injury

Since its introduction into clinical practice as life-sustaining therapy in the polio epidemic, mechanical ventilation has proved to be an important tool for the treatment of the respiratory failure. One of the main reasons for a patient's admission into the intensive care unit (ICU) is to receive ventilator support [1]. According to a recent review by Esteban and co-workers [2], 66% of patients who require mechanical ventilation suffer from acute respiratory failure, including acute respiratory distress syndrome (ARDS), heart failure, pneumonia, sepsis, complications of surgery and trauma. The remaining indications include coma (15%), acute exacerbation of chronic obstructive pulmonary disease (13%) and neuromuscular disorders (5%). The aims of mechanical ventilation are primarily to decrease the work of breathing and to reverse life-threatening hypoxaemia or acute progressive respiratory acidosis. However, over the last two decades, research in a number of animal models has shown that mechanical ventilation itself can produce acute lung injury (ALI) [3]. The classical form of iatrogenic lung injury, recognised clinically for many decades, is the well-known *barotrauma*, defined as radiological evidence of extra-alveolar air [4]. The extra-alveolar accumulation of air has several manifestations, of which the most threatening is tension pneumothorax.

There are also more subtle morphologic, structural and physiologic changes that can be induced by mechanical ventilation. A large number of studies have observed that high end-inspiratory lung stretch can lead to diffuse alveolar damage, increased fluid filtration, epithelial permeability and microvascular permeability, pulmonary oedema [3]. The term *volutrauma* was coined to indicate that the critical variable causing injury was alveolar distension, namely volume, rather than high proximal airway pressure [5]. However, it is important to point out that alveolar overdistension is due to an increased transpulmonary pressure (alveolar minus pleural pressure), such that volutrauma actually represents a form of barotrauma.

In addition to the injury caused by ventilation at high lung volumes, ventila-

U. Lucangelo, P. Pelosi, W.A. Zin, A. Aliverti (eds.) *Respiratory System and Artificial Ventilation.* © Springer 2008

tion at low lung volumes may be harmful. This injury, termed as *atelectotrauma* is related to repetitive opening and closing of lung units [6].

Ventilator-induced lung injury (VILI) is the term coined to define ALI directly induced by mechanical ventilation in animal models [7]. VILI comprises morphological, physiological and radiological features that are indistinguishable from those of the diffuse alveolar damage of ALI/ARDS [7].

Since it is ethically not possible to perform experiments on humans exposed to injurious strategies of ventilation, it is not easy to demonstrate that mechanical ventilation can cause damage to human lungs. Thus, a better term that might be used in human studies is ventilator-associated lung injury (VALI), which is defined as lung injury that resembles ARDS and occurs in patients receiving mechanical ventilation [7].

The types of injury described above are largely thought to be related to the mechanical stress placed on the pulmonary and non-pulmonary structures by mechanical ventilation. In the last few years, there has been increasing evidence that mechanical stresses produced by mechanical ventilation can lead to the up-regulation of an inflammatory response. This new mechanism of injury has been termed *biotrauma* [8]. One hypothesis that has recently been advanced is that activation and/or propagation of the inflammatory cascade, induced by mechanical ventilation, plays a pivotal role in the clinical outcomes of patients with ALI/ARDS and may also lead to the development of a systemic inflammatory response syndrome (SIRS) [8,9] and multiple systemic organ failure [10]. This hypothesis offers a reason why mortality in ARDS remains about 35–65% despite advances in critical care, and most patients with ARDS who die do so from multiple systemic organ failure rather than from hypoxia [11].

Mechanical Stress and Ventilator-Associated Lung Injury

Two distinct phenomena have been proposed as responsible for VALI: (1) high lung volume associated with elevated transpulmonary pressure and alveolar overdistension; (2) the continuous recruitment/derecruitment of collapsed alveoli due to low end-expiratory volume [12]. Other factors contribute to or aggravate injury, including pre-existing lung damage, high-inspired oxygen concentration and the local production and systemic release of inflammatory mediators [13]. Therefore, the main determinant of the degree of VALI is the interaction of the ventilator settings with patient-related factors, particularly the condition of the ventilated lung.

Alveolar Overdistension

The observation that trumpet players commonly achieve airway pressures of 150 cmH_2O without the occurrence of air leakage suggests that the degree of lung inflation is a more important determinant of lung injury than airway pressure per se [14]. Therefore, excessive alveolar volume in conjunction with increased transalveolar pressure is the deleterious factor of VALI. In fact, in patients with ARDS, there is a poor correlation between airway pressure and the occurrence of air leakage, accounting for only 8–14% of patients [15–18].

The relative contribution of pressure and volume to lung injury was assessed in several experimental settings in animals. Dreyfuss [5] demonstrated that ventilated rats whose tidal excursion was limited by strapping the chest and abdomen, i.e. high airway pressure without a high tidal volume (V_T), did not show signs of lung injury. In contrast, animals ventilated without thoracic restriction using high V_T, either with high positive inspiratory pressure or negative pressure in an iron lung, developed severe injury. These results, which have been confirmed in other species [19,20], suggest that large lung volumes, but not high intra-thoracic pressures per se, are involved in VALI.

The degree of alveolar over-distension is determined by the pressure gradient across the alveoli. This gradient is better evaluated by measurement of the difference, defined as the *transpulmonary pressure*, between the static airway pressure—estimated by the end-inspiratory plateau airway pressure (P_{plat})—and the pleural pressure. Peak airway pressure, which depends on the resistance to flow in the airways, is not a reflection of alveolar pressure. Therefore, according to recent guidelines, it is detrimental maintaining P_{plat} above 35 cmH_20 [7]. Moreover, it is necessary to contemplate factors that increase (or decrease) the degree of alveolar distension for a given alveolar pressure, such as the condition modifying chest-wall compliance (for example, increased chest-wall compliance in immaturity, reduced chest-wall compliance in patients with abdominal distension).

Shear Forces

Another mechanism sustaining VALI is the previously mentioned atelectotrauma, which is damage that is induced by increased local shear stress. Shear stress is a form of mechanical stress generated when fluids (blood or air) move across a cell surface, thereby generating a force parallel to the plasma membrane that induces a tangential distortion of the cell. In damaged lungs, the development of shear stress is related to the cyclic opening and closing of small airways induced by recruitment/derecruitment of alveolar units. Diseased lungs with a heterogeneous distribution of lesions may be subjected to a much greater regional stress than homogeneous lungs [21].

Applied airway pressure, which is useful to recruit and ventilate some lung units, may be inadequate to open atelectatic regions and can cause overdistension in the most compliant adjacent areas. Mead et al. showed that, in a non-uniformly expanded lung such as that found in ARDS, at a transpulmonary pressure of 30 cmH_2O, the forces acting on an atelectatic region surrounded by fully expanded lung could be subject to a pressure of 140 cmH_2O, thus inducing severe shear stress [22]. Therefore, ventilation at low end-expiratory lung volumes, despite adequate levels of end-inspiratory pressure and alveolar distension, can lead to atelectotrauma and then lung injury. Hence, the application of a positive end-expiratory pressure (PEEP), which increases the end-expiratory lung volume and maintains recruitment throughout the ventilatory cycle, has a protective effect, as demonstrated by several studies [5,23–25]. For example, in an ex-vivo rat lung, ventilation with small V_T (5–6 ml/kg) and low or zero PEEP caused lung injury, which was reduced by the application of higher levels of PEEP [21]. The beneficial effect of PEEP, related to the prevention of derecruitment, is counterbalanced by the detrimental effect of overdistension, if is too high and/or not associated with a reduction of V_T. Theoretically, high-frequency oscillatory ventilation represents the ideal combination of minimum V_T and maximal recruitment (the 'open lung'), providing maintenance of an adequate end-expiratory lung volume.

Other Risk Factors

Beyond V_T, airway pressure and PEEP, VALI might be affected by other factors related to the ventilator. For example, an increased respiratory frequency may augment lung injury through greater stress cycling or through the deactivation of surfactant. Oxidant stress, related to exposure to a high inspired oxygen fraction (FiO_2) and to the increased generation of reactive oxygen species, can be involved in the pathogenesis of several lung diseases, including ARDS and VALI. Therefore, the current clinical recommendation in ARDS is the use of the lowest FiO_2 ensuring an oxygen saturation of 90% [26,27].

Pre-existing damage of ventilated lungs is important in determining susceptibility to VALI. Patients without readily apparent lung injury have been treated with positive-pressure ventilation for protracted periods of time without clinically discernible VALI [28]. Otherwise, the abnormal lungs of patients with ARDS are highly susceptible to this form of lung injury.

An important factor underlying the predisposition to VALI is uneven distribution of disease and inflation, as seen in injured lungs. Computed tomography (CT) scanning showed that the lungs of ARDS patients are highly asymmetrical along the vertical axis, with a small non-dependent lung region continuously open to ventilation ('baby lung') and a dependent consolidated, atelectatic region that was not ventilated. In between, there is a region that can be recruited/derecruited, with consequent mechanical stress [29]. Thus, ALI/ARDS may be considered the most important and readily identifiable risk factor for VALI [30].

Pathological Findings in VALI

It has been recognised that the development of a pressure gradient between an alveolus and its adjacent bronchovascular sheath could disrupt the pulmonary epithelium, resulting in the typical manifestations of barotrauma [4]. Mechanical ventilation can also produce more subtle diffuse lung injury, characterised by hyaline membrane formation, interstitial and alveolar oedema and haemorrhage, and increased alveolar-capillary membrane permeability.

Animal lungs injured by mechanical ventilation with high pressure and volume display a pattern of changes in endothelial and epithelial permeability that are similar to other forms of experimental lung injury. Microscopic examination of the lungs of animals that die soon after the induction of lung injury showed severe alveolar damage, alveolar haemorrhage, hyaline membranes and neutrophil infiltration, whereas the lung of animals that survived for longer periods contained collapsed alveolar spaces and proliferating fibroblasts and alveolar type II cells.

Electron microscopy has confirmed profound alterations in the lung, including endothelial (breaks and the formation of intracapillary blebs) and epithelial (discontinuities and occasional complete destruction of type I cells) abnormalities. Alterations in the endothelium are detectable by electron microscopy within only a few minutes of high airway pressure ventilation and seem to precede damage of the epithelium [3,5]. The structural disruption caused by VALI is often associated with microvascular leakage and pulmonary oedema. Experimental studies suggested that changes at both the epithelial and endothelial barriers lead to increased permeability and to pulmonary oedema, a prominent feature of VALI [3,23,31]. Increased microvascular permeability has been assessed using the pulmonary extravascular redistribution of intravenous injected ^{125}I-labelled albumin in mechanically ventilated rats with high airway pressure [32].

Lecuona et al. showed, in an isolated-perfused rat lung model, that lung permeability increased significantly in rats ventilated for 60 min with high V_T, compared with low V_T, moderate V_T, and control rats [33]. The investigators found a decrease in Na,K-ATPase activity that paralleled the impairment in lung oedema clearance by alveolar type II cells isolated from rats ventilated with moderate V_T and high V_T. This study suggested that lung structural disruption is not only associated with pulmonary oedema but also decreases the ability of the lung to clear it by inhibiting active sodium transport and Na,K-ATPase function in the alveolar epithelium.

There is no experimental evidence for increased vascular transmural pressure and for the contribution of hydrostatic pressures to the development of pulmonary oedema in mechanical ventilation. Even if there is no large increase in vascular transmural pressure during injurious ventilation with high airway pressure, an important increase in regional transmural pressure may occur in the heterogeneous lung, adding this effect to those of altered permeability and enhancing oedema severity [22,34].

The histological features observed in VALI (increased vascular permeability, diffuse alveolar damage, inflammatory cell infiltrates, fibroproliferative changes) are not specific to VALI but can also be seen in ARDS and other forms of lung injury.

Mechanism of VALI

The mechanisms by which mechanical ventilation may induce/increase ALI include: (1) physical disruption of lung tissues and cells, caused by lung overdistension and shear stress generated by the repetitive opening and closing of atelectatic regions; (2) alteration of surfactant, leading to an increased tendency for alveolar and distal-airways collapse and an increased surface tension in the alveoli, with consequent increased transmural capillary pressure gradients; (3) aberrant activation of cellular mechanisms leading to inappropriate and harmful inflammatory responses.

Physical Disruption (Stress Failure)

The limited strength of the alveolar-capillary barrier may explain the mechanism of injury of mechanical stress. Mechanical ventilation with high distending pressures in the absence of PEEP can cause stress failure of the plasma membrane and of epithelial and endothelial barriers [35–37]. Stress failure depends on the development of excessive wall stress, defined as the ratio of alveolar wall tension to thickness. It is known that high airway pressure between the alveolus and the bronchovascular sheath during positive-pressure ventilation causes the passage of air across the epithelial surface, along the bronchovascular sheath and then into the interstitial tissues, producing manifestations of barotrauma [4].

The endothelium, which is located very close to the epithelial surface, is subject to stress failure determined by forces derived from transpulmonary and intravascular pressures [37]. Fu et al. showed that, at a constant transmural pressure, an increase of the transpulmonary pressure from 5 to 20 cmH_20 produced a significant increase in the number of epithelial and endothelial breaks. There was a further increase in number of breaks at the same transpulmonary pressure when the capillary transmural pressure was increased [38]. The local or regional stress induced by lung inflation may increase microvascular transmural pressures with subsequent capillary disruption (*capillary stress failure*), thereby determining changes in the alveolar-capillary barrier [39]. The forces generated by mechanical ventilation may therefore interact with those arising from pulmonary vascular perfusion to increase lung injury.

The occlusion of small airways by exudate or apposition of their walls requires high airway pressure to restore patency, resulting in shear stress and damage of the airways, particularly if the cycle is continuously repeated [40]. Airway collapse and the consequent recruitment/derecruitment may not occur in normal lungs, being favoured by surfactant deficiency and lung disease, which modifies interstitial support of the airways [41].

Mechanical ventilation has profound effects on the function of surfactant, inactivating it and so increasing alveolar surface tension. Surfactant dysfunction, as observed in experimental models of pneumonia and in patients with ARDS, can increase the injurious effect of mechanical ventilation [42,43]. The application of injurious ventilatory strategies (high V_T and low PEEP) reduces the pool of functional surfactant (decreased large aggregate:small aggregate ratio), particularly in injured lungs [44].

Surfactant abnormalities, i.e. increased alveolar surface tension, results in an increased tendency for distal airways and alveolar collapse, with the generation of shear stress as both structures are reopened, a need for higher airway pressure to reopen the lung and keep it open, increasing stress forces, and, last but not least, an increased transvascular filtration pressure, which favours movement of fluid into the lung and thus oedema formation [45]. In addition, surfactant may have an important immunoregulatory role, one that is impaired by mechanical ventilation [46]. The application of PEEP preserves surfactant function by maintaining an elevated end-expiratory lung volume, thus avoiding surface film collapse and subsequent inactivation during re-expansion and preventing the loss of surfactant in the airway.

In the last few years, there has been increasing evidence that mechanical factors can lead to injury, mediated by the activation of inflammatory cells and the release of soluble mediators, a type of injury called biotrauma [8]. From an anatomic and physiologic perspective, the lungs are particularly exposed to this type of injury. The lung has the largest epithelial surface of any organ (alveolar surface area of about 50–100 m^2) with an extensive capillary bed that receives the entire cardiac output and contains a large reservoir of marginated neutrophils (up to a third of all neutrophils outside the bone marrow) [47]. Moreover, the most abundant non-parenchymal cell in the lung is the alveolar macrophage, which plays a central role in maintaining normal lung structure and function by a variety of mechanisms (phagocytosis, expression of specific cell-surface receptors, synthesis and release of various mediators). These inflammatory cells can be injurious to the lung through the release of a wide range of mediators [48]. In addition, many structural cells, such as epithelial cells, endothelial cells and interstitial cells, produce numerous pro-inflammatory mediators in response to a variety of stimuli.

Mechanical stress, leading to the up-regulation of an inflammatory response, is evidenced from animal model of injurious ventilatory strategies that resulted in neutrophil infiltration of the lungs [49], increased cytokine levels in lung lavage [50] and increased cytokine levels in the systemic circulation [51,52]. The involvement of pro-inflammatory cytokines is suggested by the observation that lung damage can be attenuated by the administration of anti-tumour necrosis factor-α (TNF-α) antibodies [53] or interleukin-1(IL-1) receptor antagonist [54].

It is not clear how mechanical ventilation induces its deleterious effects. Ventilator-induced release of pro-inflammatory mediators may result from different mechanism: stress failure of the plasma membrane or of endothelial and epithelial barriers, stretch-induced mechanotransduction and effects on the pulmonary vasculature (increased vascular pressure and shear stress). It has been suggested that mechanotransduction, the conversion of mechanical stimuli, such as cell deformation, by cell membrane/receptors into biological signals, play an important role in the ventilator-induced lung inflammatory response. Lung stretch is an important factor in lung growth and development. The hypothesis is that, by alternating both the pattern and the magnitude of stretch, mechanical ventilation leads to alterations in cellular metabolism and/or gene expression [55].

Vlahakis et al. [56] have shown that transformed human type II alveolar cells (A549) subjected to 24–48 h of cyclic stretch (defined as the percent change in the length of any line element in the cell's membrane) with a larger versus a smaller strain pattern produced significantly greater amount of IL-8, a chemokine involved in granulocyte recruitment. This result suggests that cyclic deformation alone can trigger inflammatory signalling and that epithelial cells participate in the inflammatory response, even in the absence of structural damage.

A recent study showed that VILI can lead to the release of inflammatory mediators, including TNF-α, IL-6 and macrophage inflammatory protein-2 (MIP-2), into the systemic circulation, contributing to the initiation or propagation of a systemic inflammatory response and, eventually, leading to multiple systemic organ failure [10]. Clinical evidence in support of this model was provided in a randomised clinical trial by Ranieri et al. [57], who demonstrated that the concentration of pro-inflammatory mediators (IL-1β, TNF-α, IL-6) remained elevated in the bronchoalveolar lavage fluid (BALF) of patients receiving conventional mechanical ventilation, whereas a protective ventilatory strategy attenuated the increase in cytokines. These results support experimental data showing that cellular injury can be caused by mechanical ventilation. Moreover, they showed that VALI not only resulted in pulmonary inflammation but also could lead to increased plasma cytokine concentrations, indicating that injured lungs represent an important source of systemic inflammation.

Another mechanism whereby mechanical ventilation may contribute to the genesis of multiple systemic organ failure is the loss of compartmentalisation of inflammatory mediators or bacteria in the lungs, thereby promoting organ dysfunction. Experimental studies demonstrated that an adverse ventilatory strategy can induce the systemic dissemination of bacteria [58,59] or endotoxin [60] and of locally produced cytokines. These studies have led to the hypothesis that injurious strategies of mechanical ventilation end in the development of multiple systemic organ failure. If this hypothesis is true, it would explain the high mortality of patients with ARDS and perhaps lead to novel strategies to abrogate or prevent these detrimental consequences.

Clinical Evidence of VALI

The clinical manifestation of VALI consists of the worsening of respiratory function in patients with ALI/ARDS undergoing mechanical ventilation. However, VALI is hard to demonstrate clinically, since its pathological appearance is identical to that of ARDS. Furthermore, there are no clinical symptoms, signs or changes in physiological variables that are specific for VALI, as reported by the International Consensus Conference on VALI in ARDS [7]. In fact, the presence of VALI has to be distinguished from other causes of deteriorating respiratory function in patients with ALI/ARDS, such as progression of the underlying disease, infection from pulmonary or extra-pulmonary sites, fluid overload and absorption atelectasis. Moreover, ARDS has a heterogeneous and dynamic nature, characterised by an early phase in which lung oedema predominates and a later phase consisting of inflammatory and fibrotic proliferative changes. Beside the morphological changes, the pulmonary mechanics in ARDS become altered over time or, depending on the aetiology (pulmonary or extra-pulmonary), produce further difficulties in the diagnosis of VALI, whose incidence during the different phases of ARDS is still not clearly understood.

In the diagnosis of VALI, routine chest X-ray is not very helpful because there are technical difficulties, when the image is obtained in the ICU, related to the supine position of the patient and to the nature of anteroposterior films, such that their already poor sensitivity in the detection of pulmonary interstitial damage is reduced even further. More reliable, instead, is chest CT scanning, although it is not recommended as a routine method of diagnosis or of monitoring VALI due to the wide variety of problems related to patient transportation, lack of evidence of improved outcome with repeated scanning and the cost of the procedure. However, high-resolution chest CT scan can reveal the presence of lesions, such as extensive consolidation, emphysema, intraparenchymal cysts and hyper-inflated lung regions, which can be associated with VALI but are less or not detectable clinically or by chest X-ray.

Therefore, confirmation of suspected VALI requires the frequent and careful clinical evaluation of the ALI/ARDS patient undergoing mechanical ventilation as well as monitoring for the occurrence of potential risk factors, gas exchange and responses to changes in ventilator settings. For example, a decrease in PaO_2 and increase in $PaCO_2$ might suggest the presence of VALI as can an increase in peak inspiratory or P_{plat} during volume-controlled ventilation, or a decrease in V_T during pressure-controlled ventilation, even though all of these changes can be induced by several other causes.

Preventive Therapeutic Strategies for VALI

As shown above, a large body of evidence has confirmed that VALI can sustain or increase pulmonary inflammation in patients with ALI/ARDS undergoing mechanical ventilation with a traditional strategy. The inflammatory mediators released can also enter the systemic circulation, thus leading to distal non-pulmonary organ failure.

The traditional approach to mechanical ventilation was aimed at obtaining normal values of $PaCO_2$ and pH, despite the fact that a large V_T (10–15 ml/kg) or high inspiratory airway pressure induces alveolar overdistension in aerated areas of the lungs and thus an inflammatory reaction. Therefore, several alternative ventilatory strategies have been tested to determine whether the use of lower V_T in patients with ALI/ARDS improves clinical outcome, including a reduction of the incidence of VALI.

The largest trial was performed by ARDSNet, a group founded by the National Heart, Lung and Blood Institute (NHLBI) of the National Institutes of Health (NIH) to conduct clinical trials in ARDS patients [15]. The study was a multi-centred, randomised controlled trial that enrolled patients with ALI or ARDS in ten academic centres with 75 ICUs to compare a control ventilatory strategy with a V_T of 12 ml/kg, based on predicted body weight, with a lung-protective strategy using a V_T of 6 ml/kg, also based on predicted body weight. A wide spectrum of patients was enrolled in this trial, including septic and non-septic as well as patients with different degrees of lung dysfunction. The study was stopped at 861 patients because an interim analysis revealed a 22% lower mortality rate in the lung-protective group than in the control group.

Other, earlier trials compared the effect of ventilation with lower V_T vs. higher V_T, although these studies were smaller than the ARDSNet trial. Stewart et al. evaluated 120 patients at high risk for ARDS; 60 patients were enrolled in a conventional mechanical ventilation group and the other 60 patients were enrolled in a protective mechanical ventilation group on the basis of V_T and P_{plat} (7 vs. 11 ml/kg and 26.8±6.7 vs. 22.3±5.4 cmH_2O, respectively). PEEP was set as the minimal value that achieved acceptable arterial oxygen saturation (89–93%) with non-toxic FiO_2 values (≤0.5) in both the conventional and the protective ventilation groups and amounted to 7.2±3.3 and 8.6±3.0 cmH_2O, respectively. The in-hospital mortality rate was not different between the two groups: 47% in the conventional ventilation group and 50% in the protective ventilation group [17].

Brochard et al. obtained similar findings in a prospective randomised clinical trial that consisted of 116 patients, with 58 randomised to conventional ventilation and 58 to protective ventilation. After the first 24 h of treatment, P_{plat} and PEEP values were 31.7 and 10.7 cmH_2O and 25.7 and 10.7 cmH_2O in the conventional and protective ventilatory groups, respectively. Mortality rates at 60 days were not significantly different: 38% in the conventional group and 47% in the protective group [18].

The study of Brower et al. was conducted to assess the adverse effects and potential benefits of small V_T ventilation. Fifty-two patients were recruited in a prospective randomised clinical trial, 26 to conventional ventilation (V_T 10–12 ml/kg ideal body weight, reduced if inspiratory P_{plat} was >55 cmH_2O) and 26 to protective ventilation (V_T 5–8 ml/kg ideal body weight, to keep P_{plat}<30 cmH_2O). Mean V_T values during the first 5 days in traditional and small V_T

patients were 10.2 and 7.3 ml/kg, respectively ($p<0.001$), with mean P_{plat}=30.6 and 24.9 cmH_2O, respectively ($p<0.001$). There were no significant differences in the requirements for PEEP or FiO_2, fluid intake/output, requirements for vasopressors, sedatives, or neuromuscular blocking agents, percentage of patients that achieved unassisted breathing, ventilator days or mortality [61].

The ARDSNet trial was, therefore, the only study that showed a decrease in mortality. Several theories have been provided to explain the difference in the outcomes of the ARDSNet trial and the other studies [62]. The ARDSNet trial, enrolling 861 patients compared with the total of 288 patients enrolled in the three others, had a higher relative power. However, this explanation is less likely because the trend for the three negative trials was a lower mortality rate for patients in the high-V_T groups than for those in the protective arms. In fact, combining all three studies, the mortality rate was 44% in the control arm and 48% in the lung-protective arm.

In the smaller trials, the spread between the V_T and P_{plat} values that were used in the control arm and the lung-protective arm was less than that in the ARDSNet trial. In the latter, the difference between P_{plat} (on day 1) was 8 cmH_2O, compared with 4.5, 5.7 and 6.0 ml/kg in the other studies; similarly there was a greater difference in V_T between the control and intervention arms in the ARDSNet trial. On the basis of the data from these trials, a threshold in P_{plat} (as an indicator of overdistension) of 32 cmH_2O was proposed; above this level, the risk of injury due to mechanical ventilation may increase [63]. According to this theory, since the average P_{plat} values (for both groups) of the three negative trials were <32 cmH_2O, a change in mortality between groups could not be demonstrated because both received 'protective' strategies. In contrast, the ARDSNet trial had an average P_{plat} in the control arm of 33 cmH_2O, a value greater than the threshold value. However, it seems unlikely that there is a specific break point for every patient, especially considering the spatial heterogeneity of injury and the presence of a stiff chest wall, which renders a high P_{plat} difficult to interpret.

Another possible explanation for the positive ARDSNet trial is related to the different approaches used to control respiratory acidosis. All of the trials applied the concept of 'permissive hypercapnia' [64], which allows $PaCO_2$ to increase if necessary rather than increasing V_T (or pressure). However, the approach to increases in $PaCO_2$ differed substantially between the studies. In particular, the ARDSNet study was the most aggressive in terms of trying to maintain $PaCO_2$ relatively close to the normal range. It employed higher respiratory rates and a more liberal use of bicarbonate than the other studies.

There are several sources of evidence that 'permissive hypercapnia' is beneficial in the context of VALI [65,66]. For example, the effect of hypercapnia was investigated in vivo in a rat model of lung ischaemia-reperfusion [67]. The treated group of rats, with a $PaCO_2$ >100 mmHg (control group $PaCO_2$ was ~60 mmHg) and pH<7.10, had a smaller lung wet:dry ratio, less protein in the BALF and less pulmonary inflammation as assessed by BALF levels of TNF-α and lung tissue 8-isoprostane. Moreover, it is known that acidosis attenuates a number of inflammatory processes, inhibits xanthine oxidase and restricts the production of free radicals [66,68]. However, there are also potentially detrimental effects, such as increased catecholamine release, that could mitigate the potential beneficial effects of hypercapnia on lung injury. Bicarbonate infusions in the treatment of hypercapneic acidosis may result in adverse consequences, such as reduced hypoxic pulmonary vasoconstriction and reduced myocardial contractility.

As mentioned above, in the ARDSNet trial higher respiratory rates were used in the low-V_T arm of the study to minimise hypercapnia. It has been suggested that this may have had a fortuitous benefit, because of the possible development of auto-PEEP, thus minimising injury due to the recruitment/de-recruitment of lung units [69].

Beyond the ARDSNet trial, another study [70], performed by Amato et al., demonstrated a significantly lower mortality rate at 28 days in the protective group than in the conventional group (38 and 71%, respectively). Of the 53 ARDS patients included in the trial; 29 were randomised to receive protective mechanical ventilation and 24 to receive conventional mechanical ventilation. Ventilator settings in the protective ventilation group consisted of a low V_T, relatively high PEEP titrated according to the patient's own inspiratory pressure–volume (PV) curves plus intermittent continues positive airway pressure (CPAP) recruitment. This strategy resulted in P_{plat} and PEEP levels of 30.1±0.7 and 16.4±0.4 cmH_2O in the protective group vs. 34.4±1.9 and 8.7±0.4 cmH_2O in the conventional group. Conventional mechanical ventilation was defined by a V_T targeted to maintain a $PaCO_2$ level between 35 and 38 mmHg, independent of airway pressure and the minimal PEEP required, with FiO_2<0.6. Despite the lower mortality rate at 28 days in the protective group, a significant reduction in mortality was not observed at hospital discharge.

Despite the criticism of that study [71], its results suggested that analysis of the inspiratory PV curve of the respiratory system may be used in patients with ARDS to establish appropriate ventilatory strategies. The average critical pressure, i.e. that required to re-open previously collapsed peripheral airways and/or alveoli and the value at which stretching and overdistension of some alveolar units occurs, was indicated by the lower and upper inflection points of the PV curve, respectively [72]. Based on these concepts, mechanical stress and VILI might be minimised by applying PEEP above the lower inflection point and inspiratory pressure below the upper one. In the studies of Stewart and Brochard, minimal PEEP was used for both study arms, whereas in the Amato trial, the PV curve was used explicitly to adjust PEEP to values greater than the lower inflection point. This adjustment most likely leads to decreased mechanical stress because of repeated end-expiratory collapse. Conversely, PEEP may favour over-inflation if V_T is not reduced.

Thus, there are two plausible hypotheses [12] to explain the results of Amato et al. The first is that the high PEEP strategy minimised injury caused by recruitment/derecruitment, the critical factor causing VILI. The second is that the main difference in mortality rates among these studies was not in the treatment arms but in the control arms. Accordingly, patients in Amato's study had a greater chance to be exposed to mechanical injury because of the higher inflating pressures.

Individualisation of PEEP and V_T based on the lower and upper inflection points by measurement of the static PV curve to define the protective ventilatory strategy has been criticised because of the potential harm to patients [71]. Moreover, the complexity of the measurements and their interpretation has discouraged clinical use of this approach. Recently, Ranieri et al. proposed another predictive coefficient (*b-index*) to determine a non-injurious ventilatory strategy [73].

During constant flow conditions and when resistances are constant, the transpulmonary pressure (P_L) changes linearly with time—when compliance does not change with increasing lung volume. When compliance decreases, P_L is concave upward; when compliance increases, P_L is concave downward with respect to the time axis. This analysis of the pressure-time (Pt) relation is based on the assumption that during volume-controlled ventilation with constant flow inflation, the rate of change in pressure is related to changes in pulmonary compliance [74–77]. Under these circumstances, the P_L profile as function of inspiratory time (t) can be described by a power equation: $P_L = a \times t^b + c$. The coefficient a is a scaling factor, c is the pressure value at t=0, and the coefficient b describes the shape of the Pt curve: b=1 describes a straight Pt curve, b<1 a downward concavity and b>1 an upward concavity (Fig. 1).

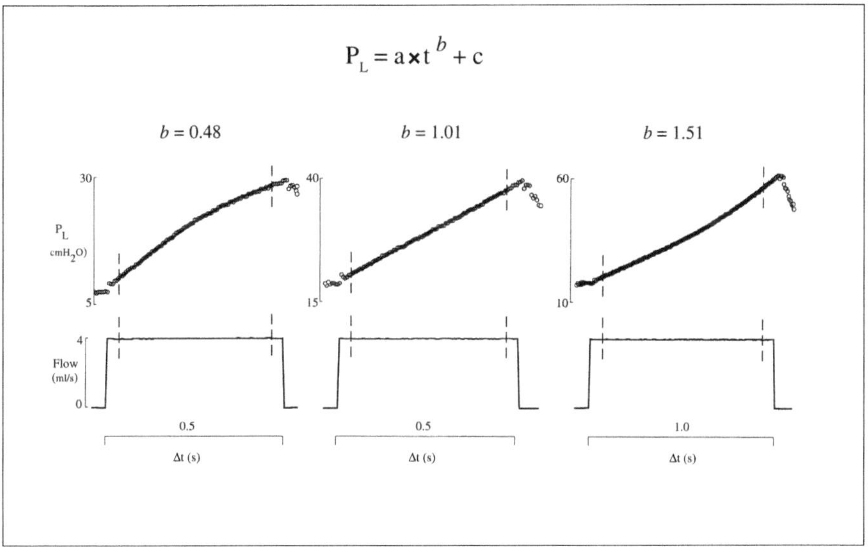

Fig. 1 Conceptual illustration of the dynamic pressure-time (Pt) curve. Based on the power equation $P_L = a \times t^b + c$; b=0.5 produces a convex Pt curve, indicating continuous recruitment; b=1 produces a straight Pt line, indicating no alveolar continuous recruitment or overdistension; and b=1.5 produces a concave Pt curve, indicating alveolar overdistension. The power equation was applied to the transpulmonary pressure (P_L) signal during constant inspiratory flow (*vertical bars*). Modified from [73]

This relationship was used in an experimental model of ALI to test the hypothesis that ventilator settings resulting in a straight Pt profile minimise the occurrence of VALI. In an isolated, non-perfused, lavaged rat model of ALI, V_T and PEEP were set to obtain: (1) a straight Pt curve (constant compliance, minimal stress); (2) a downward concavity in the Pt curve (increasing compliance, low volume stress); and (3) an upward concavity in the Pt curve (decreasing compliance, high volume stress). After 3 h, the rat lungs were analysed for histological evidence of pulmonary damage and the lavage concentration of inflammatory mediators. The threshold value for the coefficient *b* that best discriminated between lungs with and without histological and inflammatory evidence of VALI ranged between 0.90 and 1.10. A significant relationship ($p<0.001$) between values of *b* and injury score, IL-6, and MIP-2 was found. Conversely, strategies that produced values of $b<0.85$ or $b>1.15$ did not guarantee injury, although there was a significant correlation between *b* values and total airway injury score, IL-6, and MIP-2 values. These results indicate that *b* is not a reliable monitoring tool to detect VALI, but it should be considered as a therapeutic target to define a protective ventilatory strategy. Although *b* values different from 1 were, in a few cases, related to already non-injurious ventilator settings (low specificity), simple, safe, and inexpensive adjustments of PEEP and V_T leading to a straight Pt curve and to $b=1$ resulted in a ventilatory strategy that certainly minimised VALI (optimal sensitivity). However, the *b index* has been proposed on an ex-vivo experimental model. Therefore, it remains to be evaluated whether the assumptions of this model limit the use of the *b index* at the bedside.

Undoubtedly, the ventilation strategy considered as the gold standard in ARDS models is at the moment the one adopted by the ARDSNet trial, with a V_T of 6 ml/kg as calculated on the basis of predicted body weight. However, several issues remain to be clarified. For example, it has not been established whether volume-controlled ventilation with a V_T=6 ml/kg and pressure-controlled ventilation with relatively low pressures in the range of those found in the lung-protective arm (<30 cmH_2O) can be used indifferently. Physiologically a pressure-limited strategy should be as good as a volume-limited strategy, but more evidence is necessary to test whether there might be something specific to the ARDSNet strategy that is not incorporated by using pressure limitation. An example of this is the patient with a very stiff chest wall, such that limiting P_{plat} to 30 cmH_2O might limit V_T more than is necessary to minimise overdistension, and could even lead to under-recruitment of the lung, poor oxygenation and further derecruitment.

Moreover, the mechanisms that led to a lower mortality in the 6 ml/kg group in the ARDSNet trial remain to be explained in detail. The result was certainly not due to a decrease in barotrauma, as its incidence was virtually identical in the two groups (10 vs. 11%). It is tempting to speculate that it was related to a greater decrease in serum cytokines. It was previously suggested that injurious forms of mechanical ventilation lead to an increase in various mediators in the lung (biotrauma) and, owing to the increased alveolar-capillary permeability, these mediators may enter the circulation and cause organ dysfunction.

Further evidence has come from a randomised clinical trial comparing conventional mechanical ventilation as a control group with a lung-protective ventilatory strategy group made up of ARDS patients [57]. Significant differences were found between the control and the lung-protective strategy groups in V_T (11.1±1.3 vs. 7.6±1.1 ml/kg), P_{plat} (31.0±4.5 vs. 24.6±2.4 cmH_2O), and PEEP (6.5±1.7 vs. 14.8±2.7 cmH_2O) ($p<0.01$). The concentration of inflammatory mediators 36 h after randomisation was significantly higher in the control group than in the lung-protective strategy group, perhaps due to a minimising of overdistension and recruitment/derecruitment of the lung.

This conclusion suggests innovative treatments for preventing VALI. In animal models of VALI (VILI), it was demonstrated [78] that inhibition of polymorphonuclear cell adhesion by leumedins, through direct actions on leucocytes to inhibit the up-regulated expression of β_2-integrin involved in leucocyte adhesion, blocked the inflammatory response of VILI in rabbits. Treatment targeted at leumedins resulted in improved gas exchange. Moreover, pre-treatment with intratracheal instillation of high and low doses of anti-TNF-α antibody improved oxygenation and respiratory compliance, reduced leucocyte infiltration and ameliorated the pathological findings in rats undergoing injurious ventilation, suggesting that immunomodulation with anti-TNF-α antibody attenuates VALI [53].

In addition to direct immune-therapy in VALI, a role for endogenous catecholamines in the cellular response to ALI is possible. Adrenergic agents commonly used in clinical management may also have a role in attenuating the pulmonary inflammatory response. Treatment with the β-adrenoreceptor agonist isoproterenol attenuated endotoxin-induced release of TNF-α and lipid peroxidation in association with an increase in intracellular cAMP levels. The adenylate cyclase activator forskolin also inhibited endotoxin-induced changes in TNF-α and lipid peroxidation, suggesting that the pulmonary inflammatory response is regulated by stimulating β-adrenergic activity on lung cell-surface receptors [79]. Although potentially appealing, these experimental strategies need more studies and clinical evidence before they can be applied at the bedside.

Another important issue not addressed in the ARDSNet trial is the importance of recruitment manoeuvres. These are useful in preventing recruitment/derecruitment, which is crucial in animal studies on the development of VALI. The hypothesis that the effectiveness of a recruiting manoeuvre to improve oxygenation in patients with ARDS is influenced by the elastic properties of the lung and chest wall was examined [80]. Measurements of PaO_2/FiO_2 and chest-wall and lung elastance were obtained at zero PEEP, at baseline, and at 2 and 20 min after the administration of a recruiting manoeuvre (40 cmH_2O of continuous positive airway pressure for 40 s) in patients with ARDS ventilated according to the ARDSNet lung-protective strategy. Patients were classified a priori as responders and non-responders on the basis of the occurrence or non-occurrence of a 50% increase in PaO_2/FiO_2 after the recruiting manoeuvres.

Such manoeuvres increased PaO_2/FiO_2 by 20 ±3% in non-responders (n=11) and by 175±23% (n=11; mean±standard deviation) in responders. On zero PEEP, lung elastance (28.4±2.2 vs. 24.2±2.9 cmH_2O/l) and chest-wall elastance (10.4±1.8 vs. 5.6±0.8 cmH_2O/l) were higher in non-responders than in responders (p<0.01). Therefore, the application of recruiting manoeuvres seems to improve oxygenation only in patients with early ARDS who do not have impaired chest-wall mechanics and with a large potential for recruitment, as indicated by low values of lung elastance.

In summary, these results, as pointed out by the International Consensus Conference in Intensive Care Medicine [7], suggest that: high tidal volumes (12 ml/kg), resulting in high transpulmonary pressure and P_{plat}>30–35 cmH_2O, are potentially hazardous since they may increase the risk of barotrauma and mortality. A relatively simple strategy of reducing V_T to 6 ml/kg, or lower, if necessary, to reduce P_{plat} to <30 cmH_2O, appears to be safe and is associated with improved outcome. Other aspects, such as the increase in PEEP, titrated to the PV curve, and the use of recruitment manoeuvre, may, in particular situations, confer a protective effect against VALI, but they are not recommended for routine clinical management, before further experimental evidence has supported their use.

References

1. Tobin MJ (2001) Advances in mechanical ventilation. N Engl J Med 344(26):1986–1996
2. Esteban A, Anzueto A, Alìa I et al (2000) How is mechanical ventilation employed in the intensive care unit? An international utilization review. Am J Respir Crit Care Med 161(5):1450–1458
3. Dreyfuss D, Saumon G (1998) Ventilator-induced lung injury: lessons from experimental studies. Am J Respir Crit Care Med 157(1):294–323
4. Macklin MT, Macklin CC (1944) Malignant interstitial emphysema of the lungs and mediastinum as an important occult complication in many respiratory diseases and other conditions: an interpretation of the clinical literature in the light of laboratory experiment. Medicine 23:281–358
5. Dreyfuss D, Soler P, Basset G, Saumon G. High inflation pressure pulmonary edema. Respective effects of high airway pressure, high tidal volume, and positive end-expiratory pressure. Am Rev Respir Dis 137(5):1159–1164
6. Robertson B, Van Golde LMG, Batenburg JJ (eds) (1984) Pulmonary surfactant: from molecular biology to clinical practice. Elsevier, Amsterdam
7. Anonymous (1999) International Consensus Conferences in Intensive Care Medicine. Ventilator-associated lung injury in ARDS. Am J Respir Crit Care Med 160:2118–2124
8. Tremblay LN, Slutsky AS (1998) Ventilator-induced injury: from barotrauma to biotrauma. Proc Assoc Am Physicians 110(6):482–488
9. Slutsky AS (1999) Lung injury caused by mechanical ventilation. Chest 116(1 Suppl):9S-15S
10. Slutsky AS, Tremblay LN (1998) Multiple system organ failure. Is mechanical ventilation a contributing factor? Am J Respir Crit Care Med 157(6 Pt 1):1721–1725
11. Montgomery AB, Stager MA, Carrico CJ, Hudson LD (1985) Causes of mortality in patients with the adult respiratory distress syndrome. Am Rev Respir Dis 132(3):485–489

12. Ranieri VM, Zhang H (1999) Respiratory mechanics in acute respiratory distress. Curr Opin Crit Care 5:17–20
13. Whitehead T, Slutsky AS (2002) The pulmonary physician in critical care. 7: Ventilator induced lung injury. Thorax 57:635–642
14. Bouhuys A (1969) Physiology and musical instruments. Nature 221:1199–1204
15. Anonymous (2000) Ventilation with lower tidal volumes as compared with traditional tidal volumes for acute lung injury and the acute respiratory distress syndrome. The Acute Respiratory Distress Syndrome Network. N Engl J Med 342(18):1301–1308
16. Weg JG, Anzueto A, Balk RA et al (1998) The relation of pneumothorax and other air leaks to mortality in the acute respiratory distress syndrome. N Engl J Med 338(6):341–346
17. Stewart TE, Meade MO, Cook DJ et al (1998) Evaluation of a ventilation strategy to prevent barotrauma in patients at high risk for acute respiratory distress syndrome. Pressure- and Volume-Limited Ventilation Strategy Group. N Engl J Med 338(6):355–361
18. Brochard L, Roudot-Thoraval F, Roupie E et al (1998) Tidal volume reduction for prevention of ventilator-induced lung injury in acute respiratory distress syndrome. The Multicenter Trail Group on Tidal Volume reduction in ARDS. Am J Respir Crit Care Med 158(6):1831–1838
19. Hernandez LA, Peevy KJ, Moise AA, Parker JC (1989) Chest wall restriction limits high airway pressure-induced lung injury in young rabbits. J Appl Physiol 66(5):2364–2368
20. Carlton DP, Cummings JJ, Scheerer RG et al (1990) Lung overexpansion increases pulmonary microvascular protein permeability in young lambs. J Appl Physiol 69(2):577–583
21. Muscedere JG, Mullen JB, Gan K, Slutsky AS (1994) Tidal ventilation at low airway pressures can augment lung injury. Am J Respir Crit Care Med 149(5):1327–1334
22. Mead J, Takishima T, Leith D (1970) Stress distribution in lungs: a model of pulmonary elasticity. J Appl Physiol 28(5):596–608
23. Webb HH, Tierney DF (1974) Experimental pulmonary edema due to intermittent positive pressure ventilation with high inflation pressures. Protection by positive end-expiratory pressure. Am Rev Respir Dis 110(5):556–565
24. Argiras EP, Blakeley CR, Dunnill MS et al (1987) High PEEP decreases hyaline membrane formation in surfactant deficient lungs. Br J Anaesth 59(10):1278–1285
25. Sandhar BK, Niblett DJ, Argiras EP et al (1988) Effects of positive end-expiratory pressure on hyaline membrane formation in a rabbit model of the neonatal respiratory distress syndrome. Intensive Care Med 14(5):538–546
26. Chabot F, Mitchell JA, Gutteridge JM, Evans TW (1998) Reactive oxygen species in acute lung injury. Eur Respir J 11(3):745–757
27. Davis WB, Rennard SI, Bitterman PB, Crystal RG (1983) Pulmonary oxygen toxicity. Early reversible changes in human alveolar structures induced by hyperoxia. N Engl J Med 309(15):878–883
28. Nash G, Bowen JA, Langlinais PC (1971) 'Respirator lung': a misnomer. Arch Pathol 91(3):234–240
29. Gattinoni L, Pesenti A, Avalli L et al (1987) pressure–volume curve of total respiratory system in acute respiratory failure. Computed tomographic scan study. Am Rev Respir Dis 136(3):730–736
30. Gammon RB, Shin MS, Buchalter SE (1992) Pulmonary barotrauma in mechanical ventilation. Patterns and risk factors. Chest 102(2):568–572
31. Kolobow T, Moretti MP, Fumagalli R et al (1987) Severe impairment in lung function induced by high peak airway pressure during mechanical ventilation. An experimental study. Am Rev Respir Dis 135(2):312–315
32. Dreyfuss D, Basset G, Soler P, Saumon G (1985) Intermittent positive-pressure hyperventilation with high inflation pressures produces pulmonary microvascular injury in rats. Am Rev Respir Dis 132(4):880–884
33. Lecuona E, Saldias F, Comellas A et al (1999) Ventilator-associated lung injury decreases lung ability to clear edema in rats. Am J Respir Crit Care Med 159(2):603–609
34. Albert RK, Lakshminarayan S, Kirk W, Butler J (1980) Lung inflation can cause pulmonary

edema in zone I of in situ dog lungs. J Appl Physiol 49(5):815–819
35. Verbrugge SJ, Böhm SH, Gommers D et al (1998) Surfactant impairment after mechanical ventilation with large alveolar surface area changes and effects of positive end-expiratory pressure. Br J Anaesth 80(3):360–364
36. Verbrugge SJ, de Jong JW, Keijzer E et al (1999) Purine in bronchoalveolar lavage fluid as a marker of ventilation-induced lung injury. Crit Care Med 27(4):779–783
37. Mathieu-Costello OA, West JB (1994) Are pulmonary capillaries susceptible to mechanical stress? Chest 105:102S-107S
38. Fu Z, Costello ML, Tsukimoto K et al (1992) High lung volume increases stress failure in pulmonary capillaries. J Appl Physiol 73:123–133
39. West JB, Tsukimoto K, Mathieu-Costello O, Prediletto R (1991) Stress failure in pulmonary capillaries. J Appl Physiol 70(4):1731–1742
41. Gaver DP, Samsel RW, Solway J (1990) Effects of surface tension and viscosity on airway reopening. J Appl Physiol 69(1):74–85
42. Vanderzwan J, McCaig L, Mehta et al (1998) Characterizing alterations in the pulmonary surfactant system in a rat model of Pseudomonas aeruginosa pneumonia. Eur Respir J 12(6):1388–96
43. Lewis JF, Jobe AH (1993) Surfactant and the adult respiratory distress syndrome. Am Rev Respir Dis 147(1):218–233
44. Malloy J, Veldhuizen R, Yao LJ et al (1997) Alterations of the endogenous surfactant system in septic adult rats. Am J Respir Crit Care Med 156(2 Pt 1):617–623
46. Wright JR (1997) Immunomodulatory functions of surfactant. Physiol Rev 77(4):931–962
47. West JB, Mathieu-Costello O (1998) Stress-induced injury of pulmonary capillaries. Proc Assoc Am Physicians 110(6):506–512
48. Kawano T, Mori S, Cybulsky M et al (1987) Effect of granulocyte depletion in a ventilated surfactant-depleted lung. J Appl Physiol 62(1):27–33
49. Tsuno K, Miura K, Takeya M et al (1991) Histopathologic pulmonary changes from mechanical ventilation at high peak airway pressures. Am Rev Respir Dis 143(5 Pt 1):1115–1120
50. Tremblay L, Valenza F, Ribeiro SP et al (1997) Injurious ventilatory strategies increase cytokines and c-fos m-RNA expression in an isolated rat lung model. J Clin Invest 99(5):944–952
51. von Bethmann AN, Brasch F, Nusing R et al (1998) Hyperventilation induces release of cytokines from perfused mouse lung. Am J Respir Crit Care Med 157(1):263–272
52. Chiumello D, Pristine G, Slutsky AS (1999) Mechanical ventilation affects local and systemic cytokines in an animal model of acute respiratory distress syndrome. Am J Respir Crit Care Med 160(1):109–116
54. Narimanbekov IO, Rozycki HJ (1995) Effect of IL-1 blockade on inflammatory manifestations of acute ventilator-induced lung injury in a rabbit model. Exp Lung Res 21(2):239–254
55. Dos Santos CC, Slutsky AS (2000) Invited review: mechanisms of ventilator-induced lung injury: a perspective. J Appl Physiol 89(4):1645–1655
56. Vlahakis NE, Schroeder MA, Limper AH, Hubmayr RD (1999) Stretch induces cytokine release by alveolar epithelial cells in vitro. Am J Physiol 277(1 Pt 1):L167-L173
57. Ranieri VM, Suter PM, Tortorella C et al (1999) Effect of mechanical ventilation on inflammatory mediators in patients with acute respiratory distress syndrome: a randomized controlled trial. JAMA 282(1):54–61
58. Nahum A, Hoyt J, Schmitz L et al (1997) Effect of mechanical ventilation strategy on dissemination of intratracheally instilled Escherichia coli in dogs. Crit Care Med 25(10):1733–1743
59. Verbrugge SJ, Sorm V, van 't Veen A et al (1998) Lung overinflation without positive end-expiratory pressure promotes bacteremia after experimental Klebsiella pneumoniae inoculation. Intensive Care Med 24(2):172–177
60. Murphy DB, Cregg N, Tremblay L et al (2000) Adverse ventilatory strategy causes pulmonary-to-systemic translocation of endotoxin. Am J Respir Crit Care Med 162(1):27–33

61. Brower RG, Shanholtz CB, Fessler HE et al (1999) Prospective, randomized, controlled clinical trial comparing traditional versus reduced tidal volume ventilation in acute respiratory distress syndrome patients. Crit Care Med 27(8):1492–1498
62. Slutsky AS, Ranieri VM (2000) Mechanical ventilation: lessons from the ARDSNet trial. Respir Res 1(2):73–77
63. Tobin MJ (2000) Culmination of an era in research on the acute respiratory distress syndrome. N Engl J Med 342(18):1360–1361
64. Hickling KG, Henderson SJ, Jackson R (1990) Low mortality associated with low volume pressure limited ventilation with permissive hypercapnia in severe adult respiratory distress syndrome. Intensive Care Med 16(6):372–377
65. Shibata K, Cregg N, Engelberts D et al (1998) Hypercapnic acidosis may attenuate acute lung injury by inhibition of endogenous xanthine oxidase. Am J Respir Crit Care Med 158(5 Pt 1):1578–1584
67. Laffey JG, Tanaka M, Engelberts D et al (2000) Therapeutic hypercapnia reduces pulmonary and systemic injury following in vivo lung reperfusion. Am J Respir Crit Care Med 162(6):2287–2294
68. Feihl F, Perret C (1994) Permissive hypercapnia. How permissive should we be? Am J Respir Crit Care Med 150(6 Pt 1):1722–1737
69. de Durante G, del Turco M, Rustichini L et al (2002) ARDSNet lower tidal volume ventilatory strategy may generate intrinsic positive end-expiratory pressure in patients with acute respiratory distress syndrome. Am J Respir Crit Care Med 165(9):1271–1274
70. Amato MB, Barbas CS, Medeiros DM et al (1995) Beneficial effects of the 'open lung approach' with low distending pressures in acute respiratory distress syndrome. A prospective randomized study on mechanical ventilation. Am J Respir Crit Care Med 152(6 Pt 1):1835–1846
71. Hudson LD (1998) Protective ventilation for patients with acute respiratory distress syndrome. N Engl J Med 338(6):385–387
72. Brochard L (1998) Respiratory pressure–volume curves. In: Tobin MJ (ed) Principle and practice of intensive care monitoring. McGraw-Hill, New York, pp 579–616
73. Ranieri VM, Zhang H, Mascia L et al (2000) Pressure-time curve predicts minimally injurious ventilatory strategy in an isolated rat lung model. Anesthesiology 93(5):1320–1328
74. Ranieri VM, Giuliani R, Fiore T et al (1994) Volume-pressure curve of the respiratory system predicts effects of PEEP in ARDS: 'occlusion' versus 'constant flow' technique. Am J Respir Crit Care Med 149(1):19–27
75. Ranieri VM, Brienza N, Santostasi S et al (1997) Impairment of lung and chest wall mechanics in patients with acute respiratory distress syndrome: role of abdominal distension. Am J Respir Crit Care Med 156(4 Pt 1):1082–1091
76. Bates JH, Rossi A, Milic-Emili J (1985) Analysis of the behavior of the respiratory system with constant inspiratory flow. J Appl Physiol 58(6):1840–1848
77. D'Angelo E, Robatto FM, Calderini E et al (1991) Pulmonary and chest wall mechanics in anesthetized paralyzed humans. J Appl Physiol 70(6):2602–2610
78. Rimensberger PC, Fedorko L, Cutz E, Bohn DJ (1998) Attenuation of ventilator-induced acute lung injury in an animal model by inhibition of neutrophil adhesion by leumedins (NPC 15669). Crit Care Med 26(3):548–555
79. Zhang H, Kim YK, Govindarajan A et al (1999) Effect of adrenoreceptors on endotoxin-induced cytokines and lipid peroxidation in lung explants. Am J Respir Crit Care Med 160(5 Pt 1):1703–1710
80. Grasso S, Mascia L, Del Turco M et al (2002) Effects of recruiting maneuvers in patients with acute respiratory distress syndrome ventilated with protective ventilatory strategy. Anesthesiology 96(4):795–802

Controlled Mechanical Ventilation in ARDS

U. Lucangelo, S. Gramaticopolo, B. Bacer

Introduction

Acute respiratory distress syndrome (ARDS) is a severe form of hypoxaemic respiratory failure that is associated with several critical diseases, such as trauma, inhalation injury, shock and pulmonary and extrapulmonary infections. ARDS has been classified into two forms: primary (caused by an insult in the lung) and secondary (caused by an indirect insult, e.g. sepsis or acute pancreatitis, followed by an acute systemic inflammatory response). Lung disease originating from an inflammatory response has several degrees of severity. In the presence of sepsis, these range from a subclinical expression of pulmonary damage to overt respiratory failure. The most feared complication of sepsis is ARDS, a severe form of acute lung injury (ALI).

This chapter describes ventilatory strategies to deal with ALI and ARDS, as these pathologies are a major concern in everyday practice in the intensive care unit (ICU). In addition, ALI and ARDS are defined, as definitions of these conditions have had a major role in guiding therapeutic decisions and have contributed to establishing homogeneous populations in multi-centre and international trials. A brief anatomopathologic description of ARDS, with its different stages and their physiopathologic expression, is also provided. Medical therapy in ARDS has produced few positive results, whereas lung-protective strategies have had a major role in improving survival. For this reason, conventional and non-conventional ventilatory strategies are discussed in order to provide an overview of the techniques that have been made available thus far to intensive-care practitioners.

Definitions: Acute Lung Injury, Acute Respiratory Distress Syndrome

For over 20 years, experts tried to define complex nosologic entities such as sepsis and respiratory failure. In both cases the numerous overlapping definitions

U. Lucangelo, P. Pelosi, W.A. Zin, A. Aliverti (eds.) *Respiratory System and Artificial Ventilation*. © Springer 2008

made it impossible to compare international studies and epidemiological data. Today an agreement has been reached that has made available an important instrument of work, both in clinical application and research.

Since the first definition of ARDS, in 1967, criteria aimed at defining this condition have been often revised, however the hallmarks of ARDS have basically never changed: bilateral pulmonary infiltrates, acute severe hypoxaemia and no evidence of left-heart failure. The American-European Consensus Conference on ARDS published a set of diagnostic criteria that have been widely accepted and

Table 1 Diagnostic criteria for acute lung injury (*ALI*) and acute respiratory distress syndrome (*ARDS*) according to the 1994 American-European Consensus Conference on ARDS

Criteria	ALI	ARDS
Onset	Acute	Acute
Frontal chest X-ray	Bilateral infiltrates	Bilateral infiltrates
Pulmonary artery occlusion pressure	≤18 mmHg	≤18 mmHg
Cardiac function	No clinical evidence of left atrial hypertension	No clinical evidence of left atrial hypertension
PaO2/FiO2	≤300	≤200

distinguish ALI from ARDS (Table 1) [1]. Since the introduction of these criteria, homogeneous epidemiological data have been collected [2]. However, despite the introduction of commonly accepted hallmarks for the diagnosis of ARDS, the same are non-specific: ARDS and ALI are the final expression of lung inflammatory damage that is neither an isolated nor a primary condition: ARDS is often just one part of a multi-organ illness and it exemplifies the limitations of management strategies whose major focus are the lungs [3].

Epidemiology and Prognosis

The incidence of ALI/ARDS in the USA has been estimated by the National Institute of Health as 75 per 100000. Sepsis is the most frequent cause of ALI and is responsible for about 40% of all such cases. Sepsis evolves into ARDS in 25–42% of patients [4,5]. Morbidity and mortality associated with ALI and ARDS have slowly decreased in the last 10 years but nonetheless remain between 30 and 40%.

Predictors of mortality in ALI/ARDS patients are still a matter of debate. The currently available scoring systems (Acute Physiology and Chronic Health

Evaluation, Multiple Organ Dysfunction Syndrome, Sequential Organ Failure Assessment, Injury Severity Score) are unreliable in predicting outcome. A specific score for ARDS was developed but its efficacy is controversial [6]. The prognostic hallmark that remains valid for ALI patients hospitalised in the ICU is the number of organ insufficiencies associated with the main pathology; this criterion can be extended to ARDS patients. Several studies have demonstrated that, even if initially severe hypoxaemia is not a valid indicator of prognosis, an improvement or deterioration of PaO_2/FiO_2 values in the first 24 h can predict outcome [7]. Last, but not least, mortality in ARDS patients is often due to the initiating pathology (for example, sepsis) or to multi-organ failure (MOF) rather than to progressive respiratory failure [8].

Efforts to predict outcome in ARDS patients have converged on biological markers with no better success than physiological scores. However, procollagen-peptide III has been identified as a marker of fibrosis and, as such, has been shown to correlate with a worst prognosis for patient. The concentration of procollagen-peptide III can be measured in plasma and in bronchoalveolar lavage fluid. Other promising prognostic indicators are the levels of pro-inflammatory cytokines and maintenance of integrity of the epithelial barrier. In the latter case, patients with a higher protein concentration in pulmonary oedema fluid in the first 12 h (reflecting the integrity of the epithelial barrier and active fluid transport in the lymphatic system) had a better prognosis [9]. However, none of these markers has been approved as an outcome predictor for ARDS; therefore, physiopathologic consideration of a patient's clinical condition is still a cornerstone in attempts to predict recovery. In this respect, the restoration of respiratory function in a patient with ARDS within a brief period of time generally indicates a good prognosis [10] The lung will suffer permanent damage if respiratory failure (ARDS) persists for several days. Clinical improvement of respiratory function occurs within the first 3 months after an ARDS episode and the chest X-ray will be negative after a couple of weeks. Nonetheless, the patient's quality of life is almost always reduced due to residual pulmonary dysfunction [11].

Physiopathology and Anatomopathology of ARDS

Phases of ARDS

The three clinical, physiopathologic and anatomopathologic stages that characterise ARDS are generally consistent. The first phase (*exudative*) is defined by intense alveolar phlogosis and disruption of alveolar structure accompanied by collagen deposition, the accumulation of inflammatory cells and exudative oedema. The exudative phase lasts for about 5 days. During this time, apoptotic type I pneumocytes are substituted by type II pneumocytes; as a result, the alveolo-capillary barrier becomes thicker, impeding oxygen transport [12]. In addition, acute respiratory failure calls for employment of a high oxygen concentration of inhaled gases and the by-product of these, oxygen free radicals, further perpetrates alveolar damage.

In the second, *fibroproliferative* phase of ARDS (days 5–10), plasmatic proteins and cellular debris fill the alveoli. Surfactant produced by type II pneumocytes is inactive or insufficient. This phase is rapid and involves almost all of the pulmonary parenchyma.

The *fibrotic* phase starts in the second week of disease and is the result of the healing processes that intervene after acute damage. Parenchymal fibrosis is associated with vascular fibrosis of the arteriolar tunica media, thus compromising a variable percentage of the vascular bed. Dead-space ventilation increases, even if the alveolar oedema and intrapulmonary shunt resolve. Thoracic X-ray shows residual fibrosis, while spirometry is characterised by a restrictive and sometimes emphysematous pattern [13].

Pulmonary and Extrapulmonary ARDS

Two different forms of ARDS have been distinguished: the pulmonary form originates from a primary pulmonary insult (infective disease, chemical injury, embolic disease, parenchymal contusion), and the extrapulmonary or secondary form is the result of a systemic pathology (sepsis, trauma, massive transfusion, etc.). It has been suggested that the respiratory mechanics associated with primitive or secondary ARDS differ such that patients will have different responses to the ventilatory strategies applied. Animal models have shown that extrapulmonary ARDS is characterised by disruption of the vascular endothelium, which in turn is due to inflammatory mediators that circulate in the blood stream and cause abundant interstitial oedema. Pulmonary ARDS, in contrast, is characterised by primary alveolar epithelial damage that evolves into an exudative alveolar oedema, rich in fibrin, collagen and neutrophils, and only a slight interstitial oedema.

Chest X-ray in primary ARDS patients shows patchy densities, while that of patients with secondary ARDS is more likely to show diffuse lung densities representing interstitial oedema and compression atelectasis. Computed tomography scanning allows a better distinction between primary and secondary ARDS: consolidation is more frequent in the former, while ground-glass opacification characterises the latter [14,15]

Respiratory Mechanics

Mechanical alteration of the respiratory system in ALI/ARDS results in a reduced pulmonary compliance, decreased airways diameter and alveolar collapse. In the early phase of ARDS, lung volume is reduced by alveolar oedema and a surfactant deficit. These changes are consistent with the 'baby' lung recognised in the exudative phase and which must be distinguished from the 'stiff' (fibrotic) lung typical of the subsequent phase of ARDS.

The distinction is not trivial since ventilatory strategies in different stages of ARDS must be guided by the principle of protecting the lungs from barotrauma and volutrauma (by reducing stress to the alveolar walls); that is, to guide the ventilation plateau pressure, the mean and peak airway pressures must be understood. While plateau pressure is considered the best index of trans-alveolar pressure during mechanical ventilation, mean airway pressure is the best parameter to predict the overall effect of ventilation on oxygenation and haemodynamics: as the mean airway pressure increases, atelectatic areas of the lung are recruited, but the increase in mean airway pressure may hinder venous return to the left heart, thus diminishing cardiac output. In the normally compliant lungs, a plateau pressure of 35 cmH_2O mirrors total lung capacity. Thoracic tomographic scans of ARDS patients have shown that non-dependent lung lobes are almost normal; these represent alveoli with normal compliance. When plateau pressures >35 cmH_2O are reached by ventilating the ARDS patient, the risk of volutrauma is high because normal alveoli will be overstretched while pathologic alveoli are not ventilated [16]. Studies conducted on animals have shown that mechanical ventilation causes damage to alveoli due to overdistension even if barotrauma is not evident; inflation of the alveoli over total lung capacity provokes haemorrhagic oedema [17]. Since it has been recognised that excess alveolar volume is an important source of damage to the airways in ARDS patients, the term 'volutrauma' has been employed to describe this situation.

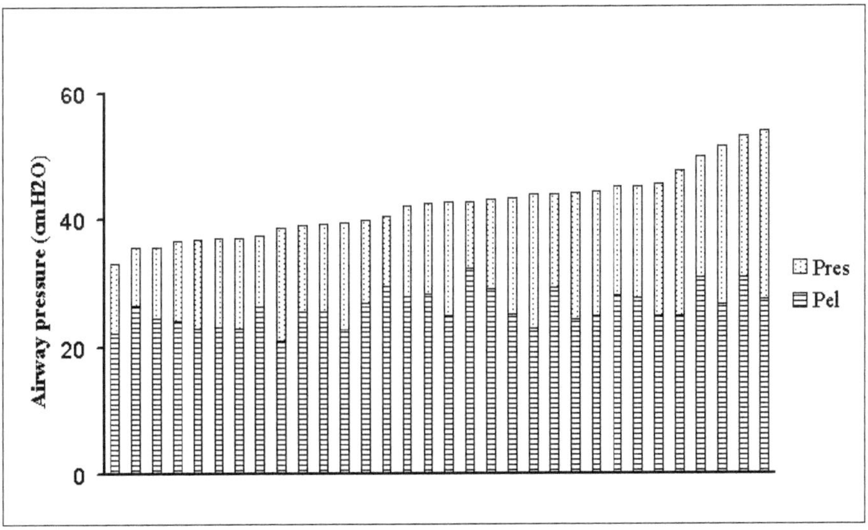

Fig. 1 Peak airway pressure partitioned into its elastic (*Pel*) and resistive (*Pres*) components in 32 ALI/ARDS patients (*bars*). Different pairs of Pel and Pers describe the heterogeneous contribute of resistive and elastic load in acute lung injury/acute respiratory distress syndrome (ALI/ARDS) during mechanical ventilation

Peak airway pressure in ARDS may sometimes reach disproportionately high values compared to plateau pressure (Fig. 1). This gap may be due to a high resistance to flow in the airways caused by oedema, secretions, bronchospasm or the calibre of the endotracheal tube; however, resistance to flow in the airways as well as pulmonary compliance have to be assessed and correlated with the actual lung volume participating in ventilatory exchange [18].

A distinction between primary and secondary ARDS implies an understanding of the role of lung and chest-wall elastance and their individual contributions in creating total respiratory system elastance. While in primary (pulmonary) ARDS the increase in elastance is due to areas of pulmonary consolidation, in secondary ARDS it is due also to an increase in thoracic-wall stiffness, as a consequence of increased intra-abdominal pressure. The latter has been thus far undervalued in bed-side monitoring; however, it is a frequent finding in critically ill patients, as a consequence of bowel-wall oedema and reactive intra-abdominal fluid, both of which are expressions of abdominal inflammatory injury. This is not a merely semantic distinction but has different consequences in the clinical setting: alveolar recruitment by PEEP will be successful in secondary but not in primary ARDS, since in the latter it leads to atelectasis due to augmented intra-abdominal pressure. At the same time, excessive PEEP value will produce lung overinflation in a patient with primary ARDS.

Thus, in the ventilatory strategy for an ARDS patient, it is important to gauge the potential for pulmonary recruitment; however, a successful recruitment manoeuvre and improvement of the oxygenation index do not correlate with better outcome: a recent clinical study evidenced that patients with a worse oxygenation index and greater potential for recruitment, even with an optimal ventilatory strategy, do not have a better outcome than other patients [19]. This result points out two considerations: (1) patients with potentially recruitable lung have a larger percentage of seriously compromised lung parenchyma and (2) improvement of oxygenation in an ARDS patient does not improve outcome, as the cause of death in most of these patients is the primary disease.

Pulmonary Fluid Balance and Pulmonary Hypertension

Inflammatory injury to the endothelium augments its permeability to proteins and disrupts arteriolar auto-regulation. Both events contribute to alterations in oncotic and hydrostatic pressures, resulting in leakage of fluid outside the capillaries. When this process takes place in the pulmonary circulation, it leads to characteristic ALI/ARDS lung interstitial oedema. As interstitial fluid collects in pulmonary tissues, it is drained by the lymphatic system, but when it is overwhelmed fluid collects in extravascular spaces.

Thus, pulmonary hypertension that develops during ARDS is multi-factorial in origin: perivascular oedema has an important role in causing pulmonary hypertension in the initial phase of ARDS, while during later stages both hypoxaemia-induced vasoconstriction and thrombotic reduction of the vascular bed contribute to a decreased compliance of the pulmonary vascular system. In the last stage of ARDS, fibrosis adds its burden by obliteration of the vascular bed. Pulmonary-artery hypertension is a characteristic finding in ARDS; however, although the pulmonary vascular resistance is normal or only moderately elevated, this is due to the reduced cardiac output [20].

ARDS and Pulmonary Shunt

In healthy subjects, pulmonary shunt is 5% of cardiac output, but during ARDS the shunt fraction may exceed 25% of cardiac output. Shunt in ARDS is due to perfusion of atelectatic or oedema-filled alveoli and to an abolished hypoxic vasoconstriction reflex. After initial lung injury, dependent lung zones, which are better perfused, consolidate and are responsible for the main part of the shunt [16]. The shunting of blood into large, non-ventilated lung areas explains why hypoxaemia is refractory to oxygen supplementation.

Management of ARDS

The management of ARDS involves intervention with respect to ventilatory strategy and pharmacotherapy. Since the recognition of ARDS as a pathologic entity, only the use of low-tidal-volume mechanical ventilation has proven effective in improving patient survival. The ventilatory strategy proposed by the ARDS-NET study decreased mortality by 9% in patients in whom the end-inspiratory plateau pressure was <30 cmH_2O [21]; lung damage due to mechanical ventilation has been abated by increasing PEEP level and reducing tidal volume. This has diminished alveolar stress and the risk of mechanical stress to alveoli (barotrauma and volutrauma).

Pharmacotherapeutic approaches have not given satisfactory results: the inhibition of specific inflammatory mediators was inconclusive, while corticosteroid therapy was effective only in selected patient groups. Care of the ARDS patient is based on supporting vital functions and promoting oxygen transport while the primary disease that caused the ARDS is resolved.

In the following sections, lung-protective ventilatory strategies involving conventional and non-conventional ventilation are discussed. Ventilatory support in ARDS has several advantages: it diminishes the work of breathing and allows better redistribution of blood flow to other vital organs; however ventilatory support is not therapeutic, but is only a supportive measure to promote oxygen transport for as long as necessary. During that time, the damage resulting from mechanical ventilation must be limited.

ARDS NET

As mentioned above, the ARDS-NET ventilatory strategy is thus far the only successful therapeutic approach to ARDS, improving mortality by limiting iatrogenic pulmonary damage. The protocol proposed by the study had three goals: employ tidal volume of 6–8 ml/kg body weight, keep plateau pressure <30 cmH_2O and avoid severe respiratory acidosis. These goals are reached by keeping the tidal volume low, by employing increasing levels of PEEP, maintaining the appropriate respiratory rate and varying FiO_2, which depends on the severity of hypoxaemia and is set to obtain SpO_2=90%.

PEEP is applied to avoid alveolar closure and parenchymal derecruitment; the optimal level of PEEP has been discussed extensively. It is generally agreed that the right PEEP for each patient is the value that prevents derecruitment of the majority of alveoli while causing minimal overdistension. PEEP is determined with pressure–volume compliance curves and set about 2 cmH_2O above the lower inflection point [22]. Plotting a pressure–volume curve is cumbersome in the clinical setting, so this procedure is often bypassed by clinicians; however, it was recently reported that deep sedation of patient facilitates the manoeuvres required to plot the curve without the need for neuromuscular paralysis [23]. Current microprocessor technology is available that allows this measurement to be accomplished routinely with the single-breath technique without the need to reduce PEEP to 0 cmH_2O. Nonetheless, the best PEEP level that should be adopted when managing patients with ARDS or ALI remains a matter of discussion. The NIH-ARDS Clinical Trials Network provided PEEP/FiO_2 tables to select such values. This is the best evidence-based practice proposed so far; however, while providing a protocol for treating this aspect of ARDS, it does not take into account extreme cases and does not differentiate between patients with low pulmonary compliance and those with low thoracic-wall compliance. The first group is well-represented by patients with primary ARDS or ARDS superimposed on already stiff lungs, who will need moderate application of PEEP as they are at major risk for barotraumas and volutrauma. Conversely, patients with low thoracic-wall compliance (obese patients, patients affected by intra-abdominal hypertension of any cause) may need levels of PEEP that are much higher than those suggested by the ARDS Clinical Trial Network PEEP/FiO_2 tables. In particular, it is the experts' opinion that PEEP settings for cases at the extremes of 'standard' ARDS should be selected based on accurate analysis of lung mechanics [24].

Despite the never-ending debate about the best PEEP level, lung-protective ventilation has brought major changes and improvements in survival for ARDS patients. A recent observational study conducted by the Mechanical Ventilation International Study Group stated that ARDS patients in whom low PEEP or no PEEP was employed in the first week of respiratory failure had a worse outcome [25].

Non-invasive Ventilation

Non-invasive positive-pressure ventilation (NIPPV) has received renewed consideration due to the improved technology and better patient comfort. As a result, it has been employed in an increasing number of clinical conditions. Clinical trials conducted in the 1990s did not show any advantage in employing NIPPV in the treatment of ARDS patients [26,27]. Indications for non-invasive ventilation are still discussed: recent studies have defined several applications, but a recent meta-analysis concluded that NIPPV in ARDS does not reduce the necessity of orotracheal intubation nor does it improve survival. It should be noted, however, that the studies on which the meta-analysis was based were probably too heterogeneous to be compared [28].

A recent prospective study of 147 ARDS patients showed encouraging results: in half of the patients who received NIPPV, respiratory exchange improved and orotracheal intubation was not necessary. As a consequence, there was a lower incidence of ventilator-associated pneumonia and mortality was reduced. The need for intubation was associated with older age, severity of the clinical condition, necessity of high-pressure support and PEEP. A SAPS II >34 and a PaO_2/FiO_2 <175 after one hour of NIPPV were independent predictors of the requirement for intubation [29].

Pressure Control Ventilation

Pressure control ventilation (PCV) is considered to be a protective ventilatory strategy for ALI and ARDS patients. Compared to volume control ventilation (VCV), the flow distribution in the lung parenchyma is more homogeneous with PCV, and for the same tidal volume PCV employs a lower airway pressure than is the case in VCV. These beneficial effects of VCV are explained by a better adaptation between PCV and the patient's respiratory pattern, while the set limit in pressure avoids the risk of barotraumas. PCV has a decelerating inspiratory flow pattern as opposed to the constant inspiratory flow rate of VCV. Inspiratory flow in PCV decreases exponentially during lung inflation to keep airway pressure at the selected value, and this flow pattern is responsible for the reduced peak airway pressure and the improved gas distribution between lung regions with different time constants. In the latter, the lower airways pressure may reduce regional overdistension in ARDS or ALI patients. The effect may be due to the partial recruitment of lung parenchyma; however, Prella et al. found little influence on gas exchange when PCV rather than VCV was administered (tidal volume, respiratory rate and PEEP held constant), even if on thoracic CT scan a more homogeneous gas distribution was noted. This suggested that there was no significant alveolar recruitment in PCV mode [30].

There is a tendency of lower insufflation volumes during PCV; thus, PCV is applied in ARDS, it may not provide adequate ventilation due to decreasing compliance in the patient's lungs.

Adaptive pressure control ventilation (APCV) was introduced to guarantee minimum tidal-volume delivery to patients receiving PCV (PCV with a volume target) and assure patient-ventilator synchrony. This is achieved by adjusting the pressure target (using a pre-set algorithm) to meet the patient's needs breath-by-breath. APCV, by guaranteeing a minimum minute ventilation around a pre-set pressure limit, allows a lower airway pressure to be employed, thus meeting the goals of the ARDS Network Trial; however further studies are needed to demonstrate the advantages of APCV in ALI and ARDS [31].

High-Frequency Ventilation

This approach was introduced in the 1960s with the aim of improving gas exchange and reducing the complications of mechanical ventilation. HFV has played a predominant role in the management of neonatal acute respiratory failure. Its application has been extended to adults with respiratory failure for whom conventional mechanical ventilation is not sufficient.

The main features of HFV are: a respiratory frequency >60 breaths per minute, a tidal volume that is less than the dead space, a large capacity for functional reserve volume, lower peak airway pressure and better oxygenation.

Several techniques to achieve HFV have been developed and they can be roughly classified by the respiratory frequency employed: high-frequency oscillation ventilation (HFOV) uses high frequencies (60–2400 cycles/min), while high-frequency positive pressure ventilation (HFPPV) has lower frequencies (60–300 cycles/min). Halfway between the two, high-frequency jet ventilation delivers small volumes (1–5 ml/kg) at 60–360 cycles/min; this produces a degree of ventilation between the lower and upper inflection points of the pressure–volume curve, thus preventing alveolar overdistension, atelectasis and shear stress due to cyclic opening and closure of the alveolar walls. Studies conducted thus far have had encouraging results, but effective CO_2 removal with HFV techniques is difficult and is therefore an important drawback to this approach [32].

Meta-analysis of the application of HFV in ARDS and ALI did not show improvements in mortality and morbidity [33]; however, some HDV techniques applied to selected groups of patients actually improve respiratory exchange and reduce the total length of ventilator days. Specifically, seriously compromised patients with risk factors for barotrauma and volutrauma benefit from HFOV and show an improved oxygenation index [34]. When HFOV is associated with recruitment manoeuvres, carried out by an easily applicable protocol, it allows for the employment of lower FiO_2 and better tolerance of HFV [35].

High-Frequency Percussive Ventilation

Here, the features of high frequency and conventional ventilation are combined. HFPV can thus be described as a mechanical ventilation time-cycled and flow-

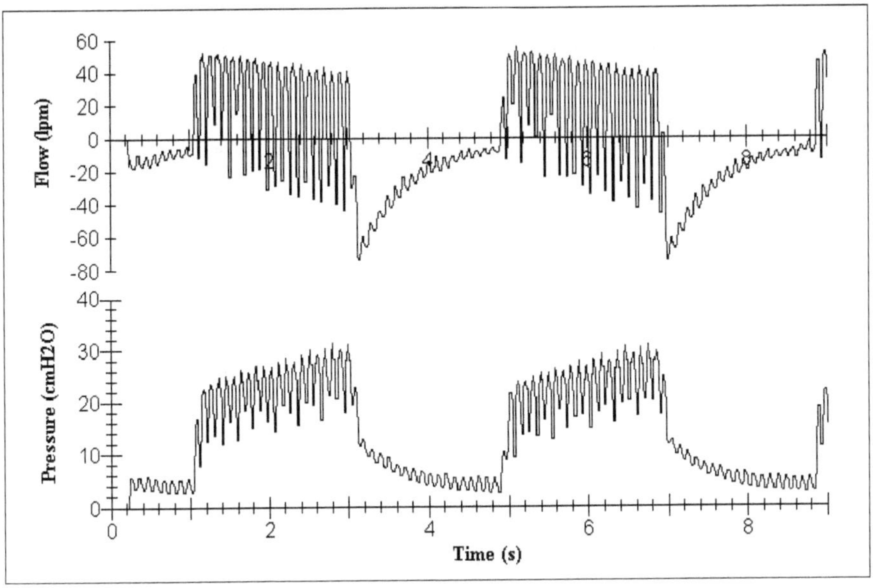

Fig. 2 Flow and pressure curves recorded during high-frequency percussive ventilation (HFPV)

limited with a high-frequency pulsatile waveform associated with the inspiratory and expiratory phases. Each respiratory act is the result of a conventional mechanical ventilation cycle upon which is superimposed the high-frequency delivery of microvolumes (Fig. 2).

When HFPV is employed, the value of Pmax measured at the airway during the inspiratory phase is close to conventional mechanical ventilation values, but since Pmed is significantly lower (due to pulsed volume delivery and an open circuit) the risk of barotrauma is negligible.

Inspiratory time and the percussion frequency setting create a convective alveolar ventilation that distributes flow homogeneously in pathologic as well as in intact alveoli, thus avoiding preferential ventilation of the latter.

PEEP can be applied to the expiratory phase with or without superimposed oscillation; this avoids alveolar derecruitment and allows for better removal of secretions. Last, but not least, at low frequencies, air trapping in alveoli with a long time-constant (that is, pathological alveoli that have lost elastic recoil and thus necessitate a longer time to exhale a given volume) is avoided [36].

HFPV (associated with conventional ventilation) has been successfully used in the ventilation of paediatric and neonatal patients [37] and in respiratory failure due to smoke-inhalation injury [38]. Thus, there is good reason to foresee a field of application in treating ARDS patients, independent of the aetiology of this syndrome.

Prone Position

Prone positioning is an adjunct to lung-protective strategies. It improves oxygenation by promoting lung recruitment, thus improving ventilation-perfusion matching and allowing regional changes in ventilation associated with varying chest-wall mechanics. Unfortunately, despite a better PaO_2/FiO_2 ratio, several studies have been unable to show a definite improvement in survival following the use of prone positioning [39]. However, encouraging results have recently been obtained and there is a suggestion that the introduction of prone positioning early in the course of acute respiratory failure may actually improve outcome. Moreover, prone positioning, although perhaps cumbersome forICU staff, has not been linked to more adverse events than is the case with patients remaining in the supine position [40]. Prone positioning has been used in trauma patients with ALI or ARDS and produced a statistically significant improvement in oxygenation but not in mortality. However, fewer cases of ventilator-associated pneumonia and progression to ARDS were noted in a prone-positioned patient group [41].

Prone position has been compared and combined with HFOV, based on the potential for pulmonary recruitment, improvement of oxygenation indices, and a decrease in circulating inflammatory cytokines. The use of HFOV in supine patients after prone positioning was shown to help in maintaining the improvement in oxygenation [42,43].

References

1. Bernard GR, Artigas A, Brigham GL et al (1994) The American-European consensus conference on ARDS. Definitions, mechanisms, relevant outcomes, and clinical trial coordination. Am J Respir Crit Care Med 149:818–824
2. Thomsen GE, Morris AH (1995) Incidence of the adult respiratory distress syndrome in the state of Utah. Am J Respir Crit Care Med 152:965–971
3. Marino PL (2007) The ICU Book. Lippincott Williams & Wilkins, Philadelphia
4. Montgomery AN, Stager MA (1985) Causes of mortality in patients with the adult respiratory distress syndrome. Am Rev Respir Dis 132:485–489
5. Murray JF, Matthay MA (1988) An expanded definition of the adult respiratory distress syndrome. Am Rev Respir Dis 138:720–723
6. Sloan PJ, Gee MH (1992) A multicenter registry of patients with acute respiratory distress syndrome: physiology and outcome Am Rev Respir Dis 142:1250–1257
7. Doyle RL, Szaflarski N (1995) Identification of patients with acute lung injury. Predictors of mortality. Am J Respir Crit Care Med 152:1818–1824
8. Demling RH (1995) The modern version of the adult respiratory distress syndrome. Annu Rev Med 46:193–202
9. Matthay MA, Wiener Kronish JP (1990) Intact epithelial barrier function is critical for the resolution of alveolar edema in humans. Am Rev Respir Dis 142:1250–1257
10. Mc Hugh LG, Milberg JA (1994) Recovery of function in survivors of the acute respiratory distress syndrome. Am J respir Crit Care Med 150:90–94
11. Davidson TA, Caldwell ES (1999) Reduced quality of life in survivors of acute respiratory distress syndrome compared with critically ill control patients JAMA 281:354–360

12. Lumb AB (ed) (2005) Nunn's applied respiratory physiology, 6th edition. Elsevier, Philadelphia
13. Steinberg KP, Milberg JA (1988) Evolution of bronchoalveolar cell populations in the adult respiratory distress syndrome. Am Rev Respir Dis 138:720–723
14. Pelosi P, Caironi P, Gattinoni L (2001) Pulmonary and extrapulmonary forms of acute respiratory distress syndrome. Semin Respir Crit Care Med 22(3)259–68
15. Pelosi P, D'Onofrio D, Chiumello D et al (2003) Pulmonary and extrapulmonary acute respiratory distress syndrome are different. Eur Respir J 22(Suppl 42):48s-56s
16. Gattinoni L, Pesenti A, Bombino M (1988) Relationships between lung computed tomographic density, gas exchange and PEEP in acute respiratory failure. Anesthesiology 69:824–832
17. Webb HH, Tierney DF (1974) Experimental pulmonary edema due to intermittent positive pressure ventilation with high inflation pressures: protection by positive and-expiratory pressure. Am Rev Respir Dis 110:556–565
18. Wright PE, Bernard GR (1989) The role of airflow resistance in patients with the adult respiratory distress syndrome. Am Rev Respir Dis 139:1169–1174
19. Gattinoni L, Caironi P, Cressoni M et al (2006) Lung recruitment in patients with the acute respiratory distress syndrome. N Eng J Med 354:1775–1786
20. Falke KJ (ed) (1992) Lung biology in heath and disease. Philadelphia, Saunders
21. The Acute Respiratory Distress Syndrome Network (2000) Ventilation with lower tidal volumes as compared with traditional tidal volumes for acute lung injury and the acute respiratory distress syndrome. N Engl J Med 342:1301–1308
22. Villar J, Kacmarek RM, Pérez-Méndex Lina et al (2006) A high positive end-expiratory pressure, low tidal volume ventilatory strategy improves outcome in persistent acute respiratory distress syndrome: a randomized controlled trial. Crit Care Med 34(5):1311–1318
23. Decailliot F, Demoule A, Maggiore SM et al (2006) Pressure–volume curves with and without muscle paralysis in acute respiratory distress syndrome. Intensive Care Med 32:1322–1328
24. Kallet RH, Branson RD (2007) Do the NIH ARDS Clinical Trials Network PEEP/FiO2 Tables provide the best evidence-based guide to balancing PEEP and FIO2 settings in adults? Respiratory Care 52(4):461–475
25. Ferguson ND, Frutos-Vivar F, Esteban A et al (2005) Airway pressure, tidal volumes and mortality in patients with acute respiratory distress syndrome Crit Care Med. 33(1):21–30
26. Alsous F, Amoateng Adjepong Y(1999) Noninvasive ventilation: experience at a community teaching hospital. Intensive Care Med 25:459–463
27. Patrick W, Webster K (1996) Noninvasive positive-pressure ventilation in acute respiratory distress without prior chronic respiratory failure. Am J Respir Crit Care Med 153:1005–1011
28. Agarwal R, Reddy C, Aggarwal AN (2006) Is there a role for noninvasive ventilation in acute respiratory distress syndrome? A meta-analysis. Respir Med 100(12):2235–2238
29. Antonelli M, Conti G, Esquinas A et al (2007) A multiple-center survey on the use in clinical practice of noninvasive ventilation as a first-line intervention for acute respiratory distress syndrome Crit Care Med 35(1):18–25
30. Prella M, Feihl F, Domenighetti G (2002) Effect of short-term pressure-controlled ventilation on gas exchange, airway pressures and gas distribution in patients with acute lung injury/ARDS. Comparison with volume-controlled ventilation. Chest 122:1382–1388
31. Branson RD, Catburn RL (2007) Should adaptive pressure control modes be utilized for virtually all patients receiving mechanical ventilation? Respir Care 52(4):478–485
32. Merker D, Groll JR (2001) Prospective trial of high-frequency oscillation in adults with acute respiratory distress syndrome Crit Care Med 29:1360–1369
33. Wunsch H, Mapstone J, Takala J (2005) High-frequency ventilation versus conventional ventilation for the treatment of acute lung injury and acute respiratory distress syndrome: a systematic review and Cochrane analysis. Anesth Analg 100(6):1765–1772
34. Bollen CW, van Well GTJ, SherryT et al (2005) High frequency oscillatory ventilation com-

pared with conventional mechanical ventilation in adult respiratory distress syndrome: a randomized controlled trial. Critical Care 9:R430-R439
35. Ferguson ND, Chicche JD, Kacmarek RM et al (2005) Combining high-frequency oscillatory ventilation and recruitment maneuvers in adults with early acute respiratory distress syndrome: the Treatment with Oscillation and an Open Lung Strategy (TOOLS) trial pilot study. Crit Care Med 33(3):479–486
36. Lucangelo U, Fontanesi L (2003) High frequency ventilation, principles and technique. Minerva Anesthesiol 69:841–851
37. Birnkrant DJ, Pope JF (1996) Persistent pulmonary consolidation treated with intrapulmonary percussive ventilation: a preliminary report. Pediatr Pulomonol 21:246–249
38. Reper P, Dankaert R(1998) The usefulness of high frequency percussive ventilation during acute respiratory failure after smoke inhalation. Burns 24:34–38
39. Gattinoni L, Tognoni G, Pesenti A et al (2001) Effect of prone positioning on the survival of patients with acute respiratory failure. N Engl J Med 345(8):568–573
40. Mancebo J, Fernández R, Blanch L et al (2006) A multicenter trial of prolonged prone ventilation in severe acute respiratory distress syndrome. Am J Respir Crit Care Med 173:1233–1239
41. Voggenreiter G, Aufmkolk M, Stiletto RJ et al (2005) Prone positioning improves oxygenation in post-traumatic lung injury–a prospective randomized trial. J Trauma 59(2):333–341
42. Papazian L, Gainnier M, Marin V et al (2005) Comparison of prone positioning and high-frequency oscillatory ventilation in patients with acute respiratory distress syndrome. Crit Care Med 33(10):2162–2171
43. Demory D, Michelet P, Arnal JM et al (2007) High-frequency oscillatory ventilation following prone positioning prevents a further impairment in oxygenation. Crit Care Med 35(1):106–111

The Open Lung Concept in Cardiac Surgery Patients

C. Preis, D. Gommers, B. Lachmann

Introduction

Cardiac surgery is associated with a pulmonary and systemic inflammatory response. The pulmonary effects of this inflammatory reaction are often modest: decreased lung compliance, pulmonary oedema, increased intrapulmonary shunt fraction and decreased functional residual capacity (FRC) [1]. Less than 2% of the patients undergoing cardiac surgery develop a full-blown respiratory failure, i.e. acute respiratory distress syndrome (ARDS) [1]. For example, after cardiac surgery, FRC is reduced up to 40–50% during the first 24 h after extubation [2]. However, after general anaesthesia, FRC is only decreased by 20–30% [3]. The exaggerated disturbance of pulmonary function is not yet fully understood. It has been suggested that this impaired pulmonary function is the result of pulmonary inflammation, triggered by cardiopulmonary bypass (CPB), ischaemia-reperfusion injury, the surgical procedure itself or by mechanical ventilation.

The ARDS network trial has shown that mechanical ventilation with smaller tidal volumes (V_T) leads to a reduction in mortality in patients with ARDS [4]. This result was somewhat surprising because the most common cause of death in ARDS is not pulmonary failure but rather multi-organ dysfunction (MOD). There is increasing evidence that conventional mechanical ventilation itself can cause damage to the lung in critically ill patients, a phenomenon also known as ventilator-induced lung injury (VILI) [5]. Recent studies suggested that this may also occur in cardiac surgery patients, in whom CPB provides sufficient inflammation to sensitise the lungs to the harmful effects of conventional mechanical ventilation [6–8]. This indicates that the exaggerated pulmonary dysfunction, as seen after cardiac surgery, is the result of two noxious hits on the lung: (1) the cardiac surgical procedure, with or without the use of CPB and (2) mechanical ventilation of the lungs in an inflammatory environment. In this review, we discuss the beneficial effects of open lung ventilation in cardiac surgery patients.

U. Lucangelo, P. Pelosi, W.A. Zin, A. Aliverti (eds.) *Respiratory System and Artificial Ventilation.* © Springer 2008

Two-Hit Model

First Hit: Cardiac Surgery

Activation of the inflammatory response during cardiac surgery is an extremely complex process and has various triggers, such as CPB, ischaemia and surgical trauma [9]. Despite the fact that CPB does not seem to have a significant effect on pulmonary dysfunction, it triggers an important amount of cytokine release and mediator release [10,11]. Further, ischaemia-reperfusion injury contributes to inflammation mainly from the myocardium and less from the lung, as the bronchial circulation seems to meet pulmonary oxygen demands [12]. And finally, the surgical procedure itself causes a significant inflammatory response. In patients undergoing CABG without the use of CPB, complement and interleukin levels were higher following median sternotomy than after anterolateral thoracotomy [13].

Second Hit: Mechanical Ventilation

Pulmonary inflammation induced by mechanical ventilation is the result of mechanical trauma and biotrauma [5]. Mechanical trauma reflects lung injury because of atelectasis, volume or pressure; biotrauma reflects pulmonary and systemic inflammation caused by mediators airborne from the ventilated lung.

Atelectasis results in the repetitive opening and closure of alveoli and is therefore a major source of pulmonary inflammation [14,15]. Roughly three zones can be identified (Fig. 1): (A) alveoli that do not open even during inspiration, (B) alveoli that remain open and (C) alveoli that open during inspiration and collapse during expiration. Alveoli in zone C (Fig. 1) will be subjected to repetitive opening and closure, which is known to be a major cause of pulmonary inflammation [16]. As alveoli in zone A (Fig. 1) do not participate in V_T ventilation, V_T is distributed over alveoli in the other two zones. This may increase the risk of regional overdistention. Finally, the co-existence of atelectatic and open alveoli may results in shear forces that exceed transpulmonary pressures, as predicted by Mead and colleagues [17]. Shear forces act on the fragile alveolar membrane in alveoli undergoing cyclic opening and closure. In a mathematical model, transpulmonary pressures of 30 cm H_2O will result in shear forces between atelectatic and aerated lung areas of 140 cm H_2O [17]. These shear forces, rather than end-inspiratory overstretching, may be of importance for epithelial disruption and the loss of barrier function of the alveolar epithelium.

To further explore the role of V_T and pressure on mechanical trauma on the lung, Dreyfuss and colleagues [18] applied high inspiratory pressures in combination with high volumes in an experimental model. These authors concluded that: (1) high pressures together with high V_T resulted in increased alveolar permeability; (2) combining low pressure with high volume (iron lung ventilation) resulted again in increased alveolar permeability; (3) when high pressure was

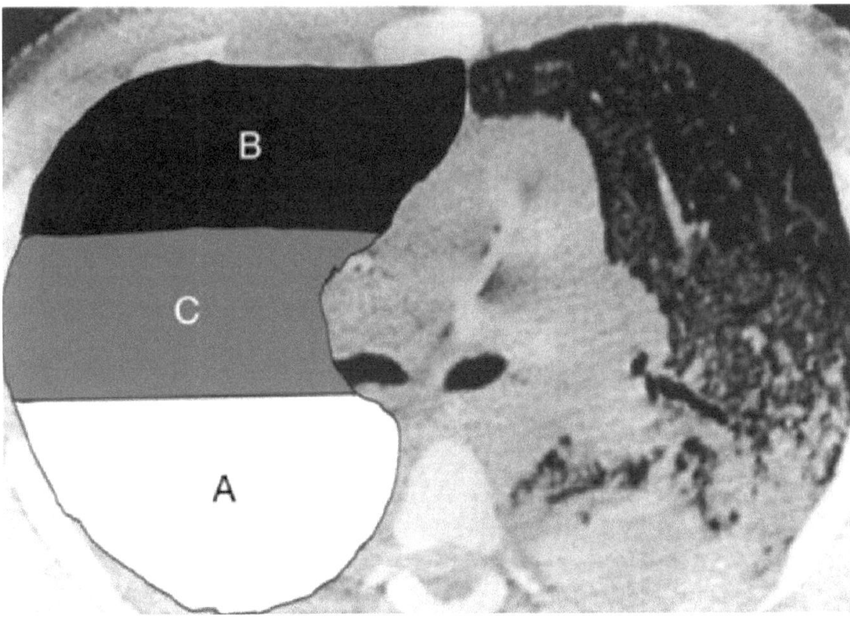

Fig. 1 Computed tomography (CT) slice of the lung showing atelectasis on the dorsal side. Roughly three zones can be identified: (*A*) alveoli that do not open even during inspiration, (*B*) alveoli that remain open and (*C*) alveoli that open during inspiration and collapse during expiration

associated with low V_T (chest-wall strapping) the alveolar permeability of the study group did not differ from that of the control group. The authors concluded that (high) V_T ventilation, not pressure, is the main determinant for lung injury.

Mechanical forces such as shear forces between open and closed alveoli or alveolar overdistention cause an inflammatory response called biotrauma. Although it is not clear how mechanical forces are converted to biochemical signals, several pathways have been suggested such as: stretch-sensitive channels, mechanoreceptors, stress-activated signalling cascade of the MAPK [14,19] and activation of the transcription of NF-κB [20]. In ARDS patients, Ranieri and colleagues [21] have shown that cytokine levels (TNF-α, IL-6 and IL-8) in bronchoalveolar lavage fluid (BAL) were attenuated by a protective ventilation strategy. This strategy consisted of a V_T of 7 ml/kg applied with 10 cm H_2O of positive end-expiratory pressure (PEEP). In the control group, a V_T of 11 ml/kg was applied with 6 cm H_2O of PEEP. The authors conclude that mechanical ventilation induces a cytokine response, which can be reduced by minimising overdistention and repetitive alveolar collapse. In a large multi-centre study in 861 ARDS patients (ARDS Network trial), low V_T ventilation (6 ml/kg) led to lower plasma IL-6 concentrations and a significant decrease in 28-day mortality in

ARDS patients [4]. Stüber et al. [22] have shown that switching from a lung protective ventilation strategy of low V_T and high PEEP to a conventional strategy with high V_T and low PEEP in patients with acute lung injury (ALI) leads to an increase of plasma cytokines within one hour and a decrease to baseline after switching back to lung-protective ventilation. In addition, Imai et al. [23] have shown that injurious ventilation can induce apoptosis in distal organs (kidney and small intestine) in a rabbit model of ARDS. Protective ventilation in that study was associated with much lower levels of plasma cytokines, very little apoptosis, and only minimal changes in biochemical markers. The authors concluded that protective ventilation could in fact protect distal organs from ventilator-induced end-organ dysfunction. They also suggested that this mechanism explains the decrease in mortality observed in the ARDS Network trial of low V_T ventilation [4]. The results of plasma measurements of cytokines of patients enrolled in this latter trial [4] showed that the highest cytokine levels are measured in patients with ARDS due to sepsis and pneumonia and that the beneficial effect of protective ventilation was better in those patients. This provides further evidence that the pre-existing inflammatory process present at the diagnosis of ARDS can be modulated by the early application of low V_T ventilation.

Therefore, it is also conceivable that the exaggerated pulmonary dysfunction after cardiac surgery is due to two hits on the lung: the inflammatory response following cardiac surgery combined with conventional mechanical ventilation of the lung in an inflammatory environment. In particular, a mechanical ventilation strategy allowing atelectasis and high V_T ventilation seems to cause extended pulmonary inflammation.

Protective Ventilation in non-ARDS

From ARDS studies it has become clear that high V_T ventilation can induce a systemic inflammatory response and that protective ventilation attenuates this response. Therefore, several investigators studied the effect of protective ventilation on the cytokine network in patients without ALI/ARDS. Wrigge et al. [24,25] carried out two studies in patients with normal pulmonary function who underwent elective surgery and found no difference between injurious and non-injurious ventilation. These authors concluded that a protective effect of non-injurious ventilation on the release of cytokines does not occur in healthy lungs during major non-cardiac surgery in which the surgery-induced systemic inflammatory response is relatively small. This suggests that protective ventilation modulates the cytokine network only in the presence of a more significant primary inflammatory stimulus, such as CPB. This was shown by Ranieri and coworkers [6], who observed lower IL-6 and IL-8 concentrations in BAL fluid (6 h after CPB) in a lung protective group (V_T 7 ml/kg, PEEP 9 cm H_2O) than in a control group (V_T 11 ml/kg, PEEP 3 cm H_2O). However, Koner et al. [7] and Wrigge et al. [8] found no or only a minor effect of protective ventilation on systemic and pulmonary inflammatory responses in patients with healthy lungs after uncomplicated CPB surgery.

The open lung concept (OLC) is another protective ventilation strategy that combines low V_T ventilation with high levels of PEEP [26]. To open up collapsed alveoli, a recruitment manoeuvre is performed and a sufficient level of PEEP is used to keep the lung open. The smallest possible pressure amplitude is applied in order to prevent lung overdistention; this results in low V_T (4–6 ml/kg) ventilation.

We applied the OLC in cardiac surgery patients and found that OLC ventilation (V_T 6 ml/kg, PEEP 14 cm H_2O), applied immediately after intubation, significantly decreased plasma IL-8 and IL-10 compared to conventional ventilation (V_T 8 ml/kg, PEEP 5 cm H_2O) [27]. Application of the OLC was accompanied by a significantly higher PaO_2/FiO_2 ratio during mechanical ventilation, suggesting a significant reduction of atelectasis [28]. We could also demonstrate that ventilation according to the OLC leads to significantly better preservation of FRC and better oxygenation several days after extubation when compared to conventional ventilation [29]. A decreased FRC is associated with post-operative pulmonary dysfunction. After cardiac surgery, respiratory dysfunction accounts for 40% of readmissions to the ICU [30,31]. Chung et al. [32] have shown that each percent increase of inspired oxygen fraction on discharge from the ICU increases significantly the risk of readmission. Several other attempts to preserve FRC after extubation in cardiac patients have been without success.

Consistent with the two-hit model, OLC should be started immediately after CPB and continued until extubation in order to obtain the great beneficial effects, such as decreased interleukin release [27], increased PaO_2/FiO_2 ratio during mechanical ventilation [28] attenuated FRC decrease after extubation and fewer episodes of hypoxaemia [29]. Three days after extubation, patients did not require additional oxygen when ventilated according to the OLC peri-operatively [29]. This may allow earlier hospital discharge.

How To Perform the Open Lung Concept

The basic principle is shown in the pressure–volume curve in Fig. 2, where P_o is the pressure needed to open the lung. Once the lung has been opened, we can operate in the area between D and C to keep the lung open (Fig. 2). If the pressure decreases below the closing pressure Pc, the lung will collapse again. This principle describing the management of the open lung consists of three steps: (1) finding the opening pressure and the collapse pressure for the patient's lung, (2) opening the lung and (3) keeping the lung open. The openings pressure is reached with peak inspiratory pressure (PIP), collapse pressure is determined by PEEP [26].

Recruitment manoeuvres should not be performed in patients with hypovolaemia; preferentially, hypovolaemia is monitored in relation to the respiratory cycle. During hypovolaemia, systolic arterial pressure decreases by >5 mmHg

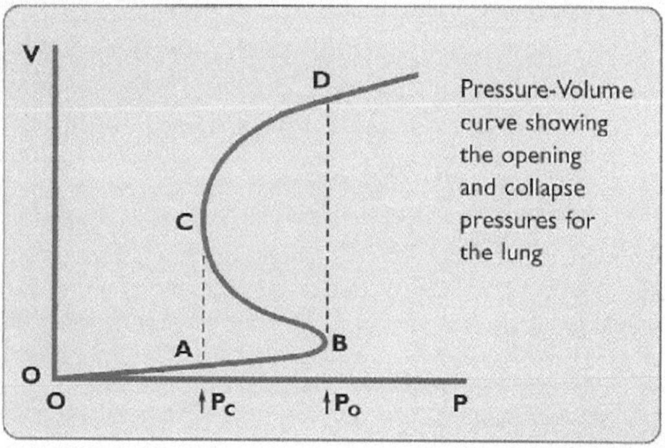

Fig. 2 In this theoretical pressure–volume curve, *Po* is the pressure that is needed to open the lung. Once the lung has been opened, we can operate in the area between *D* and *C* to keep the lung open. If the pressure decreases below the closing pressure P_c, the lung will collapse again. This principle describing the open lung concept consists of three steps: (1) finding the opening pressure and the collapse pressure for the patient's lung, (2) opening the lung and (3) keeping the lung open

during inspiration [30,31]. Hypovolaemia can also be monitored using transoesophageal echocardiography: a 35% collapse of the vena cava superior during inspiration indicates hypovolaemia [32,33]. The inferior vena cava can also be used as a discriminator of hypovolaemia: an 18% increase in the diameter of the vena cava inferior reflects hypovolaemia. When hypovolaemia is present but fluid administration is not desirable for clinical reasons, α- or β-mimetic agents should be used to avoid a large decrease in cardiac output during a recruitment manoeuvre. In the latter, attention is given to the heart rate and the arterial pressure. It should be noted that a decrease in arterial pressure is normal and usually self-limiting. Minimal arterial pressures accepted during a recruitment manoeuvre should be fixed on a case-by-case basis.

A recruitment manoeuvre can be performed with high, normal or low V_T. If the lung is recruited with high V_T, the respiratory frequency is set between 6 and 10/min, PEEP is set at 15 cm H_2O and an I/E ratio of 1:1. PIP is gradually increased in approximately 3 s to 40 cm H_2O for three breaths and thereafter gradually decreased in approximately 3 s to a PIP, resulting in a V_T of approximately 6 ml/kg. If the lung is not open yet (see 'Monitoring an open lung'), PIP is increased by 5 cm H_2O. In several OLC studies in cardiac surgery patients, we used a maximal recruitment pressure of 60 cm H_2O [29]. When the lung is recruited with a normal V_T, the respiratory frequency is set between 20 and 40/min, PEEP is set at 15 cm H_2O, I/E ratio of 1:1 and a driving pressure to obtain a V_T of 6 ml/kg. During recruitment, the driving pressure is kept constant and PEEP set on the ventilator is gradually increased in approximately 3 s until PIP reaches 40 cm H_2O for a few seconds and then PEEP is again gradually decreased in 3 s to the original setting. This manoeuvre is easily applicable with ventilators in which PIP is set as inspiratory pressure above PEEP. If actual PIP is set on the ventilator, both PEEP and PIP have to be increased in order to maintain a constant driving pressure. If the lung is not open yet, PIP is increased by 5 cm H_2O. If the lung is recruited with low V_T, PEEP is set at 15 cm H_2O, respiratory frequency is set between 120 and 150/min and I/E ratio at 4:1. In this case, PIP is gradually increased in 3 s to 40 cm H_2O for a few seconds and then gradually decreased in 3 s to the previous setting. Respiratory frequency and I/E ratio are then restored to the previous setting. During the recruitment manoeuvre, care should be taken that the V_T is well below 6 ml/kg.

After a recruitment manoeuvre, the lung is ventilated in a pressure-controlled mode with sufficient PEEP levels to maintain the lung open: just above P_c (Fig. 2). The ventilator is set to obtain the lowest possible airway pressure, driving pressure and V_T [34]. Ideally, driving pressure is below 10 cm H_2O with a V_T between 4 and 6 ml/kg. This is done in order to avoid shear forces and to ensure proper elimination of CO_2 from the lung. CO_2 elimination while ventilating with low V_T can be improved by optimalisation of respiratory frequency and inspiratory time. Respiratory frequency can be increased as long as the inspiratory flow reaches zero. If the inspiratory flow does not reach zero, a less than optimal V_T for the given driving pressure is delivered. This results in inappropriate CO_2 elimination. If with increasing respiratory frequency the inspiratory flow is interrupted prematurely, respiratory frequency can be increased if the inspiration time is increased. While inspiration time increases, expiration time decreases, with a possible increase of intrinsic PEEP. In this case, external PEEP is lowered to maintain total PEEP constant. Intrinsic PEEP probably offers the best method of CO_2 elimination [35].

Monitoring of an Open Lung

In the OLC, the opening or closure of lung units is monitored by gas exchange. However, at the same time, it should be kept in mind that the determination of lung collapse by gas exchange assumes a minimal extrapulmonary shunt. The opening pressure is recorded when the PaO_2 reaches its maximum value and does not increase any further with increasing airway pressure. Usually, a PaO_2/FiO_2ratio >50 kPa is obtained as an open lung status, but in consolidated or fibrotic lungs this may be less. Therefore, ideally, blood gas is monitored continuously. A second solution is to set the FiO_2 level such that peripheral saturation is between 90 and 93% before a recruitment manoeuvre is performed. During this manoeuvre, PIP is increased until pulse oxygen saturation (SpO_2) reaches its maximum value (98–100%). At this level, FiO_2 is lowered again and a new recruitment manoeuvre is performed until SpO_2 again reaches its maximum value. SpO_2 is a rougher parameter than PaO_2 in the determination of opening pressure.

A much better, albeit more cumbersome technique is the use of computer tomography or magnetic resonance imaging, both of which allow optimal visualisation of individual lung areas. However, neither technique is readily available on the ICU and both demand transportation of the patient to the radiology department, with increased risk of complications.

Another parameter that can help in managing the OLC is to determine FRC. Recently, GE Healthcare and Dr Ola Stenqvist have developed a technology to measure the FRC of a mechanically ventilated patient. The technique measures nitrogen washout after a step change in the inspired-gas O_2 fraction. Calculation of FRC is based on the values of VCO_2, EtO_2, and $EtCO_2$. With this method, there is no need to use supplementary gases or specialised gas-monitoring devices, but the patient's breathing pattern has to be constant in order to achieve a valid VCO_2. FRC measurements may be used to measure increases in lung volume after a recruitment manoeuvre and help to find the lowest PEEP level without loss of lung volume (Fig. 3). However, an increase of FRC will not always be due to an increase of recruitable lung area (e.g. atelectasis); rather, it can also be due to overinflation of the already ventilated lung.

Another bedside technique is electrical impedance tomography (EIT) [36]. EIT generates cross-sectional images (i.e. scans) of the internal distribution of electrical impedance (i.e. resistance to alternating electrical current) and enables detection of changes in impedance during a physiological process, e.g. breathing. Although this technique is currently used mostly in experimental settings, preliminary clinical studies have shown its great promise as a bedside tool to optimise PEEP [37]. In cardiac surgery patients, we use EIT to monitor the effect of a recruitment manoeuvre in order to open up the lung (Fig. 4).

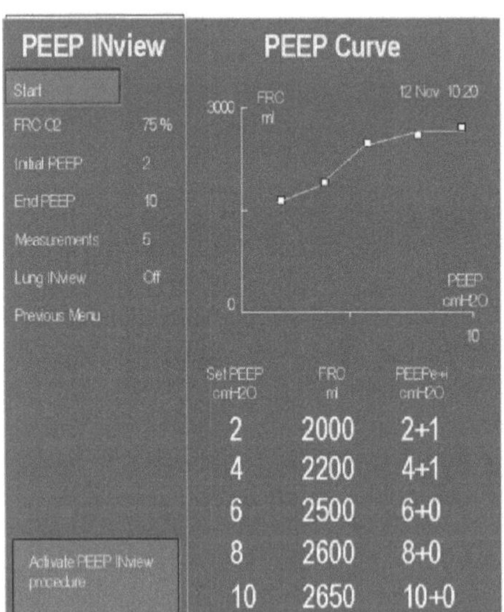

Fig. 3 Functional residual capacity (FRC) (ml) measured at five different positive end-expiratory pressure (*PEEP*) levels (2, 4, 6, 8 and 10 cm H_2O). According to these measurements, the best PEEP for this patient is 6 cm H_2O

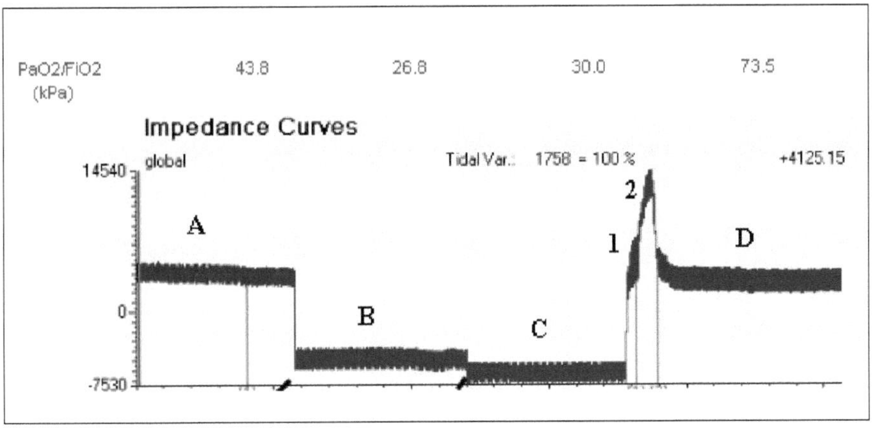

Fig. 4 Electrical impedance tomography curves of a cardiac surgical patient. Global impedance is displayed on the vertical axis. High impedance reflects the presence of air; low impedance reflects the presence of liquid. Time is displayed on the horizontal axis. Note that the time axis is not continuous. The total time displayed on the time axis is 25 min. *A* is the time axis starts with 5 min of spontaneous breathing, before induction of anaesthesia. *B* indicates the phase after surgery, after closure of the sternum. *C* denotes the arrival at the ICU, after manual bagging without PEEP during transport from operating room to intensive care. Thereafter, the patient is recruited twice (*1*, *2*). *D* is the phase after recruitment and 15 cm H_2O PEEP

Conclusions

Pulmonary dysfunction after cardiac surgery is probably a two-hit process: the first hit is due to the surgical procedure, the second to mechanical ventilation of the lung in an inflammatory environment. Pulmonary inflammation is aggravated by non-optimal mechanical ventilation of the lung. We have shown that, by applying the open lung concept in cardiac surgery patients, pulmonary dysfunction can be decreased. The beneficial effect of this ventilation strategy is best when applied immediately after intubation. In addition, new bedside techniques (FRC, EIT) have been introduced to monitor the patient's lung function. These may be of particular importance during application of the open lung concept.

Acknowledgements. The authors thank Laraine Visser-Isles for English-language editing.

References

1. Ng CS, Wan S, Yim AP et al (2002) Pulmonary dysfunction after cardiac surgery. Chest 121:1269–1277

2. Nicholson DJ, Kowalski SE, Hamilton GA et al (2002) Postoperative pulmonary function in coronary artery bypass graft surgery patients undergoing early tracheal extubation: a comparison between short-term mechanical ventilation and early extubation. J Cardiothorac Vasc Anesth 16:27–31
3. Hedenstierna G, Rothen HU (2000) Atelectasis formation during anesthesia: causes and measures to prevent it. J Clin Monit Comput 16:329–335
4. The ARDS Network Group (2000) Ventilation with lower tidal volumes as compared with traditional tidal volumes for acute lung injury and the acute respiratory distress syndrome. N Engl J Med 342:1301–1308
5. Pinhu L, Whitehead T, Evans T et al (2003) Ventilator-associated lung injury. Lancet 361:332–340
6. Zupancich E, Paparella D, Turani F et al (2005) Mechanical ventilation affects inflammatory mediators in patients undergoing cardiopulmonary bypass for cardiac surgery: a randomized clinical trial. J Thorac Cardiovasc Surg 130:378–383
7. Koner O, Celebi S, Balci H et al (2004) Effects of protective and conventional mechanical ventilation on pulmonary function and systemic cytokine release after cardiopulmonary bypass. Intensive Care Med 30:620–626
8. Wrigge H, Uhlig U, Baumgarten G et al (2005) mechanical ventilation strategies and inflammatory responses to cardiac surgery: a prospective randomized clinical trial. Intensive Care Med 31:1379–1387
9. Paparella D, Yau TM, Young E (2002) Cardiopulmonary bypass induced inflammation: pathophysiology and treatment. An update. Eur J Cardiothorac Surg 21:232–244
10. Ascione R, Lloyd CT, Underwood MJ et al (2000) Inflammatory response after coronary revascularization with or without cardiopulmonary bypass. Ann Thorac Surg 69:1198–1204
11. Diegeler A, Doll N, Rauch T et al (2000) Humoral immune response during coronary artery bypass grafting: a comparison of limited approach, 'off-pump' technique, and conventional cardiopulmonary bypass. Circulation 102:III95-III100
12. Loer SA, Kalweit G, Tarnow J (2000) Effects of ventilation and nonventilation on pulmonary venous blood gases and markers of lung hypoxia in humans undergoing total cardiopulmonary bypass. Crit Care Med 28:1336–1340
13. Gu YJ, Mariani MA, Boonstra PW et al (1999) Complement activation in coronary artery bypass grafting patients without cardiopulmonary bypass: the role of tissue injury by surgical incision. Chest 116:892–898
14. Uhlig U, Haitsma JJ, Goldmann T et al (2002) Ventilation-induced activation of the mitogen-activated protein kinase pathway. Eur Respir J 20:946–956
15. Haitsma JJ, Uhlig S, Goggel R et al (2000) Ventilator-induced lung injury leads to loss of alveolar and systemic compartmentalization of tumor necrosis factor-alpha. Intensive Care Med 26:1515–1522
16. Taskar V, John J, Evander E et al (1997) Surfactant dysfunction makes lungs vulnerable to repetitive collapse and reexpansion. Am J Respir Crit Care Med 155:313–320
17. Mead J, Takishima T, Leith D (1970) Stress distribution in lungs: a model of pulmonary elasticity. J Appl Physiol 28:596–608
18. Dreyfuss D, Soler P, Basset G et al (1988) High inflation pressure pulmonary edema. Respective effects of high airway pressure, high tidal volume, and positive end-expiratory pressure. Am Rev Respir Dis 137:1159–1164
19. Dos Santos CC, Slutsky AS (2000) Invited review: mechanisms of ventilator-induced lung injury: a perspective. J Appl Physiol 89:1645–1655
20. Kyriakis JM, Avruch J (2001) Mammalian mitogen-activated protein kinase signal transduction pathways activated by stress and inflammation. Physiol Rev 81:807–869
21. Ranieri VM, Suter PM, Tortorella C et al (1999) Effect of mechanical ventilation on inflammatory mediators in patients with acute respiratory distress syndrome: a randomized controlled trial. JAMA 282:54–61
22. Stuber F, Wrigge H, Schroeder S et al (2002) Kinetic and reversibility of mechanical ventilation-associated pulmonary and systemic inflammatory response in patients with acute lung injury. Intensive Care Med 28:834–841

23. Imai Y, Parodo J, Kajikawa O et al (2003) Injurious mechanical ventilation and end-organ epithelial cell apoptosis and organ dysfunction in an experimental model of acute respiratory distress syndrome. JAMA 289:2104–2112
24. Wrigge H, Zinserling J, Stuber F et al (2000) Effects of mechanical ventilation on release of cytokines into systemic circulation in patients with normal pulmonary function. Anesthesiology 93:1413–1417
25. Wrigge H, Uhlig U, Zinserling J et al (2004) The effects of different ventilatory settings on pulmonary and systemic inflammatory responses during major surgery. Anesth Analg 98:775–781
26. Lachmann B (1992) Open up the lung and keep the lung open. Intensive Care Med 18:319–321
27. Reis Miranda D, Gommers D, Struijs A et al (2005) Ventilation according the open lung concept attenuates pulmonary inflammatory response in cardiac surgery. Eur J Cardiothorac Surg 28:889–895
28. Reis Miranda D, Gommers D, Struijs A et al (2004) The open lung concept: effects on right ventricular afterload after cardiac surgery. Br J Anaesth 93:327–332
29. Reis Miranda D, Struijs A, Koetsier P et al (2005) Open lung ventilation improves functional residual capacity after extubation in cardiac surgery. Crit Care Med 33:2253–2258
30. Pizov R, Cohen M, Weiss Y et al (1996) Positive end-expiratory pressure-induced hemodynamic changes are reflected in the arterial pressure waveform. Crit Care Med 24:1381–1387
31. Preisman S, Pfeiffer U, Lieberman N et al (1997) New monitors of intravascular volume: a comparison of arterial pressure waveform analysis and the intrathoracic blood volume. Intensive Care Med 23(6):651–657
32. Vieillard-Baron A, Augarde R, Prin S et al (2001) Influence of superior vena caval zone condition on cyclic changes in right ventricular outflow during respiratory support. Anesthesiology 95(5):1083–1088
33. Vieillard-Baron A, Chergui K, Rabiller A et al (2004) Superior vena caval collapsibility as a gauge of volume status in ventilated septic patients. Intensive Care Med 30(9):1734–1739
34. Haitsma JJ, Lachmann B (2006) Lung protective ventilation in ARDS: the open lung maneuver. Minerva Anestesiol 72:117–132
35. Olegard C, Sondergaard S, Houltz E et al (2005) Estimation of the functional residual capacity at the bedside using standard monitoring equipment: a modified nitrogen washout/washin technique requiring a small change of the inspired oxygen fraction. Anesth Analg 101:206–212
36. Frerichs J, Scholz J, Weiler N (2006) Electrical impedance tomography. Neth J Crit Care 10:487–494
37. Erlandsson K, Odenstedt H, Lundin S, Stenqvist O (2006) Positive end-expiratory pressure optimization using electric impedance tomography in morbidly obese patients during laparoscopic gastric bypass. Acta Anaesthesiol Scand 50:833–839

Nosocomial Pneumonia

Diagnosis and Treatment of Nosocomial Pneumonia

A. Liapikou, M. Valencia, A. Torres

Definition and Classification

The usual concept of nosocomial pneumonia (NP) includes pneumonias in non-critically immunosuppressed patients initiating more than 48 h after hospital admission. Due to the differences in the clinical picture, microbial patterns, diagnostic strategies and antibiotic therapy, NP is divided into three types [1]: (1) hospital-acquired pneumonia (HAP) is defined as a new infection of the lung parenchyma while the patient is hospitalised. (2) Ventilator-associated pneumonia (VAP) refers to pneumonia that arises more than 48–72 h after endotracheal intubation. By contrast, ventilator-associated tracheobronchititis (VAT) is characterised by the presence of signs of respiratory infection, such as an increase in the volume and purulence of respiratory secretions, fever and leucocytosis in patients undergoing mechanical ventilation; however, unlike VAP, radiological infiltrates suggestive of consolidation on chest X-ray are not observed. (3) Health-care-associated pneumonia (HCAP) is a recently described term referring to patients who contract pneumonia while receiving health care in an outpatient facility. In an important study, Friedman et al. [2] showed that health-care-associated bloodstream infections are more similar to nosocomial infections than to community-acquired infections. Kollef and colleagues [3] carried out a retrospective cohort study based on a large inpatient database of 4543 patients and found that the mortality of HCAP was 19.8%, similar that of HAP (18.8%), but not to that of CAP (10%). Risk factors for HCAP are admission in an acute-care hospital facility for 2 or more days within 90 days of infection, residence in a nursing home or long-term-care facility, having received recent intravenous antibiotic therapy, chemotherapy or wound care within the past 30 days or having attended a hospital or haemodialysis clinic [1].

Data from The National Nosocomial Infection Surveillance showed that 27% of all nosocomial infections in ICUs in the USA and Canada were due to pneumonia, with 86% of NPs associated with mechanical ventilation [4]. According to the microbial pattern and the clinical outcome, NP or VAP can be divided into:

U. Lucangelo, P. Pelosi, W.A. Zin, A. Aliverti (eds.) *Respiratory System and Artificial Ventilation*. © Springer 2008

(1) early-onset NP/VAP, which occurs during the first 4 days of hospitalisation and is caused by community microorganisms such as *Streptococcus pneumoniae, Haemophilus influenzae, Moraxella catarrhalis* and methicillin-sensitive *Staphylococcus aureus* and (2) late-onset pneumonia, which occurs >5 days after hospital admission and is usually due to resistant microorganisms such as *Pseudomonas aeruginosa, Acinetobacter* spp., *Enterobacter* spp. and methicillin-resistant *Staphylococcus aureus* (MRSA) and is associated with increased mortality [1,4–6].

Another classification used to classify pneumonia is based on the presence of microorganisms isolated in cultures of epidemiologic surveillance samples. It includes the following categories [7]:

- Primary endogenous pneumonia: The causative pathogenic microorganisms are isolated in surveillance cultures obtained upon patient admission to the hospital.
- Secondary endogenous pneumonia: This is caused by nosocomial pathogens, not present in the patient on admission, that colonise the oropharynx, stomach and/or the intestine, where they multiply and thereafter invade the lower respiratory tract.
- Exogenous pneumonia: In this form, microorganisms that are not isolated in the surveillance cultures are the infectious agents. Patients are not previously carriers; rather, material of the artificial airway (ventilation tubes, humidifiers) is colonised due to the infection of invasive devices (e.g. bronchoscopes). Infection following nebulisation or inhalation plays an important role in this category.

Epidemiology

Nosocomial pneumonia is the second most common nosocomial infection and the leading cause of death in critically ill patients. The incidence of NP is age-dependent, with 5/1000 cases among hospital admissions <35 years of age and up to 15/1000 in those >65 years old [5]. In earlier reports, NP increased hospital stay by 7–9 days per affected patient, accounting for up to 25% of all ICU infections and for more than 50% of the antibiotics prescribed [1,4].

A Spanish study by Sopena et al. [8] analysed the epidemiology of HAP in 186 non-ICU patients from 12 hospitals. The results showed that HAP was observed mostly in elderly patients with underlying diseases, with the most frequent aetiological diagnosis being *S. pneumoniae, Legionella pneumophila, Aspergillus* spp., and *P. aeruginosa*. The mortality rate was 26%, with an attributable mortality of 13%.

A French study estimated that the risk of VAP was 1% per day of mechanical ventilation, but Cook et al. [9] demonstrated that risk changes over time, being 3% the first 5 days, 2% at days 5–10 and 1% for every additional day of mechanical ventilation. Considering that the intubation period is short, nearly half of the cases of VAP occur during the first few days of mechanical ventilation [1,4].

The crude mortality of VAP may be as high as 30–70%, although the difficulty in determining the exact cause of death in critically ill patients prevents this figure from being established with certainty. Mortality attributable to VAP has been defined as the percentage of deaths that would not have occurred in the absence of infection. Several case-matching studies have estimated that one-third to one-half of all VAP-related deaths are the direct result of infection, with a higher attributable mortality in cases of bacteraemia or in which the aetiological agent is *P. aeruginosa* or *Acinetobacter* spp. [3,10,11]. The presence of NP was shown to lead to a 1.8- to 4-fold increase in the risk of death. A multicentre cohort French study [6] evaluated the attributable mortality in late-onset pneumonia. Risk factors for death were evaluated in 764 patients admitted to the ICU for >96 h. A 47% mortality in late-onset pneumonia vs. 22% in the total population was found. The percentage of the former was dependent on the appropriateness of the initial empirical therapy. Luna et al. [12] focussed on the appropriateness of the therapy and the consequences of its delay in therapy in VAP. They used the clinical pulmonary infection score (CPIS) as a reference tool and estimated an overall mortality of 52.6%.

A reasonable conclusion is that attributable mortality cannot accurately be measured due to differences in patients, microbial patterns, antibiotic treatment and diagnostic methods and strategies.

Pathogenesis

The pathogenesis of bacterial pneumonia requires the entry of an inoculum of bacteria with specific virulence factors into the lower respiratory tract and the failure of the host defences to combat it, resulting in colonisation, tracheobronchitis and pneumonia [13]. Microorganisms gain access by one of four routes: (1) aspiration of secretions, either from the oropharynx or by reflex from the stomach; (2) direct extension of contiguous infection (pleural effusion); (3) inhalation of contaminated air or nebulised aerosols and (4) haematogenous spread from a site of local infection (catheter, trauma). Both the haematogenous and contiguous routes of invasion are rare [7,14].

A major factor in the pathogenesis of NP is colonisation of the respiratory tract, especially the oropharynx [1,7]. The source of the bacteria colonising the upper airway is most likely the patients own intestinal flora, although medical staff can transmit their flora to patients [14]. Antimicrobial treatment favours colonisation with potentially multiresistant pathogens by elimination of the community of endogenous flora. The role of the stomach and sinuses as reservoirs of contaminated secretions that are aspirated into the airways has been examined in many studies in recent years [11,14]. Torres et al. found that colonisation of the stomach depends on the gastric pH [15]. Prophylactic medications for gastric ulcers, which increase the pH >4.6, may facilitate colonisation with NP-inducing bacteria. Additionally, nasogastric tubes reduce the oesophageal reflex while the supine position promotes aspiration [16,17].

Aspiration is the main route leading to VAP. A number of host-related and treatment-related colonisation factors, such as the severity of the underlying disease, previous surgery, exposure to antibiotics and other medications and exposure to invasive respiratory devices, are important in the pathogenesis of VAP.

Intubation is another most important risk factor for developing VAP, as it allows direct entry of bacteria into the lung [18]. The endotracheal tube (ETT) maintains the vocal cords of sedated patients in the open state, which prevents the patient from coughing up secretions and instead promotes their aspiration. Once aspirated, the secretions pool above the cuff of the ETT [18]. Changes in cuff pressure allow the secretions to be transported around the cuff by capillary action and they may be aspirated if the ETT is left in place for several days. Recent studies have suggested that microorganisms can adhere to the surface of the ETT [19]. Some species may produce an exopolysaccharide that acts as a slime-like bacterial adhesive, referred to as a bacterial biofilm [20].

Biofilm formation seems to be independent of the duration of mechanical ventilation. Endoluminal biofilms form either more rapidly or more frequently at the distal end of the ETT. Biofilm-covered bacteria in the inner lumen of ETT are less susceptible to antibiotic drugs [21,22]. Recent research indicates that bacterial biofilms form more frequently in the ETTs of patients with VAP [23]. Nevertheless, this may represent contamination and the magnitude of the contribution of endoluminal bacterial biofilm to the pathogenesis of VAP may be minimal when other risk factors are taken into account [24]. However, bacterial biofilms of ETTs may play an important role as persistent sources of infectious material, leading to recurrent episodes of VAP [25].

An additional factor is probably a disturbance of alveolar integrity by stress (ventilator-induced lung injury). In particular, VAP displays a pattern of multifocal spread that frequently has a polymicrobial aetiology.

Diagnostic Evaluation

For more than 20 years, the diagnosis of HAP, particularly VAP, has been one of the most crucial and difficult issues in the care of critically ill patients. The major problem is the lack of a gold standard for comparing the different techniques used to confirm suspicion of an infectious process. The diagnostic evaluation of NP has three objectives:

- To grade the severity of the disease: According to the American Thoracic Society (ATS) guidelines of NP, acute respiratory failure, septic shock with or without organ failure and multilobular infiltrates should be considered as severity criteria. However, the criteria for diagnosing severe NP remain to be validated.

- To confirm the presence of NP using clinical and microbiological approaches: These are discussed in detail below.
- To identify causative pathogens.

Confirming the Presence of NP: Clinical Approach

The presence of VAP is defined by the following clinical criteria:

- New or progressive radiographic infiltrate
- Plus at least two of the following:
  1. Temperature>38°C or hypothermia <36°C
  2. Leucocytosis (>12x10^3/l) or leucopaenia (<4x10^3/l)
  3. Purulent tracheobronchial secretions

Unfortunately, these criteria are of little diagnostic value in establishing the presence of VAP. In a postmortem study by Fabregas et al. [26] using lung culture samples obtained immediately after death of the patient and histological analysis, the presence of two of the previously mentioned criteria were shown to have a sensitivity of 69% and a specificity of 75% [14].

In an attempt to improve the specificity of clinical diagnosis, Pugin et al. [27] developed the clinical pulmonary infection score (CPIS), which combines different clinical, radiological, physiological, laboratory and microbiological data in a numerical result. A CPIS score of >6 correlates well with the presence of pneumonia. The results of several studies give to the CPIS a sensitivity of 77% and a specificity of 42%. In a series of 102 patients with VAS, Ibrahim et al. [28] used the CPIS as a clinical guideline for the severity of VAP, managed to increase the initial adequate antibiotic treatment and to shorten the duration of hospital stay; however, this did not reduce the mortality rate. In another study, Fartoukh et al. [29] found the CPIS to be inaccurate (sensitivity 60%, specificity 59%), but the accuracy of diagnosis increased with the addition of Gram staining of bronchial alveolar lavage (BAL) secretions of the respiratory tract, resulting in a sensitivity of 85% and a specificity of nearly 49%. Luna et al. [30] measured the CPIS during pneumonia at days –3 (before VAP), 0 (onset of VAP), +3, +5 and +7 (after VAP) in 742 intubated patients. In 63 of those patients, the presence of VAP was confirmed based on the results of BAL cultures. The CPIS rose from day –3 to the onset of VAP and then progressively decreased in all patients. The decline was significant in 31 survivors and not significant in 32 non-survivors. The authors concluded that serial measurements of CPIS can define the clinical course of VAP resolution and is able to identify patients with a good outcome as early as day 3 of hospital admission.

Typical radiological signs of NP include:

- Alveolar opacities
- Opacities following the main bronchi
- Changes in the silhouette of adjacent mediastinal structures or the hemidiaphragm
- Positive pneumobronchogram

- Shadows in the interlobar fissures
- Cavitation

In the erect or semi-recumbent body position, the medial and the posterior basal lung segments are most frequently affected. However, in the supine position, all dependent lung areas may be affected [31].

Markers in the blood or in the BAL of the pneumonia patients are an important new diagnostic tool for VAP. Soluble TREM-1 is a member of the immunoglobulin superfamily and its expression on phagocytes is specifically up-regulated by microbial products [15].

Gibot and coworkers [32] used a rapid immunoblot technique in BAL fluid and found that the levels of soluble triggering receptor expressed on myeloid cells (sTREM-19) were the strongest independent predictor of pneumonia (sensitivity 98% and specificity 90%).

Another serum marker is procalcitonin, which is the precursor molecule of calcitonin, a 116-amino acid peptide. Procalcitonin levels have been associated with prognosis during sepsis and septic shock. Dufflo et al. [33] recently reported that serum procalcitonin could be used as a diagnostic marker of VAP, with serum levels being higher in non-survivors than in survivors. Another study, by Chastre et al. [34], investigated the kinetics of procalcitonin in 63 patients with VAP at days 1, 3 and 7 and found that levels of the peptide paralleled the severity and evolution of VAP, thus making it an early indicator of VAP outcome.

Confirming the Presence of NP: Microbiological Approach

Aetiological diagnosis generally requires a culture obtained from the lower respiratory tract but may, on rare occasions, be achieved with blood or pleural-fluid cultures. Although the sensitivity of blood cultures is less than 25%, positivity indicates that the microorganisms originate from another site of infection. Respiratory tract cultures can be obtained by:

1. Non-invasive diagnostic tools include sputum from endotracheal aspiration (ETA) and 'blind' samples of distal-airways secretions released via the endobronchial catheter. Blind bronchial sampling (BBS), protected specimen brush (PSB), protected telescopic catheter (PTC), BAL and protected BAL (mini-BAL) samples can be obtained with the latter method. Campell [35] reviewed 15 studies evaluating the accuracy of blind methods. A total of 654 episodes of VAP were included in the population analysed and the sensitivity of BBS, mini-BAL and PSB was 74–97%, 63–100% and 58–86%, and the specificity ranged from 74–100%, 66–96% and 71–100% for PSB, respectively [36].

   Marik and Brown [37] compared blind PSB to PSB obtained by bronchoscopy. Fifty-five paired PSB specimens were taken from 53 patients, and an 85% quantitative agreement between the two methods was determined. The sensitivity of blind PSB was 86% with a specificity of 85% and a negative predictive value of 90%.

2. Invasive techniques mainly include bronchoscopy with retrieval of lower respiratory secretions by PSB or BAL. However, bronchoscopy has been systematically investigated, mainly in mechanically ventilated patients.

Sputum should be validated microscopically by estimating neutrophil and epithelial cell counts. Antimicrobial pretreatment significantly reduces the diagnostic yield. The sensitivity of blood cultures is around 5–10 %, with a specificity of 50–90%. Thoracocentesis is clearly indicated in patients with large effusions causing symptoms or on suspicion of empyema. Transthoracic needle aspiration (TTA) of the lung is rarely used, although the diagnostic yield obtained with a 25-G needle is reportedly high (sensitivity 60%, specificity 90–100%) [38].

In ventilated patients, respiratory secretions are of crucial importance. Qualitative cultures of tracheobronchial secretions offer a high sensitivity (>90%) but a very low specificity (<25%) [45]. The high sensitivity may be explained by the fact that pneumonia tends to spread multifocally and preferably in depending lung areas. The low specificity may be the result of frequent colonisation of the respiratory tract with pathogenic microorganisms that do not necessarily cause pneumonia. The results of qualitative cultures are reported according to the growth of the microorganism, light, moderate or heavy, and are most useful when negative and the patient has not received any antibiotics for the last 72 h [1].

For these reasons the quantitative culture technique was developed. Quantitative cultures claim to differentiate colonisation from infection based on a predefined threshold. The rationale behind these thresholds is that a higher bacterial load should reflect true pneumonia. Quantitative tracheobronchial aspirates (threshold $>10^5$ CFU/ml) have a higher specificity than qualitative samples, although at the expense of sensitivity. Sensitivity and specificity both reach around 70%.

The technique of quantitative culture of bronchoscopically retrieved respiratory secretions, including PSB and BAL, has been evaluated by five different approaches:

1. In experimental animal studies.
2. In healthy non-ventilated patients and in mechanically ventilated patients without suspicion of VAP, in a study evaluating the specificity of these techniques.
3. In mechanically ventilated patients with suspicion of VAP; this study did not use strictly independent references to define true cases and controls.
4. In postmortem studies of mechanically ventilated patients, using histology or lung cultures as independent references.
5. In comparative diagnostic studies of mechanically ventilated patients; these analyses focussed on clinically meaningful outcome measures using techniques other than the associated diagnostic indices.

The results of these studies can be summarised as follows:

Bronchoscopically retrieved PSB (threshold $>10^3$ CFU/ml) achieves a higher specificity (80–90%) whereas the sensitivity usually does not surpass 70%

and is usually less (and may still be an effective measure below this level).

The specificity of BAL (threshold >10^4 CFU/ml) does not exceed 80%, whereas the sensitivity may reach 70%. Similar results can be achieved by modified non-bronchoscopic, 'blind' BAL sampling techniques (i.e. mini-BAL using the Ballard catheter). The reasons for the limited yield of these tools are summarised in Table 1.

For many years, the diagnostic performance of invasive vs. non-invasive techniques has been under debate [39]. In three randomised, controlled, Spanish studies [40–42] no differences were found in mortality and morbidity when either invasive (PSB or BAL) or ETT techniques were used to diagnose VAP [26]. In a large French study [43] comprising 413 patients with suspicion of VAP and comparing quantitative cultures of PSB and BAL with qualitative cultures of ETT, empirical antibiotic therapy was initiated in one group of patients based on direct examination of tracheal aspirates while a second group was treated based on the results of BAL or PSB. The patients in the second (invasive) group had less antibiotic use, a lower mortality rate on day 14 (25 vs. 16%) and lower sepsis-related organ failure assessment scores on days 3 and 7.

A few months ago, a Canadian Group [44] published a study consisting of 740 patients in 28 ICUs. The patients were intubated longer than 4 days before pneumonia was suspected and underwent either BAL with quantitative culture of the BAL fluid or endotracheal aspiration without quantitative culture of the aspirate. Empirical antibiotic therapy was started in all patients until culture results

Table 1 Reasons for false-negative and false-positive results in the diagnostic evaluation of ventilator-associated pneumonia (VAP)

Both false-negative and false-positive results
- Variability of diagnostic technique (demonstrated by protected specimen brush)
- Limitations of quantitative culture technique

False-negative results
- Sampling errors due to the multifocal evolution of VAP
- Prior antimicrobial treatment, particularly:
  (a) in the presence of core organisms
  (b) when new antimicrobial agents have been introduced 72 h prior to diagnostic evaluation
- Borderline results in an early stage of infection

False-positive results
- Contamination of the sample:
  (a) during bronchoscopy (lack of adherence to requirements for the retrieval of uncontaminated samples of the distal respiratory tract)
  (b) in the laboratory
- Colonisation rather than infection (i.e. bronchitis rather than pneumonia), particularly in patients with pulmonary comorbidity
- Bronchiolitis

Table 2 Comparison of randomised studies evaluating the impact of quantitative culture technique and bronchoscopic sampling of respiratory secretions on defined outcome variables

	Sole-Violan et al. [15]	Fagon et al. [13]	Ruiz et al. [14]	Canadian Group [44]
Number of patients	91	413	76	740
Uni-/multicentre	Unicentre	Multicentre	Unicentre	Multicentre
Comparison	QC of bronchoscopic or non-bronchoscopic sampling vs. clinical results and qualitative TBAS	QC of bronchoscopic sampling vs. clinical results and qualitative TBAS	QC of bronchoscopic sampling vs. QC of TBAS	QC of bronchoscopic sampling vs. non-QC of TBAS
Use of antimicrobial treatment in patients with negative culture results	Not discontinued	Discontinued in the absence of severe sepsis	Not discontinued	Discontinued when cultures were negative
Length of ICU stay (days)	24±3 vs. 22±3 (*p*=n.s.)	19±9 vs. 18±9 (*p*=n.s.)	21±15 vs. 21±18 (*p*=n.s.)	12.3 vs. 12.2
Length of mechanical ventilation (days)	20±3 vs. 19±3 (*p*=n.s.)	Not reported	19±15 vs. 20±24 (*p*=n.s.)	8.8 vs. 8.9
Mortality (%)	22 vs. 21 (*p*=n.s.)	16 vs. 26 at day 14 (*p*=0.022)	38 vs. 46 (*p*=n.s.)	18.7%

U, Use of antimicrobial treatment in patients with negative culture results; *QC*, quality control; *TBAS*, tracheobronchial aspirates

were available. No significant differences were observed between the groups in the 28-day mortality rate (20%), in the rates of target therapy (74.2 and 74.6%), in days alive without antibiotics (10.4 vs.10.6) or in the ICU and hospital length-of-stay (12.3 vs. 12.2 days). The authors concluded that endotracheal aspiration with non-quantitative culture is associated with clinical outcomes and antibiotic use similar to those associated with BAL and quantitative culture. These studies are compared in Table 2.

In view of these results, the following conclusions may be made:

1. Nowadays, the use of qualitative or quantitative cultures of respiratory secretions is acceptable according to evidence-based medicine.
2. Non-invasive and invasive bronchoscopic tools have comparable diagnostic yields and share similar methodological limitations.
3. The introduction of microbiological criteria to correct for false-positive clinical results does not result in more reliable diagnoses of VAP, since the microbiological correction of false-positive results is countered by the misclassification of correctly positive results.

In contrast, bronchoscopy allows macroscopic assessment of the tracheobronchial tree, which may provide important additional information. 'Blind' methods can be a valuable aid in patients in whom bronchoscopy is not indicated. Table 3 shows the methodological principles that should be followed to ensure valid and reliable results from these costly methods.

Table 3 Factors to consider in the successful use of diagnostic tools for nosocomial pneumonia

Factor	Enhancement of diagnostic performance
Pre-test probability	Patients with a high pre-test probability High prevalence of multiresistant pathogens in the ICU itself
Patient selection	Patients without preexisting lung disease or acute pneumonia Patients with cerebral involvement Surgical patients
Antimicrobial pretreatment	Patients not receiving antimicrobial pretreatment Patients receiving antimicrobial treatment but with no change in the antimicrobial regimen within the last 72 h
Material collection	Adequate sedation No aspiration through the working channel before sampling
Material transport	<2 before work-up of the samples
Material work-up	Validation of sputum and BAL[a]

ICU, Intensive care unit; *BAL*, bronchial alveolar lavage

[a]Criteria for valid sputum collection: >25 neutrophils/visual field; criteria for valid BAL-fluid collection: <3 epithelial cells/ visual field

Bacterial colony counts should be strictly interpreted in the context of the patient's clinical situation. Since the results of bacterial cultures are usually not available until 24–48 h after sampling, rapid testing may provide supplementary support for the selection of antimicrobial drugs. Assessment of the amount of intracellular organisms in phagocytic cells shows a sensitivity and specificity similar to that of PSB. However, sensitivity decreases considerably in the presence of pre-treatment with antimicrobials [45].

Treatment of Nosocomial Pneumonia

Initial Empirical Treatment

Patients in whom NP is suspected should be administered initial empirical treatment after samples for microbiological cultures are collected. A fundamental aspect to take into account at this time is to ensure that this initial treatment is appropriate and adequate [1]. Appropriate empirical treatment refers to the use of an antibiotic to which the most probable microorganism(s) are sensitive while adequate treatment refers to the use of correct doses of an appropriate antibiotic with good penetration at the site of the infection and in combination when indicated. Several studies have demonstrated the importance of initiating appropriate empirical treatment. In 132 patients evaluated by bronchoscopy within the first 24 h of the evolution of pneumonia, Luna and colleagues [46] showed that the mortality rate of patients treated appropriately was 38% compared to 91% in those treated inappropriately ($p<0.001$). The mortality in the group not receiving treatment was 60%. Alavarez-Lerma et al. [47] reported data from a study comprising 284 patients. Significant differences were found with respect to attributable mortality (16 vs. 25%), complicated pneumonia, shock and gastrointestinal haemorrhage among patients with appropriate empirical treatment and those receiving inappropriate treatment. Correction of the latter on receipt of culture results of respiratory secretions does not reduce the mortality [48], thus, all efforts should be aimed at ensuring that the initial treatment is appropriate and adequate. In addition, the initiation of empirical treatment should not be delayed by situations such as waiting for special procedures for obtaining microbiological samples. Logistic regression analysis performed in a study of 107 patients with VAP found that an elevated APACHE II score (adjusted OR, 1.14, CI 95%, 1.09–1.18, $p<0.001$), the presence of neoplasm (adjusted OR, 3.20, CI 95%, 1.79–4.71, $p=0.044$), and the administration of late initial treatment (>24 h) (adjusted OR, 7.68, CI 95%, 4.50–3.09, $p<0.001$) were independent risk factors associated with hospital mortality [49].

When treatment of a patient with VAP is initiated, the possible microorganisms causing the infection should be considered in accordance with the different epidemiological characteristics, risk factors for the colonisation of potentially multiresistant microorganisms and–a very important aspect–the local pattern of resistance to antibiotics of each ICU. A French study of 135 patients with VAP found that nearly 60% of the microorganisms tested were potentially multiresistant microorganisms (PMM), being particularly high in patients who had received ventilation for >7 days and in those receiving antibiotic treatment prior to the development of VAP [50]. Each ICU should therefore have data on the microbiological isolates isolated from the unit and on the patterns of resistance in order to develop specific protocols for effective initial empirical therapy. It is necessary to emphasise that every ICU has its own bacteriology and that the dominant resistant organism may vary from hospital to hospital even in patients presenting with similar risk factors [51]. Additionally, the patterns of antimicrobial resistance are often unique to a particular ICU within the same hospital and may vary between medical and surgical ICUs [52]. With these aspects in mind, a fundamental point in implementing appropriate empirical treatment is to maintain and frequently update in-depth knowledge of the local, microbiological setting.

Independent of the local microbiological setting, the two main factors determining the type of antibiotics to be administered are the time course of the patient's hospitalisation, which allows pneumonia to be classified as early-onset (<5 days) or late-onset (≥5 days) and the presence of risk factors for infections by PMM (Table 4). In patients with NP of early onset without risk factors for

Table 4 Risk factors for infection by potentially multiresistant microorganisms (*PMM*)

Risk factors for PMM
– Antibiotic treatment within the last 90 days (>5 days)
– Current hospital admission or within the last 90 days >5 days
– Immunosuppressive disease and/or treatment
– Chronic dialysis within the last 30 days
– Epidemic outbreak of multiresistant organisms in the intensive care unit

PMM, pathogens that are generally of community origin and with a low probability of multiresistance should be covered (Table 5). Patients with late-onset NP with risk factors for PMM should receive broad-spectrum initial empirical treatment in combination to guarantee coverage of most of the causal microorganisms (Table 6). Several studies have demonstrated that the microorganisms leading to inappropriate treatment in these patients are *Pseudomonas aeruginosa,* MRSA, *Acinetobacter* spp., *Klebsiella pneumoniae* and *Stenotrophomonas maltophilia* [50,51].

Table 5 Initial empirical antibiotic treatment of early-onset nosocomial pneumonia (NP) and ventilator-associated pneumonia (VAP) in patients without risk factors for infection by potentially multiresistant microorganisms (PMM) and with any degree of severity

Probable microorganism
Streptococcus pneumonia
Haemophilus influenzae
Methicillin-resistant *Staphylococcus aureus*
Enteric gram-negative bacilli
Escherichia coli
Klebsiella pneumoniae
Enterobacter spp.
Proteus spp.

Recommended empirical antibiotic
Ceftriaxone
or
Levofloxacin
or
Ertapenem

Table 6 Initial empirical antibiotic treatment of late-onset nosocomial pneumonia (NP) and ventilator-associated pneumonia (VAP) or in patients with risk factors for infection by potentially multiresistant microorganisms (PMM) and with any degree of severity

Probable microorganism	Combined antibiotic treatment
Microorganisms listed in Table 3 plus:	
Pseudomonas aeruginosa *Klebsiella pneumoniae* (extended-spectrum β-lactamase+) *Serratia marcescens* *Acinetobacter* spp. Methicillin-resistant *Staphylococcus aureus* *Legionella pneumophila* Other non-fermentative gram-negative bacteria	Antipseudomonic cephalosporin (ceftazidime or cefepime) *or* carbapenem (imipenem, meropenem) *or* β-lactamic/ β-lactamase inhibitor (piperacillin/tazobactam) + antipseudomonic fluoroquinolone (ciprofloxacin, levofloxacin) *or* aminoglycoside (amikacin) ± linezolid or vancomycin

Monotherapy or Combined Treatment

The objectives of combined treatment are to search for synergy between different groups of antibiotics, widen the spectrum to ensure appropriate treatment against gram-negative microorganism and avoid the development of resistance. The synergistic effect between antibiotics has mainly been demonstrated in vitro and in animal models [53] as well as in its vivo utility in immunosuppressed patients and in those with endocarditis [54]. Nonetheless, the clinical guidelines published by the ATS/IDSA for the diagnosis and treatment of NP recommend combined treatment of an antipseudomonic β-lactamic and an aminoglycoside or fluoroquinolone in patients with suspicion of infection by potentially multiresistant gram-negative bacilli [1].

A meta-analysis of the use of β-lactamics alone or in combination with aminoglycosides for the treatment of sepsis in immunocompetent patients [55] did not demonstrate a beneficial effect in terms of overall patient mortality, clinical failure, microbiologic failure or mortality of the subgroup of patients with *P. aeruginosa* infections, but it did find a greater nephrotoxicity when the combined therapy included an aminoglycoside [56]. However, in a meta-analysis evaluating the role of combined therapy in patients with bacteraemias caused by gram-negative bacilli, the authors found benefits of combined treatment only in the subgroup of patients with *P. aeruginosa* infections. With respect to the appearance of antibiotic resistance, a meta-analysis by Bliziotis et al. [57] (including different types of severe nosocomial infections) showed that the use of β-lactamics in monotherapy was not associated with a higher rate of resistance development than obtained with the β-lactam/aminoglycoside combination (OR, 0.90; CI 95%, 0.56–1.0).

The studies included in this meta-analysis had serious methodological difficulties in responding to the question of the superiority of combined therapy compared with monotherapy in the treatment of NP. First, many studies included patients with different aetiologies of infection, such as pneumonias, intra-abdominal infections, bacteraemias, etc. Second, most studies compared a new β-lactamic in monotherapy with a combination of a different and older β-lactamics plus an aminoglycoside. Third, the dose of the aminoglycosides used in the combined-treatment arm was administered at a schedule of 12 h [58] and at doses lower than those currently used, which affects the efficacy of treatment for this group of antibiotics [59]. Monotherapy or the use of low doses of aminoglycosides administered every 12 h in combination with a β-lactamic may be considered in patients with pneumonia because of the low penetration of these drugs in pulmonary and bronchial tissue. Based on these considerations, current guidelines for the treatment of NP recommend combined treatment with an antipseudomonic β-lactam and an aminoglycoside or quinolone.

Length of Antibiotic Treatment

The length of antibiotic treatment has traditionally been 7–10 days for early-onset NPs caused by generally sensitive microorganisms of community origin. For late-onset NPs, the recommendations consider treatment times of up to 3 weeks (21 days) in patients with infection by multiresistant bacteria, such as *P. aeruginosa* and *Acinetobacter baumanni* [60]. However, in current clinical practice, based on clinical studies, the length of treatment has been shortened.

The most important, prospective, randomised and double-blind study, published by Chastre et al., evaluated two treatment periods in patients with VAP. The study was carried out in several ICUs in France [61]. Its main aim was to compare the duration of 8 vs. 15 days of antibiotic treatment. A total of 401 patients with clinical and microbiological diagnoses (according to samples of respiratory secretions obtained by bronchoscopy) of VAP were included. One interesting aspect of the study was the requirement that study patients receive adequate treatment to be eligible to participate in the efficacy analysis of the two groups. Neither patients with early-onset VAP (<5 days) nor those who had not received antibiotic treatment in the 15 previous days were included because of the likelihood of these patients having infections by microorganisms sensitive to the antibiotics. The treating physician selected antibiotic treatment and modification was allowed according to the results of the microbiological data. The 401 patients were randomised (197 to the 8-day treatment group and 204 to the 15-day group) with no significant differences being observed between the two groups with regard to demographic variables. The 28-day mortality was 18.8% in the 8-day group vs. 17.2% in the 15-day treatment group. No differences were observed with respect to the number of days on mechanical ventilation, disease severity, days of organ failure or the presence of bacteraemia, ARDS or shock. The rate of recurrence of microbiologically confirmed pulmonary infection was 28.9% in the patients treated during 8 days vs. 26% for those treated for 15 days. However, an analysis of recurrence in the subgroup of patients with primary infections caused by non-fermenting gram-negative bacilli, showed that recurrence was significantly higher in patients in the 8-day group (40.6 vs. 25.4%), but differences in mortality were not observed. Nonetheless, the fact that multiresistant microorganisms were more frequent in recurrent pneumonia patients who received 15-day treatment (42.1 vs. 62.3% of recurrent infections, $p=0.04$) is, perhaps, of greater importance. Finally, the number of antibiotic-free days and of broad-spectrum antibiotic-free days between days 1 and 28 were significantly lower in the shorter treatment group (13.1 vs. 8.7 days; $p<0.01$).

The latest ATS guidelines for the treatment of adults with NP [1] recommend that the duration of antibiotic treatment be shortened (7 days) in patients receiving appropriate initial empirical treatment, except in patients in whom the aetiological agent is *P. aeruginosa* or in those with an unsatisfactory evolution of the clinical parameters of infection. Nonetheless, further studies are necessary to validate these recommendations in the general population and in subgroups of patients with specific aetiologies, purulent complications (i.e. empyema) or other clinical situations.

Down-scaling or Reduction of Treatment

This type of treatment name refers to therapeutic strategies of NP that begin with an initial broad-spectrum empirical antibiotic treatment that generally includes a combination of two or three antibiotics. On the third day of treatment, the number of antibiotics and the spectrum is reduced or the drug(s) are discontinued [62]. At present, the problem of multiresistant microorganisms has reached worrisome levels in most of the ICUs in Spain [63], making it necessary to administer broad-spectrum antibiotics and in combination, resulting in the overuse of antibiotics and thus an increase in the prevalence of multiresistant bacteria. The down-scaling strategy attempts to break this vicious circle without compromising patient safety while protecting the hospital environment.

The first step in the reduction strategy is the collection of secretions from the lower respiratory tract for microbiologic analysis, including Gram staining and cultures. Invasive or non-invasive procedures may be carried out, and the results are important for the down-scaling phase. Cultures taken in patients not receiving antibiotic treatment are of greatest utility during sample collection from patients who have received the same treatment regimen in the last 72 h [64]. In patients in whom the initial treatment schedule was aimed against multiresistant microorganisms, if the results of cultures of valid respiratory secretion samples (see above) do not show growth of this type of microorganism then the spectrum of treatment may be reduced. If the culture result is negative and the patient had not been receiving antibiotics during sample collection, treatment may be discontinued based on the clinical parameters of disease evolution as well as the temperature and analytical parameters, such as leucocyte count, C-reactive protein and procalcitonin levels and oxygenation measurements [30,65]. These decisions are generally made on day 3, when the results of the cultures and data regarding the clinical evolution of the disease are available. Down-scaling of monotherapy when the results of the cultures demonstrate microorganisms such as *P. aeruginosa* and *Acinetobacter* spp., remains controversial. Even if *P. aeruginosa* was isolated in the cultures, the maximum benefit conferred by an associated aminoglycoside occurs after the first 5 days of combined therapy. Thus, if this is the causative germ, the reduction strategy may still involve discontinuation of the aminoglycoside after 5 days of combined treatment, especially if disease evolution in the patient is favourable.

Studies Evaluating the Efficacy of Down-scaling

To date, few studies have evaluated the strategy of down-scaling antibiotic administration, although several have demonstrated that the application of the treatment principles described above may provide adequate coverage and limit the use of antibiotics without affecting patient survival. Ibrahim and colleagues carried out a study involving 50 patients with VAP who were treated prior to the initiation of an antibiotic protocol and 52 patients with VAP who were treated with this protocol, but incorporating elements of down-scaling [28]. The protocol required an initial combined antibiotic treatment with imipenem, ciprofloxacin and vancomycin, which was modified after 48 h according to the culture results. With the application of this protocol, 94% of the patients received adequate initial empirical treatment compared with <50% of patients treated in the period of time prior to the application of the protocol. Due to the high number of initially adequate treatments, down-scaling could be frequently implemented. Only 2% of patients needed to continue treatment with a complete course of the three medications, while in 36% one of the drugs could be discontinued and in 61.5% two drugs were withdrawn. This protocol could be followed despite the fact that 25% of the microorganisms isolated were *P. aeruginosa* and 15% were MRSA. The use of the protocol was associated with a significant reduction in the development of secondary episodes of VAP produced by PMM; the total duration of antibiotic treatment ranged from 14.8±8.1 days up to 8.1±5.1 days. Mortality was not affected by the down-scaling strategy.

Micek and coworkers used a treatment protocol involving initial empirical treatment with broad-spectrum antibiotics in patients with suspected VAP. The antibiotics cefepime, ciprofloxacin or gentamicin and vancomycin or linezolid were administered [66]. Initial treatment was adequate in 93% of the patients. The protocol recommended discontinuation of the antibiotics when a non-infectious cause of the pulmonary infiltrates was determined or in patients in whom the clinical signs of pneumonia resolved. This allowed 94.7% of the patients studied (n=142) to discontinue therapy. The recommendation was followed in 88.7% of patients within 48 h after it was made.

Rello et al. published a study comprising 121 episodes of VAP, evaluated by quantitative cultures of tracheal aspirates or bronchoscopic techniques, in patients initially treated with a broad-spectrum regimen [67]. The patients underwent re-evaluation according to the clinical and microbiological responses. A reduction or down-scaling strategy was carried out in 34.4% of patients with episodes diagnosed by bronchoscopy and in 29.3% of those who were diagnosed by tracheal aspirates (non-significant difference). However, the down-scaling was carried out in only 2.7% of patients whose VAP episodes were due to non-fermenting gram-negative bacilli and other multiresistant microorganisms, compared with 49.3% of patients with episodes produced by other pathogens.

In a recently published observational study on clinical characteristics and treatment patterns, Kollef and coworkers evaluated 398 patients fulfilling predefined criteria of VAP [68]. Pathogens were identified in 49.5% of the patients, with the most frequent being MRSA and *P. aeruginosa*. The mean duration of treatment was 11.8±5.9 days and, in most cases (61.6%), treatment was neither reduced nor down-scaled. Down-scaling was possible in 22.1% of the patients.

The mortality rate was lower in patients who underwent down-scaling (17%) than in those undergoing reduction (42.6%) or in whom neither reduction nor down-scaling was performed (23.7%; χ^2=13.25, p=0.001).

Another study that evaluated the role of down-scaling strategy was that of Singh et al. [69]. The protocol was aimed at discontinuing antibiotics in patients with a low suspicion of pneumonia as determined by the CPIS on the third day of treatment. Patients with an initial CPIS of <6 with conventional treatment or ciprofloxacin during 3 days were randomised and then re-evaluated; if the CPIS continued to be <6, antibiotic treatment was discontinued. With this protocol, 42 patients with a score of ≤6 received conventional treatment and 39 were randomised to the ciprofloxacin arm for 3 days. Only 11 of these 39 patients required antibiotics for more than 3 days (increase in CPIS <6). The two groups showed the same clinical course and mortality. However, antibiotic resistance and treatment discontinuation were more frequent in the short-term group treated with ciprofloxacin.

Finally, a recently published study evaluated the role of a down-scaling based on the use of carbapenem in the treatment of NP [70]. A total of 244 patients were included, 91% of whom had late-onset pneumonia. Microbiological isolation was performed in 131 patients (54%) by tracheal aspiration (82%), PBS (33%) and BAL (4%). Nine percent of the patients received adequate initial treatment. Down-scaling was implemented in only 23% of the patients with multiresistant microorganisms compared with 68% of the patients with pneumonias caused by other pathogens (p<0.001). The authors suggested that the previous use of antibiotics and the relatively infrequent use of bronchoscopic techniques as causes of the low-level implementation of down-scaling.

Evaluation of the Clinical Guidelines for Treatment

In contrast with the guidelines for the diagnosis and treatment of community-acquired pneumonia [71] which have been validated in several studies [72], very few studies have evaluated the guidelines for treating NP issued by the main scientific societies, such as those published by the ATS [73]. One study, by Ioanas et al. [74], retrospectively evaluated the capacity of the 1996 ATS guidelines to predict the aetiological microorganisms of NP in 71 patients admitted to the ICU. In addition, the authors analysed whether the recommendation of empirical treatment, suggested by the guidelines, was adequate based on the in vitro sensitivity of the microorganism isolated. These recommendations were found to have a precision of 91% in predicting the aetiological microorganisms, In addition, the treatment suggested by the guidelines was adequate in 79% of the patients. The pathogens implicated in the recommendation of inadequate treatment were: *P. aeruginosa, A. baumanni, S. maltophilia* and MRSA.

Guidelines on the treatment of NP, based on the local resistance patterns and ATS recommendations, were evaluated in a group of 58 patients after the guidelines were implemented (GUIDE group) and in 48 patients pre-implementation

[75]. Patients in the GUIDE group has a higher percentage of adequate treatment (81 vs. 46%, $p<0.01$), as reflected by a lower 14-day mortality rate, than the pre-implementation group (8 vs. 23%, $p=0.03$).

Conclusions

Nosocomial pneumonias, and especially VAPs, are infections characterised by an elevated incidence, mainly in ICUs. Despite advances in our knowledge of the physiopathology, diagnosis and prevention of this disease, mortality continues to be unacceptably high. On suspicion of NP, samples of respiratory secretions should be taken for cultures and microbiological studies and an adequate and appropriate empirical treatment must be immediately started. If necessary, treatment should include a combination of broad-spectrum antibiotics targeted to the characteristics of the patient's condition and the specific epidemiology of the ICU. Re-evaluation on the third day of treatment is of vital importance and this is the point at which down-scaling or reduction of antibiotics should be implemented, in agreement with the results of the cultures of the respiratory secretions. At present, the length of antibiotic treatment is shorter than was the case several years ago; in general, 7 days of treatment should be adequate in patients without infections by high-risk microorganisms or in those with a poor clinical evolution.

References

1. Niederman M, Craven D (2005) Guidelines for the management of adults with hospital-acquired, ventilator-associated, and healthcare-associated pneumonia. Am J Respir Crit Care Med 171:388–416
2. Friedman ND, Kaye KS, Stout JE et al (2002) Health care-associated bloodstream infections in adults: a reason to change the accepted definition of community-acquired infections. Ann Intern Med 137(10):791–797
3. Kollef M, Shorr A, Tabak Y et al (2005) Epidemiology and outcomes of health-care-associated pneumonia. Chest 128:3854–3862
4. Mehta RM, Niedermann MS (2003) Nosocomial pneumonia in the intensive care unit: controversies and dilemmas. J Inten Care Med 18:175
5. Ewing S, Bauer T, Torres A (2002) Nosocomial pneumonia. Thorax 57:366–371
6. Moine P, Timsit JF, Lassence A et al (2002) Mortality associated with late-onset pneumonia in the intensive care unit: results of a multi-center cohort study. Intensive Care Med 28:154–163
7. Alcon A, Fabregas N, Torres A (2005) Pathophysiology of pneumonia. Clin Chest Med 26(1):35–46
8. Sopena N, Sabria M; Neumos 2000 Study Group (2005) Multicenter study of hospital-acquired pneumonia in non-ICU patients. Chest 127:213–219
9. Cook DJ, Walter SD, Cook RJ (1998) Incidence and risk factors of ventilator associated pneumonia in critically ill patients. Ann Internal Med 129(6):433–444

10. Valles J, Pobo A, Garcia-Esquirol O et al (2007) Excess ICU mortality attributable to VAP: the role of early vs. late onset. Intensive Care Med 33:1363–1368
11. Bonten M, Kollef M, Hall J (2004) Risk factors for ventilator-associated pneumonia: from epidemiology to patient management. Clin Infectious Dis 38:1141–1149
12. Luna CM, Aruj P, Niederman MS et al for the GANAR group (2006) Appropriateness and delay to initiate therapy in ventilator-associated pneumonia. Eur Res J 27:158–164
13. Craven D, De Rosa D, Thornton D (2002) Nosocomial pneumonia: emerging concepts in diagnosis, management and prophylaxis. Curr Op Crit Care 8:421–429
14. Safdar N, Crnich CJ, Maki DJ (2005) The pathogenesis of ventilator-associated pneumonia: its relevance to developing effective strategies for prevention. Resp Care 50:725–739
15. Torres A, El-Ebiary M, Soler N et al (1996) Stomach as a source of colonization of the respiratory tract during mechanical ventilation in association with VAP. Eur Respir J 8:1729–1735
16. Torres A, Serra-Batlles J, Ros E (1992) Pulmonary aspiration of gastric contents in patients receiving mechanical ventilation: the effect of body position. Ann Intern Med 116:540–543
17. Bonten MJM, Gaillard CA, van der Geest S et al (1995) The role of intragastric acidity and stress ulcer prophylaxis on colonization and infection in mechanically ventilated patients: a stratified, randomised, double blind study of sucralfate versus antacids. Am J Res Crit Care Med 152:1825–1834
18. Diaz E, Rodriguez A, Rello J (2005) Ventilator associated pneumonia: issues related to the artificial airway. Resp Care 50:900–906
19. Costerton JW, Cheng KJ, Geesey GG et al (1987) Bacterial biofilms in nature and disease. Annu Rev Microbiol 41:435–464
20. Consterton JW (1999) Introduction to biofilm. Int Antimicrob Agents 11:217–221
21. Gorman SP, McGovern JG, Woolfson AD et al (2001) The concomitant development of poly(vinyl chloride)-related biofilm and antimicrobial resistance in relation to ventilator-associated pneumonia. Biomaterials 22:2741–2747
22. Vorachit M, Lam K, Jayanetra P, Costerton JW (1993) Resistance of Pseudomonas pseudomallei growing as a biofilm on silastic discs to ceftazidime and co-trimoxazole. Antimicrob Agents Chemother 37:2000–2002
23. Koerner RJ (1997) Contribution of endotracheal tubes to the pathogenesis of ventilator-associated pneumonia. J Hosp Infect 35:83–89
24. Van Saene HKF, Damjanovic V, Williets T et al (1998) Pathogenesis of ventilator-associated pneumonia: is the contribution of biofilm clinically significant? J Hosp Infect 38:231–240
25. Feldman C, Kassel M, Cantrell J et al (1999) The presence and sequence of endotracheal tube colonization in patients undergoing mechanical ventilation. Eur Respir J 13:546–551
26. Fabregas N, Ewig S, Torres A et al (1999) Clinical diagnosis of ventilator associated pneumonia revisited: comparative validation using immediate post-mortem lung biopsies. Thorax 54:867–73
27. Pugin J, Auckenthaler R, Mili N et al (1991) Diagnosis of ventilator-associated pneumonia by bacteriologic analysis of bronchoscopic and nonbronchoscopic 'blind' bronchoalveolar lavage fluid. Am Rev Respir Dis 143:1121–1129
28. Ibrahim EH, Ward S, Sherman G et al (2001) Experience with a clinical guideline for the treatment of ventilator-associated pneumonia. Crit Care Med 29:1109–1115
29. Fartoukh M, Maitre B, Honore S et al (2003) Diagnosing pneumonia during mechanical ventilation: the clinical pulmonary infection score revisited. Am J Respir Crit Care Med 168:173–179
30. Luna CM, Blancazo D, Niederman MS et al (2003) Resolution of ventilator-associated pneumonia: prospective evaluation of the clinical pulmonary infection score as an early clinical predictor of outcome. Crit Care Med 31:676–682
31. Lipchik RJ, Kuzo RS (1996) Nosocomial pneumonia. Radiol Clin North Am 34:47–58
32. Gibot S, Gravoisy A, Levy B et al (2004) Soluble triggering receptor expressed on myeloid cells and the diagnosis of pneumonia. N Engl J Med 350:451–458

33. Duflo F, Debon R, Monneret G et al (2002) Alveolar and serum procalcitonin: diagnostic and prognostic value in ventilator-associated pneumonia. Anesthesiology 96:74–79
34. Luyt CE, Guerin V, Combes A et al (2005) Procalcitonin kinetics as a prognistic marker of ventilator-associated pneumonia. Am J Resp Crit Care Med 171:48–53
35. Campell GD Jr (2000) Blinded invasive diagnostic procedures in ventilator-associated pneumonia. Chest 117:207S-211S
36. Koenig S, Truwit J (2006) Ventilator-associated pneumonia: diagnosis, treatment and prevention. Clin Microbiol Rev 19:637–657
37. Marik PE, Brown WJ (1995) A comparison of bronchoscopic vs. blind protected specimen brush sampling in patients with suspected ventilator-associated pneumonia. Chest 108:203–207
38. Dorca J, Manresa F, Esteban L et al (1995) Efficacy, safety, and therapeutic relevance of transthoracic aspiration with ultrathin needle in nonventilated nosocomial pneumonia. Am J Respir Crit Care Med 151:1491–1496
39. Klompas M (2007) Does the patient have ventilator-associated pneumonia? JAMA 297:1583–1593
40. Ruiz M, Torres A, Ewig S et al (2000) Noninvasive versus invasive microbial investigation in ventilator-associated pneumonia. Am J Respir Crit Care Med 162:119–125
41. Sanchez-Nieto JM, Torres A, Garcia-Cordoba F et al (1998) Impact of invasive and noninvasive quantitative culture sampling on outcome of ventilator-associated pneumonia. Am J Respir Crit Care Med 157:371–376
42. Solé Violán J, Arroyo J, Bordes A et al (2000) Impact of qualitative diagnostic techniques in the management and outcome of mechanically ventilated patients with suspected pneumonia. Crit Care Med 28:2737–2741
43. Fagon JY, Chastre J, Wolff M et al (2000) Invasive and noninvasive strategies for management of suspected ventilator-associated pneumonia. Ann Intern Med 132:621–630
44. The Canadian Critical Care Trials Group (2006) A randomised trial of diagnostic techniques for ventilator-associated pneumonia. N Engl J Med 355:2619–2630
45. Torres A, De La Bellacasa JP, Xaubet A et al (1989) Diagnostic value of quantitative cultures of bronchoalveolar lavage and telescoping plugged catheters in mechanically ventilated patients with bacterial pneumonia. Am Rev Respir Dis 140:306–310
46. Luna CM, Vujacich P, Niederman MS et al (1997) Impact of BAL data on therapy and outcome of VAP. Chest 111:676–687
47. Alvarez-Lerma F; ICU-acquired Pneumonia Study Group (1996) Modification of empiric antibiotic treatment in patients with pneumonia acquired in the intensive care unit. Intensive Care Med 22:387–394
48. Kollef MH, Ward S (1998) The influence of mini-BAL cultures on patient outcomes: implications for the antibiotic management of ventilator-associated pneumonia. Chest 113:412–420
49. Iregui MS, Ward G, Sherman VJ et al (2002) Clinical importance of delays in the initiation of appropriate antibiotic treatment for ventilator-associated pneumonia. Chest 122:262–268
50. Trouillet JL, Chastre A, Vuagnat ML et al (1998) Ventilator-associated pneumonia caused by potentially drug-resistant bacteria. Am Rev Respir Dis 157:531–539
51. Rello J, Sa-Borges M, Correa H et al (1999) Variations in etiology of ventilator-associated pneumonia across four treatment sites: implications for antimicrobial prescribing practices. Am J Respir Crit Care Med 160:608–613
52. Namias NL, Samiian D, Nino E et al (2000) Incidence and susceptibility of pathogenic bacteria vary between intensive care units within a single hospital: implications for empiric antibiotic strategies. J Trauma 49:638–645
53. Pechere JC, Marchou B, Michea-Hamzehpour M, Auckenthaler R (1986) Emergence of resistance after therapy with antibiotics used alone or combined in a murine model. J Antimicrob Chemother 17(Suppl A):11–18
54. Karchmer AW, Archer GL, Dismukes WE (1995) Rifampin treatment of prosthetic valve endocarditis due to Staphylococcus epidermidis. Rev Infect Dis Suppl 3:S543-S548

55. Safdar N, Handelsman J, Maki DG (2004) Does combination antimicrobial therapy reduce mortality in Gram-negative bacteraemia? A meta-analysis. Lancet Infect Dis 4:519–527
56. Paul M, Uri-Silbiger I, Soares-Weiser K, Leibovici L (2004) Beta lactam monotherapy versus beta lactam-aminoglycoside combination therapy for sepsis in immunocompetent patients: systematic review and meta-analysis of randomised trials. BMJ 328:668
57. Bliziotis IA, Samonis G, Vardakas KZ et al (2005) Effect of aminoglycoside and beta-lactam combination therapy versus beta-lactam monotherapy on the emergence of antimicrobial resistance: a meta-analysis of randomized, controlled trials. Clin Infect Dis 41:149–158
58. Cometta A, Baumgartner JD, Lew D (1994) Prospective randomized comparison of imipenem monotherapy with imipenem plus netilmycin for treatment of severe infections in nonneutropenic patients. Antimicrob Agents Chemother 38:1309–1313
59. Munckhof WJ, Grayson ML, Turnidge JD (1996) A meta-analysis of studies on the safety and efficacy of aminoglycosides given either once daily or as divided doses. J Antimicrob Chemother 37:645–663
60. Rello J, Diaz E (2003) Pneumonia in the intensive care unit. Crit Care Med 31:2544–2551
61. Chastre J, Wolff M, Fagon JY et al (2003) Comparison of 8 vs. 15 days of antibiotic therapy for ventilator-associated pneumonia in adults: a randomized trial. JAMA 290:2588–2598
62. Niederman MS (2006) De-escalation therapy in ventilator-associated pneumonia. Curr Opin Crit Care 12:452–457
63. Alvarez-Lerma F (2002) Neumonía relacionada con la ventilación mecánica. In: Grupo de trabajo de enfermedades infecciosas de la SEMICYUC,1 ed. Estudio nacional de vigilancia de infección nosocomial en UCI (ENVIN-UCI), Madrid, pp 53–72
64. Souweine B, Veber B, Bedos JP et al (1998) Diagnostic accuracy of protected specimen brush and bronchoalveolar lavage in nosocomial pneumonia: impact of previous antimicrobial treatments. Crit Care Med 26:236–244
65. Dennesen PJ, van der Ven AM, Kessels GH et al (2001) Resolution of infectious parameters after antimicrobial therapy in patients with ventilator-associated pneumonia. Am J Respir Crit Care Med 163:1371–1375
66. Micek S, Ward TS, Fraser VJ, Kollef MH (2004) A randomized controlled trial of an antibiotic discontinuation policy for clinically suspected ventilator-associated pneumonia. Chest 125:1791–1799
67. Rello J, Vidaur L, Sandiumenge A et al (2004) De-escalation therapy in ventilator-associated pneumonia. Crit Care Med 32:2183–2190
68. Kollef MH, Morrow LE, Niederman MS et al (2006) Clinical characteristics and treatment patterns among patients with ventilator-associated pneumonia. Chest 129:1210–1218
69. Singh N, Rogers P, Atwood CHW et al (2000) Short course empiric therapy for patients with pulmonary infiltrates in the intensive care unit. Am J Respir Crit Care Med 162:505–511
70. Alvarez-Lerma F, Alvarez B, Luque P et al (2006) Empiric broad-spectrum antibiotic therapy of nosocomial pneumonia in the intensive care unit: a prospective observational study. Crit Care 10:R78
71. Niederman MS, Mandell LA, Anzueto A et al (2001) Guidelines for the management of adults with community-acquired pneumonia. Diagnosis, assessment of severity, antimicrobial therapy, and prevention. Am J Respir Crit Care Med 163:1730–1754
72. Mortensen EM, Restrepo M, Anzueto A, Pugh J (2004) Effects of guideline-concordant antimicrobial therapy on mortality among patients with community-acquired pneumonia. Am J Med 117:726–731
73. Campbell DG, Niederman MS, Broughton W et al (1006) Guidelines for the initial management of adults with hospital-acquired pneumonia. Am J Respir Crit Care Med 153:1711–1725
74. Ioanas M, Cavalcanti M, Ferrer M et al (2003) Hospital-acquired pneumonia: coverage and treatment adequacy of current guidelines. Eur Respir J 22:876–882
75. Soo Hoo GW, Wen YE, Nguyen TV, Goetz MB (2005) Impact of clinical guidelines in the management of severe hospital-acquired pneumonia. Chest 128:2778–2787

Prone Ventilation

Prone Ventilation To Prevent Ventilator-Associated Pneumonia

P. Beuret

Introduction

Ventilator-associated pneumonia (VAP) refers to pneumonia that arises more than 48 h after endotracheal intubation. VAP is the most common hospital-acquired infection among patients requiring mechanical ventilation and is associated with high morbidity, mortality and health-care costs [1,2], emphasising the need of risk-reduction strategies. Some strategies are strongly recommended by recent guidelines: general infection control measures, use of non-invasive ventilation whenever possible, semirecumbent position and continuous aspiration of subglottic secretions [1]. Prone positioning has repeatedly been shown to improve arterial oxygenation in patients with hypoxaemic respiratory failure who receive mechanical ventilation. Unfortunately, three randomised studies failed to show an improvement in survival [3–5]. However, prone positioning might interfere with the mechanisms involved in the pathogenesis of VAP.

Aspiration Around the Cuff

The aspiration of subglottic secretions around high volume-low pressure tracheal tube cuffs is usually considered as a key mechanism of bacterial tracheal colonisation and the subsequent development of VAP [1,2]. It is related to the longitudinal folds that always occur within the cuff wall when it is inflated within the trachea at the recommended pressure level [6]. Few studies investigated specifically the effect of position on the incidence of aspiration around the cuff. In the supine position, aspiration has been observed early after the instillation of dye in the subglottic space in patients undergoing general anaesthesia for surgery [7,8]. The semirecumbent position reduces the aspiration of gastric content through gastro-oesophageal reflux, when compared with supine position [9], but this effect is only partial [10]. Prone positioning may offer protection from the

U. Lucangelo, P. Pelosi, W.A. Zin, A. Aliverti (eds.) *Respiratory System and Artificial Ventilation*. © Springer 2008

aspiration of subglottic secretions, by enhancing their spontaneous drainage through the oral cavity, because of the orientation of the trachea.

To verify this hypothesis, we conducted a study comparing the incidence of aspiration of subglottic secretions in mechanically ventilated patients in semirecumbent and prone positions [11]. The patients were ventilated either in volume-controlled mode or pressure support, according to the free choice of the physicians caring for the patient. A positive end-expiratory pressure (PEEP) of 5 cm H_2O was always used. The patients were sedated if needed with continuous infusion of fentanyl and midazolam. They were eligible for the study if they required prone positioning, either because of severe hypoxaemia due to lung injury with $PaO_2/FIO_2 \leq 150$, or as prevention of lung worsening in comatose patients [12]. The position, in which each patient was studied for 4 h, was randomised: either semirecumbent at a 30° angle of head and trunk elevation (SP group, n=15) or in a horizontal prone position (PP group, n=16). At baseline, blue dye was instilled into the subglottic space via the additional lumen of the endotracheal tube (HI-LO Evac, Mallinckrodt Laboratories, Athlone, Ireland). The cuff pressure was checked every hour and reset at 30 cm H_2O if needed. The issue of blue dye by the oral cavity or the proximal tip of the endotracheal tube was checked every hour. Four hours after instillation of the dye, fiberoptic bronchoscopy was performed to search for the presence of blue dye in the trachea and/or the bronchi. During the procedure, the patient remained in the position to which he or she had been randomised. The characteristics of the patients in the SP and PP groups at baseline were similar. Blue dye was drained through the oral cavity from the first hour more frequently in the PP group (13/16) than in the SP group (4/15; $p<0.01$). During the 4 h of the study, blue dye was never drained by the proximal tip of the endotracheal tube. Fiberoptic bronchoscopy during the fourth hour never showed blue dye in the trachea and/or the bronchi of any of the patients in the two groups. The absence of aspiration in the semirecumbent position might have been related to the protective effect of PEEP maintained at ≥5 cm H_2O throughout the study in all patients, as suggested in a benchtop model [13].

In patients in the prone position, this study confirmed that subglottic secretions are frequently spontaneously drained through the oral cavity, protecting against aspiration. It was previously shown that enteral nutrition is poorly tolerated by patients in the prone position, i.e. positioned flat on the bed, and is associated with a high rate of vomiting [14]. Our results suggest that these regurgitations drain through the oral cavity and do not expose the patient to aspiration.

Colonisation of Distal Airways

Tracheal colonisation may lead to the development of pneumonia, if the normal host-defence mechanisms of cough reflex, mucociliary clearance and, below the terminal bronchioles, the cellular and humoral immune systems, are overwhelmed. Intubation and sedation impair the cough reflex, and the cuffed tracheal tube depresses bronchial mucus transport velocity [15]. To date, no study has investigated the influence of body position on mucociliary clearance. However, the trachea and main bronchi are directed backwards in patients in the supine position. Prone positioning might therefore enhance gravitational bronchial drainage, as suggested by a computed tomography study [16].

Development of Pneumonia

Recent experimental studies have focused on the effect of ventilatory settings in the development of pneumonia from tracheal bacterial inoculation. It has been demonstrated that recruitment manoeuvres using individual PEEP settings reduce the growth of bacteria in the lungs when compared with conventional ventilation with low PEEP level [17]. Moreover, this strategy reduced bacterial translocation, evaluated by the time to bacteraemia, when compared either with conventional ventilation with low PEEP or ventilation with fixed high PEEP after recruitment manoeuvres. Prone positioning has been shown to induce homogenisation of the regional distribution of ventilation, with alveolar recruitment in dependent collapsed regions [18]. Since the lesions of VAP are mainly located in dependent regions and associated with loss of aeration [19], prone positioning might interfere with the development of pneumonia in dependent lung regions. However, to date no study has investigated the effect of placing patients in the prone position on bacterial growth in the lung.

Impact of the Prone Position on the Occurrence of VAP

Three randomised studies have reported VAP rates in patients receiving prone versus supine positioning [4,5,12]. We conducted a randomised controlled trial consisting of patients who required mechanical ventilation because of a coma, except if caused by acute poisoning [12]. Exclusion criteria were contraindications to prone positioning, notably intracranial hypertension. The patients randomised into the prone position (PP) group were positioned prone for 4 h once daily, with the first period required to begin within 24 h after intubation. The mean total duration in PP was 23.9±14.6 h for patients in the PP group. The VAP rate was lower in the PP group (5/25, 20%) than in the supine position group (10/26, 38%), but the difference did not reach statistical significance (0.14). However, the study was likely under-powered regarding this criterion. This study showed a significant beneficial effect of prone compared to supine position regarding the main evaluation criteria, the occurrence of lung worsening, which was assessed by the evolution of the lung injury score. Therefore, we decided to introduce this strategy in the routine care of comatose patients. Progressive implementation of this approach provided us with the opportunity to compare the effects of daily prone positioning and supine positioning on VAP rate, out of the context of a randomised clinical trial, on a cohort of 104 comatose patients [20]. The analysis again showed a non-significant reduction in the incidence of VAP in the prone position group. Moreover, periods in the prone position had to be stopped because of the occurence of intracranial hypertension in 17% of these patients. The French multicentre trial randomised patients with hypoxaemic respiratory failure from various causes [4]. Patients were assigned to prone positioning (PP) for at least 8 h daily or supine positioning. Patients of the PP group were in the prone position for a median of 4 days. The incidence of VAP, expressed per 100 patient-days of invasive ventilation, was significantly lower in the PP group (16.6/1000 days) than in the supine position group (21.4/1000 days) (p=0.045). Conversely, the incidences of pressure sores, selective intubation and endotracheal tube obstruction were higher in the prone group. The Spanish multicentre trial enrolled patients with ARDS [5]. Patients assigned to the PP group remained in the prone position an average of 10.1±10.3 days and for an average of 17 h/day. The VAP rate was similar in the PP (14/76, 18.4%) and supine groups (9/60, 15%; p=0.65). This study was stopped before the planned sample size was reached due to decreased patient accrual and was therefore underpowered. Complications related to the prone position were few, but eventual complications were not recorded in the supine position group. A comparison of the results of these three studies with respect to the occurrence of VAP is difficult, because of the various clinical situations, duration in the prone position and time elapsed from intubation to the first prone period. The French multicentre trial was the only study to show a significant reduction in the incidence of VAP; however, the magnitude of the effect was relatively weak, and the balance between the benefit and harms is uncertain [4].

References

1. The American Thoracic Society and the Infectious Diseases Society of America guideline Committee (2005) Guidelines for the management of adults with hospital-acquired, ventilator-associated, and healthcare-associated pneumonia. Am J Respir Crit Care Med 171:388–416
2. Craven D (2006) Preventing ventilator-associated pneumonia in adults. Chest 130:251–260
3. Gattinoni L, Tognoni G, Pesenti A et al (2001) Effect of prone positioning on the survival of patients with acute respiratory failure. N Engl J Med 345:568–573
4. Guerin C, Gaillard S, Lemasson S et al (2004) Effects of systematic prone positioning in hypoxemic acute respiratory failure. JAMA 292:2379–2387
5. Mancebo J, Fernandez R, Blanch L et al (2006) A multicenter trial of prolonged prone ventilation in severe acute respiratory distress syndrome. Am J Respir Crit Care Med 173:1233–1239
6. Dullenkopf A, Gerber A, Weiss M (2003) Fluid leakage past tracheal tube cuffs: evaluation of the new Microcuff endotracheal tube. Intensive Care Med 29:1849–1853
7. Blunt MC, Young PJ, Patil A, Haddock A (2001) Gel lubrication of the tracheal tube cuff reduces pulmonary aspiration. Anesthesiology 95:377–381

8. Seegobin RD, Van Hasselt GL (1986) Aspiration beyond endotracheal cuffs. Can Anaesth Soc J 33:273–279
9. Orozco-Levi M, Torres A, Ferrer M et al (1995) Semirecumbent position protects from pulmonary aspiration but not completely from gastroesophageal reflux in mechanically ventilated patients. Am J Respir Crit Care Med 152:1387–1390
10. Orozco-Levi M, Félez M, Martinez-Miralles E et al (2003) Gastro-oesophageal reflux in mechanically ventilated patients: effects of an oesophageal balloon. Eur Respir J 22:348–353
11. Beuret P, Carton MJ, Nourdine K et al (2007) Inhalation de sécrétions oropharyngées autour du ballonnet des sondes d'intubation: comparaison de la position dorsale demi-assise et du décubitus ventral. Réanimation 16(Suppl 1):SP18
12. Beuret P, Carton MJ, Nourdine K et al (2002) Prone position as prevention of lung injury in comatose patients: a prospective, randomized, controlled study. Intensive Care Med 28:564–569
13. Young PJ, Rollinson M, Downward G, Henderson S (1997) Leakage of fluid past the tracheal tube cuff in a benchtop model. Br J Anaesth 78:557–562
14. Reignier J, Thenoz-Jost N, Fiancette M et al (2004) Early enteral nutrition in mechanically ventilated patients in the prone position. Crit Care Med 32:94–99
15. Keller C, Brimacombe J (1998) Bronchial mucus transport velocity in paralyzed anesthetized patients: a comparison of the laryngeal mask airway and cuffed tracheal tube. Anaesth Analg 86:1280–1282
16. Priolet B, Tempelhoff G, Millet J et al (1993) Ventilation assistée en décubitus ventral: evaluation tomodensitométrique de son efficacité dans le traitement des condensations pulmonaires. Réan Urg 2(2):81–85
17. Lachmann RA, Van Kaam AH, Haitsma JJ, Lachmann B (2007) High positive end-expiratory pressure levels promote bacterial translocation in experimental pneumonia. Intensive Care Med [Epub ahead of print]
18. Richard JC, Lavenne F, Lebars D et al (2005) Effets du décubitus ventral et du niveau de PEP sur le recrutement et la distribution de la ventilation alvéolaire étudiés en tomographie par emission de positons. Réanimation 14(Suppl 1):SP136
19. Rios Vieira SR, Goldstein I, Lenaour G et al (2003) Experimental ventilator-associated pneumonia: distribution of lung infection and consequences for lung aeration. Braz J Infect Dis 7(3):216–223
20. Beuret P, Nourdine K, Carton MJ et al (2007) Pneumopathies acquises sous ventilation mécanique chez les patients comateux: absence d'impact du décubitus ventral précoce. Réanimation 16(Suppl 1):SOE9

Prone Positioning of Patients with ARDS

L. Blanch, U. Lucangelo

Introduction

Acute respiratory distress syndrome (ARDS) is characterised by non-cardiogenic pulmonary oedema that increases ventilation/perfusion heterogeneity, causes intrapulmonary shunt and severely impairs oxygenation. Amato et al. [1] demonstrated for the first time in an adult population with ARDS that the open-lung approach has an impact on outcome. The strategy of these authors was to achieve and maintain maximal aeration of collapsed dependent lung regions (dorsal regions in a supine patient), since lung-recruitment strategies may be an important tool in the reduction of ventilator-induced lung injury (VILI) [2,3]. In this respect, prone positioning has been safely used to improve oxygenation in a wide population of patients with ARDS [5–15].

Physiology of the Prone Position: Regional Ventilation

In the supine position, regional inflation exponentially decreases along the vertical axis, from non-dependent to dependent regions, and the vertical inflation gradient depends on the local transpulmonary pressure. At functional residual capacity (FRC), when alveolar pressure equals atmospheric pressure, differences in transpulmonary pressure are due to regional changes in Ppl. The vertical gradient of Ppl in healthy subjects is approximately 0.2–0.3 cm H_2O/cm. The Ppl gradient depends upon lung weight, the shape and mechanical properties of the chest wall and shape of the thorax with respect to the lung [16–19]. Pelosi et al. [20] investigated lung regional inflation by obtaining CT scans of patients with normal lungs and with ARDS. They found that the ARDS lung is characterised by decreased gas volume and increased tissue volume, whereas total lung volume was similar in the two groups. Also, the vertical inflation gradient decreases from non-dependent to dependent lung regions. Consequently, in ARDS patients ventilated without PEEP in the supine position, almost total alveolar collapse occurs in the posterior zones of the lungs because gas volume decreases with alveolar flooding and tissue compression. The effect on specific lung compliance, however, is minimal because the elastic properties of oedematous lungs and normal lungs are the same [21,22].

Several groups have shown that the gravitational distribution of pleural pressure is much more uniform when animals are in a prone rather than in a supine position, both under basal conditions and in the presence of lung oedema [23–25]. Mutoh et al. [26], in an experimental study with pigs, found that the Ppl gradient is smaller in prone position, suggesting that regional inflation is more homogeneously distributed in animals in a prone than in a supine position. After volume-infusion-induced pulmonary oedema, Ppl was positive in the dependent lung regions in supine animals but much less positive in those in the prone position. Moreover, in the supine position some pulmonary regions are below their closing volume, i.e., where transpulmonary pressure at end-inspiration does not exceed airway opening pressure; thus, these regions do not receive any alveolar ventilation. This phenomenon is potentially reversible in the prone position with improved alveolar ventilation because alveolar collapse and airway closure are reduced in dorsal lung regions [27,28]. Lastly, the interaction between the heart and the lungs also influences the distribution of ventilation in supine and prone positions. In the supine position, the heart compresses the lung in dependent regions whereas this effect is offset in the prone position because the heart rests on the sternum and exerts much less effect on regional lung expansion [22].

Hydrostatic and anatomic mechanisms influence the pattern of diaphragmatic movement affecting the distribution of ventilation in patients in the prone position [29]. Froese and Bryan [30] evaluated the position and pattern of movement of the diaphragm in healthy adults during spontaneous ventilation and after muscle paralysis and mechanical ventilation. They found that, during spontaneous ventilation, the dependent part of the diaphragm had the greatest displacement and thus greater ventilation of the dependent lung. They also showed that, during anaesthesia in humans, a cephalad shift of the diaphragm was largely confined to the dependent (dorsal) portions of the lung. Under mechanical ventilation, the non-dependent regions of the diaphragm move preferentially such that ventilation is greater in non-dependent regions [31,32]. Neither the application of PEEP nor an increasing tidal volume restored ventilation to that area, which could only be accomplished by use of the prone position [30]. Therefore, in patients with ARDS, the prone position is optimal to ventilate dorsal regions of the lung with positive pleural pressure [28].

Interestingly, the presence of abdominal distension may influence the improvement in arterial oxygenation with the prone position. Mure et al. [33] found that when the abdomen of normal pigs was distended, the prone position resulted in a greater improvement in PaO_2 and a decrease in VA/Q heterogeneity. The authors speculated that the distribution of perfusion is more uniform and the decrease in pleural pressure in the dependent lung near the diaphragm is greater in the presence of abdominal distension. The interactions between positive end-expiratory pressure (PEEP) and posture on regional distribution of ventilation were examined by Johansson et al. [34]. In anaesthetised mechanically ventilated sheep, the redistribution of ventilation with 10 cmH_2O of PEEP differed between postures, shifting the mode in animals in the supine position toward dependent lung regions while eliminating the dorsal-to-ventral gradient in prone animals. The regional heterogeneity in ventilation was greater in supine sheep at both levels of PEEP, and this was due mostly to greater isogravitational heterogeneity in the supine than in the prone position. These markedly different effects of 10 cmH_2O on PEEP administered to subjects in supine vs. prone positions may have important implications for gas exchange, both in non-injured and injured lungs.

Physiology of the Prone Position: Regional Perfusion

In the supine position, lung perfusion in normal lungs is distributed according to gravity; however, the vertical perfusion gradient is diminished by prone positioning. In oedematous lungs, several studies have evaluated the effect of prone position on lung perfusion [35–38]. Wiener et al. [36] quantified regional lung perfusion in dogs using radiolabelled microspheres. Regional perfusion was quantified in three different lung regions in animals in the supine and prone positions before and after acute lung injury was induced with oleic acid. The authors found that regional perfusion followed a gravitational gradient before and after lung injury that was more uniformly distributed in the prone position, preferentially to non-dependent regions. Thus, perfusion was distributed preferentially to the dorsal lung, even in the non-dependent position. Glenny et al. [39] examined flow on a much smaller scale than had previously been attempted and found that perfusion in supine animals was strongly correlated with that observed when the animals were prone. This observation is the opposite of what would be expected if variations in perfusion distribution were the consequence of gravity. In further investigations, Lamm et al. [37] analysed the mechanisms of improved oxygenation, as determined by regional perfusion and ventilation, by using single photon emission computed tomography before and after lung injury in animals. After lung injury: (1) animals in the supine position has a decrease or cessation of ventilation to dorsal areas while perfusion was maintained, (2) in animals placed in the prone position, dorsal lung ventilation improved while perfusion was generally unchanged. These changes resulted in a decrease in relative ventilation/perfusion (V/Q) heterogeneity, thus improving intrapulmonary shunt in the prone position.

Recently, Richter et al. [40] investigated the regional mechanism by which the prone position improves gas exchange in acutely injured lungs. They used positron emission tomography imaging to assess the regional distribution of pulmonary shunt, aeration, perfusion, and ventilation in seven surfactant-depleted sheep in supine and prone positions. With animals in the supine position, the dorsal lung regions had a high shunt fraction, high perfusion and poor aeration.

The prone position was associated with an increase in lung gas content and with a more uniform distribution of aeration, as the increase in aeration in dorsal lung regions was not offset by the loss of aeration in ventral regions. Consequently, the shunt fraction decreased in dorsal regions in the prone position without a concomitant impairment of gas exchange in ventral regions, thus leading to a significant increase in the fraction of pulmonary perfusion participating in gas exchange. In summary, the prone position improves gas exchange by restoring aeration and decreasing shunt while preserving perfusion in dorsal lung regions, and by making the distribution of ventilation more uniform. In ARDS patients, Pappert et al. [38] assessed the V/Q relationships using the multiple gas elimination technique and also found that the improvement in oxygenation was associated with an improvement in V/Q matching.

Ventilator-Induced Lung Injury and Prone Position

Computed tomography (CT) studies performed on humans have shown that with the prone position lung inflation is distributed more homogeneously than occurs in the supine, suggesting a more homogeneous distribution of stress and strain throughout the lung parenchyma [41]. Valenza et al. [42] studied mechanically ventilated rats in the supine or prone position until a similar ventilator-induced lung injury was achieved. Interestingly, they found that the time taken to achieve the target ventilator-induced lung injury was longer in animals in the prone than in the supine position. Computed tomography scan analysis prior to lung injury revealed that, at end-expiration, the lung was wider in prone animals despite similar lung volumes. Moreover, lung density along the vertical axis increased significantly only in the supine position and lung strain was greater in the supine than in the prone position. Clearly, the study of Valenza et al. [42] showed a delay in the progression of ventilator-induced lung injury. In fact, the results of those authors confirmed previous data from Broccard et al. [43]. They ventilated ten normal dogs (5 prone, 5 supine) for 6 h with identical ventilatory patterns and found that wet weight/dry weight ratios and histological scores were greater in the supine than in the prone group. It was concluded that the prone position resulted in a less severe and more homogeneous distribution of ventilator-induced lung injury.

Mentzelopoulos et al. [44] tested the hypothesis that following PEEP optimisation, prone positioning may reduce overall lung parenchymal stress, assessed by measuring the relationship between plateau/peak transpulmonary pressure and tidal volume as a function of end-expiratory lung volume in patients with severe ARDS. Compared with a semi-recumbent pre-prone condition, pronation resulted in reduced peak/plateau pressures and lung elastance, thus suggesting that the prone position under PEEP optimisation reduces ventilator-induced lung injury. Finally, Galiatzou et al. [45] studied the effect of the prone position when applied after a recruitment manoeuvre in patients with acute lung injury. Prone positioning recruited the oedematous lung further than recruitment manoeuvres and reversed overinflation, without any indication of end-expiratory derecruitment, resulting in a more homogeneous distribution of aeration. The effects of the prone position were more pronounced in patients with lobar acute lung injury. Taken together, these studies support the idea that the prone position, when performed after a recruitment manoeuvre or after PEEP optimisation, is an effective method of recruiting non-aerated alveolar units and preventing overinflation, especially in lobar acute lung injury or in ARDS. This approach could further protect the lung tissue, possibly alleviating direct mechanical injury to the lung parenchyma.

Clinical Studies

After the pioneering studies of Piehl and Brown [4] and Douglas et al. [5], other investigations confirmed earlier findings showing that gas exchange was improved in patients with ARDS who were turned from the supine to the prone position [6–15]. Additionally, prone positioning was remarkably well-tolerated and clinically relevant complications were not detected during the turn or afterwards in any of the reported studies. Studies that examined the effects of the prone position on respiratory-system mechanics in obese humans [46] found no changes in the components of respiratory-system compliance, either the chest wall or the lung, whereas both FRC and PaO_2 significantly increased from the supine to the prone position. Since these patients were positioned to assure free abdominal and chest movements, the authors hypothesised that the predominant motion of non-dependent diaphragmatic regions during ventilation in the prone position caused non-dependent lung regions to receive more ventilation.

Studies in humans with ARDS showed that compliance of the respiratory system (Crs) improved with prone positioning. Servillo et al. [13] measured P-V curves of the respiratory system and found a mean increase of 7 ml/cmH_2O in Crs when patients were prone. However, these authors did not measure end-expiratory lung volume, and P-V curves obtained in the supine and prone positions cannot be placed in the same plot, since the volumes corresponding to FRC were probably not the same. Consequently, it was unclear whether the changes in Crs corresponded to a modification of the mechanical characteristics of the respiratory system or tidal breathing taking place in another segment of the P-V curve. However, Pelosi et al. [14] found a reduction in chest-wall compliance without modifications in lung compliance in ARDS patients positioned in the prone vs. the supine position. The authors argued that a different distribution of tidal volume occurred in the prone position. In other words, the stiffness of the dorsal aspect in a given position regulated the regional distribution of tidal volume. The same group [14] also found that basal chest-wall compliance and its changes played a role in determining the oxygenation response in prone positioned patients (lower chest-wall compliance in supine, less improvement in oxygenation). In addition, the magnitude of the decrease in thoracoabdominal compliance with the turn was associated with a greater improvement in oxygenation. This finding in humans with ARDS is similar to the data of Mure et al. [33] in their study of normal pigs and highlights the importance of the interactions between rib cage, lungs and abdomen during prone positioning. Also, these data suggest that free abdominal protrusion and motion during prone positioning in humans with ARDS need not occur. In a study conducted by our group [12], PaO_2/FiO_2 improvements were >15% in the prone position in 70% of patients, together with a significant increase in respiratory system compliance in those patients who responded to the prone position. Interestingly, we found that the time elapsed since the onset of ARDS was shorter in responders than in patients who did not show improved oxygenation in the prone position. This suggests that prone positioning should be applied as early as possible after the onset of the disease.

Recently, Vieillard-Baron et al. [47] tested the hypothesis that ventilation in the prone position might improve homogenisation of tidal ventilation by reducing time-constant inequalities, thus improving alveolar ventilation. Interestingly, they found that the prone position significantly reduced the expiratory time constant from baseline with ZEEP, and significantly decreased $PaCO_2$ from 55 mmHg at baseline with ZEEP to 50 mmHg. This improvement in alveolar ventilation was accompanied by a significant improvement in respiratory-system mechanics and in arterial oxygenation. The study provided indirect evidence for a reduction in time-constant heterogeneity, thus suggesting a more even distribution of tidal volume in ARDS patients ventilated in the prone position.

Prone Position and Adjuncts of Mechanical Ventilation

Mechanical ventilation is a life-saving treatment for patients with acute respiratory failure. Over the past decade, there has been interest to identify other therapeutic options or adjuncts that, together with the mechanical ventilation, improve both clinician's understanding of the pathophysiology of respiratory failure and patient outcome. The combination of prone positioning with, e.g., nitric-oxide (NO) inhalation, recruitment manoeuvres and high-frequency oscillatory ventilation has been tested but the results have been controversial. Martinez et al. [48] assessed the combined effects of NO and prone position in ARDS patients. In the prone position, PaO_2/FIO_2 increased significantly and venous admixture decreased in 60% of the patients; however, in both cases the combination of NO therapy and prone positioning was only additive. This combination also yielded a positive oxygenation response in 13 of the 14 patients treated, compared to supine patients who were not administered NO. Furthermore, NO-induced changes in PaO_2/FIO_2 correlated with changes in pulmonary vascular resistance only in prone patients, indicating that the combination of NO and prone positioning has additive effects on oxygenation because the prone position allows NO to reach previously shunted pulmonary vessels. Similar results were reported by Rialp et al. [49].

Recruitment manoeuvres can be useful to improve oxygenation in patients with ARDS receiving mechanical ventilation with low PEEP and low tidal volume. However, in patients with ARDS receiving mechanical ventilation with high PEEP levels the beneficial effects of recruitment manoeuvres are less clear. Cakar et al. [50] showed that, when recruitment is achieved with posture in experimental animals, better oxygenation after recruitment manoeuvres is obtained in the prone than in the supine position, and importantly, the benefit is sustained at lower PEEP. Oczenski et al. [51] evaluated the interaction of recruitment manoeuvres and prone positioning on gas exchange and venous admixture in patients with early extrapulmonary ARDS ventilated with high levels of positive end-expiratory pressure. They found that sustained inflation performed after 6 h of prone positioning induced sustained improvement of oxygenation and venous admixture in both responders and non-responders to prone positioning. Therefore, recruitment manoeuvres as an adjunct to improve oxygenation in ARDS during prone position could be used in selected severe hypoxaemic patients.

Improvement in oxygenation related to the prone position is not persistent in most patients when they are returned to the supine position. Therefore, in non-persistent responders to prone positioning, a strategy of prolonged periods in this position can be proposed but much greater attention has to be paid to avoid or decrease risks of skin lesions. Recently, Demory et al. [52] randomized 44 ARDS patients with a PaO_2/FIO_2 ratio <150 at PEEP >5 cmH_2O to receive one of the following three treatments: (a) conventional lung-protective mechanical ventilation in the prone position followed by a period of conventional lung-protective mechanical ventilation in the supine position; (b) conventional lung-protective mechanical ventilation in the supine position followed by high-frequency oscillatory ventilation (HFOV) in the supine position; or (c) conventional lung-protective mechanical ventilation in the prone position followed by HFOV in the supine position. Compared with the other groups, PaO_2/FIO_2 was higher and venous admixture lower at the end of the study period in the conventional lung-protective mechanical ventilation in the prone position followed by HFOV in the supine position. HFOV maintained the improvement in oxygenation related to prone positioning when ARDS patients were returned to the supine position. HFOV appears valuable, at least theoretically, because pressure swings are dampened during transmission to the alveoli, and the sustained high mean airway pressure may open slow-recruiting compartments while keeping fast-collapsing portions of the lungs open [53]. Therefore, the combination of HFOV with prone positioning could be synergic.

Randomised Multi-centre Clinical Trials on the Use of Prone Position in ARDS Patients

Four clinical studies have evaluated the impact on outcome after prone positioning of adult patients with ARDS. Although the increase in PaO_2/FIO_2 was consistently and repeatedly greater in the prone than in the supine groups, no effect was detected regarding clinical outcome. Gattinoni et al. [54] compared conventional treatment (in the supine position) with a predefined strategy of placing patients in a prone position for ≥6 h daily for 10 days. The study comprised 304 patients (152 in each group) but no differences in mortality were found at 10 days, at the time of discharge from the intensive care unit, or at 6 months. The relative risk of death in the prone group compared with the supine group was 0.84 at the end of the study period (95% CI, 0.56–1.27), 1.05 at the time of discharge from the intensive care unit (95% CI, 0.84–1.32), and 1.06 at 6 months (95% CI, 0.88–1.28). Guerin et al. [55] randomly assigned patients with acute respiratory failure to prone positioning (n=413), applied as early as possible for at least 8 h per day on standard beds, or to supine positioning (n=378). The 28-day mortality rate was 32.4% for the prone group and 31.5% for the supine group [relative risk (RR), 0.97; 95% CI 0.79–1.19; p=0.77]. However, for patients with hypoxaemic ARF, prone positioning lowered the incidence of ventilator-associated pneumonia, although the incidences of pressure sores, selective intubation and endotracheal-tube obstruction were higher in the prone group. Voggenreiter et al. [56] studied the effect of prone positioning on the duration of mechanical ventilation in multiple trauma patients who were ventilated for at least 8 h and a maximum of 23 h per day; these patients were compared with those ventilated in the supine position. The authors found that the duration of ventilatory support did not differ significantly but the prone group showed a reduction in the prevalence of pneumonia. Finally, Mancebo et al. [57] enrolled 136 patients within 48 h of tracheal intubation for severe ARDS; 60 were randomised to supine and 76 to prone ventilation. Guidelines were established for ventilator settings and weaning, and the prone group was targeted to receive continuous prone ventilation treatment for 20 h/day. Interestingly, mortality in the intensive care unit was 58% (35/60) in patients ventilated supine and 43% (33/76) in those ventilated prone (p=0.12). Multivariate analysis showed that the simplified acute physiology score II at inclusion (OR, 1.07; p<0.001), number of days elapsed between ARDS diagnosis and inclusion (OR, 2.83; p<0.001), and randomisation to supine position (OR, 2.53; p=0.03) were independent risk factors for mortality. After a total of 718 turning procedures only 28 complications were reported, and most were rapidly reversible. The study authors concluded that prone ventilation is feasible, safe and may reduce mortality in patients with severe ARDS when it is initiated early and applied for most of the day.

Decades of use of the prone position has confirmed it to be a safe procedure that increases oxygenation in the majority of ARDS patients when properly applied [58]. Moreover, in experienced hands, proning of ARDS patients is not associated with major complications. Detailed examination of the four multicentre randomised trials on the use of prone positioning in ARDS suggests that the four trials cannot be compared and are not conclusive on the use of this adjunct of mechanical ventilation. Major differences between those studies are that neither the day-average (hours) prone time nor the total (days) of prone time duration was the same, many patients randomised to the prone group missed several periods of pronation, there were numerous different diagnoses at study entry, ventilatory and weaning guidelines were not systematically employed, routine care differed between studies and, finally, some studies were limited by the fact that they were stopped due to decreased patient accrual and were thus underpowered. Therefore, an appropriately powered trial is needed to re-evaluate whether prone ventilation reduces mortality in patients with ARDS.

References

1. Amato MBP, Barbas CS, Medeiros DM et al (1998) Effect of a protective-ventilation strategy on mortality in the acute respiratory distress syndrome. N Engl J Med 338:347–354
2. Tremblay L, Valenza F, Ribeiro SP et al (1997) Injurious ventilatory strategies increase cytokines and c-fos m-RNA expression in an isolated rat lung model. J Clin Invest 99:944–952
3. Marini JJ, Amato MBP (1998) Lung recruitment during ARDS. In: Marini JJ, Evans TW (eds) Acute lung injury. Springer, Berlin, pp 236–257
4. Piehl MA, Brown RS (1976) Use of extreme position changes in respiratory failure. Crit Care Med 4:13–14
5. Douglas WW, Rehder K, Beynen FM et al (1977) Improved oxygenation in patients with acute respiratory failure: the prone position. Am Rev Respir Dis 115:559–566
6. Langer M, Mascheroni D, Marcolin R, Gattinoni L (1988) The prone position in ARDS patients. Chest 94:103–107
7. Flaatten H, Aardal S, Hevroy O (1998) Improved oxygenation using the prone position in patients with ARDS. Acta Anaesthesiol Scand 42:329–334
8. Priolet B, Tempelhoff JM, Cannamela A et al (1993) Ventilation assistée en decubitus ventral: évaluation tomodensitométrique de son efficacité dans le traitement des condensations pulmonaires. Rean Urg 2:81–85
9. Gattinoni L, Pelosi P, Vitale G et al (1991) Body position changes redistribute lung computed-tomographic density in patients with acute respiratory failure. Anesthesiology 74:15–23
10. Chatte G, Sab JM, Dubois JM et al (1997) Prone position in mechanically ventilated patients with severe acute respiratory failure. Am J Respir Crit Care Med 155:473–478
11. Vollman KM, Bander JJ (1996) Improved oxygenation utilizing a prone positioner in patients with acute respiratory distress syndrome. Intensive Care Med 22:1105–1111
12. Blanch Ll, Mancebo J, Perez M et al (1997) Short-term effects of prone position in critically ill patients with acute respiratory distress syndrome. Intensive Care Med 23:1033–1039
13. Servillo G, Roupie E, De Robertis E et al (1997) Effects of ventilation in ventral decubitus position on respiratory mechanics in adult respiratory distress syndrome. Intensive Care Med 23:1219–1224
14. Pelosi P, Tubiolo D, Mascheroni D et al (1998) Effects of the prone position on respiratory mechanics and gas exchange during acute lung injury. Am J Respir Crit Care Med 157:387–393
15. Mure M, Martling CR, Lindahl GE (1997) Dramatic effect on oxygenation in patients with severe acute lung insufficiency treated in the prone position. Crit Care Med 25:1539–1544
16. Milic-Emili J, Henderson JAM, Dolovich MB et al (1966) Regional distribution of inspired gas in the lung. J Appl Physiol 21:749–759

17. Anthonisen NR (1985) Gravity. In: Roussos C, Macklem PT (eds) The thorax, part B. Marcel Dekker, New York, pp 737–749
18. Pelosi P, Croci M, Calappi E et al (1995) The prone positioning during general anesthesia minimally affects respiratory mechanics while improving functional residual capacity and increasing oxygen tension. Anesth Analg 80:955–960
19. Gattinoni L, Pelosi P, Valenza F, Mascheroni D (1994) Patient positioning in acute respiratory failure. In: Tobin MJ (ed) Principles and practice of mechanical ventilation. McGraw-Hill, New York, pp 1067–1076
20. Pelosi P, D'Andrea L, Vitale G et al (1994) Vertical gradient of regional lung inflation in adult respiratory distress syndrome. Am J Respir Crit Care Med 149:8–13
21. Cook DC, Mead J, Schreiner GL et al (1975) Pulmonary mechanics during induced pulmonary edema in anesthetized dogs. J Appl Physiol 38:681–687
22. Albert RK (1998) The effect of body position on perfusion, ventilation, and gas exchange in normal and injured lungs. In: Marini JJ, Slutsky AS (eds) Physiological basis of ventilatory support. Marcel Dekker, New York, pp 1093–1112
23. Wiener-Kronish JP, Gropper MA, Lai-Fook SJ (1985) Pleural liquid pressure in dogs measured using a rib capsule. J Appl Physiol 59:597–602
24. Yang QH, Kaplowitz MR, Lai-Fook SJ (1989) Regional variations in lung expansion in rabbits prone vs. supine positions. J Appl Physiol 67:1371–1376
25. Yang QH, Lai-Fook SJ (1991) Effect of lung inflation on regional lung expansion in supine and prone rabbits. J Appl Physiol 71:76–82
26. Mutoh T, Guest RJ, Lamm WJE, Albert RK (1992) Prone position alters the effect of volume overload on regional pleural pressures and improves hypoxemia in pigs in vivo. Am Rev Respir Dis 146:300–306
27. Albert RK (1994) One good turn. Intensive Care Med 20:247–248
28. Albert RK (1998) Permissive hypercapnia or the prone position. In: Marini JJ, Evans TW (eds) Acute lung injury. Springer, Berlin, pp 329–337
29. Froese A (1989) Anesthesia-paralysis and the diaphragm: in pursuit of an elusive muscle. Anesthesiology 70:887–890
30. Froese AB, Bryan AC (1974) Effects on anesthesia and paralysis on diaphragmatic mechanics in man. Anesthesiology 41:242–255
31. Rehder K, Knopp TJ, Sessler AD (1978) Regional intrapulmonary gas distribution in awake and anesthetized-paralyzed prone man. J Appl Physiol 45:528–535
32. Krayer S, Rehder K, Vetterman J et al (1989) Position and motion of the human diaphragm during anesthesia-paralysis. Anesthesiology 70:891–898
33. Mure M, Glenny RW, Domino KB, Hlastala MP (1998) Pulmonary gas exchange improves in the prone position with abdominal distension. Am J Respir Crit Care Med 157:1785–1790
34. Johansson MJ, Wiklund A, Flateba T et al (2004) Positive end-expiratory pressure affects regional redistribution of ventilation differently in prone and supine sheep. Crit Care Med 32:2039–2044
35. Albert RK, Leasa D, Sanderson M et al (1987) Prone position improves arterial oxygenation and reduces shunt in oleic acid-induced acute lung injury. Am Rev Respir Dis 135:628–635
36. Wiener CM, Kirk W, Albert RK (1990) Prone position reverses gravitional distribution of perfusion in dogs with oleic acid-induced injury. J Appl Physiol 68:1386–1392
37. Lamm WJE, Graham MM, Albert RK (1994) Mechanism by which the prone position improves oxygenation in acute lung injury. Am J Respir Crit Care Med 150:184–193
38. Pappert D, Rossaint R, Slama K et al (1994) Influence of positioning on ventilation-perfusion relationships in severe adult respiratory distress syndrome. Chest 106:1511–1516
39. Glenny RW, Lamm WJE, Albert RK, Robertson HT (1991) Gravity is a minor determinant of pulmonary blood flow distribution. J Appl Physiol 71:620–629
40. Richter T, Bellani G, Scott Harris R et al (2005) Effect of prone position on regional shunt, aeration, and perfusion in experimental acute lung injury. Am J Respir Crit Care Med 172:480–487

41. Gattinoni L, Carlesso E, Cadringher P et al (2003) Physical and biological triggers of ventilator-induced lung injury and its prevention. Eur Respir J 47(Suppl):15s-25s
42. Valenza F, Guglielmi M, Maffioletti M et al (2005) Prone position delays the progression of ventilator-induced lung injury in rats: does lung strain distribution play a role? Crit Care Med 33:361–367
43. Broccard A, Shapiro RS, Schmitz LL et al (2000) Prone positioning attenuates and redistributes ventilator-induced lung injury in dogs. Crit Care Med 28:295–303
44. Mentzelopoulos SD, Roussos C, Zakynthinos SG (2005) Prone position reduces lung stress and strain in severe acute respiratory distress syndrome. Eur Respir J 25:534–544
45. Galiatsou E, Kostanti E, Svarna E et al (2006) Prone position augments recruitment and prevents alveolar overinflation in acute lung injury. Am J Respir Crit Care Med 174:187–197
46. Pelosi P, Croci M, Calappi E et al (1996) Prone positioning improves pulmonary function in obese patients during general anesthesia. Anesth Analg 83:578–583
47. Vieillard-Baron A, Rabiller A, Chergui K et al (2005) Prone position improves mechanics and alveolar ventilation in acute respiratory distress syndrome. Intensive Care Med 31:220–226
48. Martinez M, Diaz E, Joseph D et al (1999) Improvement in oxygenation by prone position and nitric oxide in patients with acute respiratory distress syndrome. Intensive Care Med 25:29–36
49. Rialp G, Betbese AJ, Perez-Marquez M, Mancebo J (2001) Short-term effects of inhaled nitric oxide and prone position in pulmonary and extrapulmonary acute respiratory distress syndrome. Am J Respir Crit Care Med 164:243–249
50. Cakar N, der Kloot TV, Youngblood M et al (2000) Oxygenation response to a recruitment maneuver during supine and prone positions in an oleic acid-induced lung injury model. Am J Respir Crit Care Med 161:1949–1956
51. Oczenski W, Hormann C, Keller C et al (2005) Recruitment maneuvers during prone positioning in patients with acute respiratory distress syndrome. Crit Care Med 33:54–61
52. Demory D, Michelet P, Arnal JM et al (2007) High-frequency oscillatory ventilation following prone positioning prevents a further impairment in oxygenation. Crit Care Med 35:106–111
53. Papazian L, Gainnier M, Marin V et al (2005) Comparison of prone positioning and high-frequency oscillatory ventilation in patients with acute respiratory distress syndrome. Crit Care Med 33:2162–2171
54. Gattinoni L, Tognoni G, Pesenti A et al.; Prone-Supine Study Group (2001) Effect of prone positioning on the survival of patients with acute respiratory failure. N Engl J Med 345:568–573
55. Guerin C, Gaillard S, Lemasson S et al (2004) Effects of systematic prone positioning in hypoxemic acute respiratory failure: a randomized controlled trial. JAMA 292:2379–2387
56. Voggenreiter G, Aufmkolk M, Stiletto RJ et al (2005) Prone positioning improves oxygenation in post-traumatic lung injury: a prospective randomized trial. J Trauma 59:333–341
57. Mancebo J, Fernandez R, Blanch L et al (2006) A multicenter trial of prolonged prone ventilation in severe acute respiratory distress syndrome. Am J Respir Crit Care Med 173:1233–1239
58. Nakos G, Tsangaris I, Kostanti E et al (2000) Effect of the prone position on patients with hydrostatic pulmonary edema compared with patients with acute respiratory distress syndrome and pulmonary fibrosis. Am J Respir Crit Care Med 161:360–368

Prone Ventilation in Trauma Patients

G. Voggenreiter

Introduction

Patients in extremis because of trauma-related massive chest injury require expedient evaluation and prompt intervention. The initial pathophysiology relates to the significant intrapulmonary shunting caused by disruption of pulmonary capillaries and extravasation into the alveolar spaces. Disproportionate or unilateral lung involvement needs measures more technical than general supportive care. Independent lung ventilation (mostly with unilateral lung involvement) and other strategies, such as inhaled nitric oxide, prone positioning, partial liquid ventilation, and extracorporeal membrane oxygenation (ECMO), have had good results. Intensivists confronted with this clinical subset may consider using these strategies as alternative/adjunctive options for optimising respiratory and haemodynamic status in the supportive management of trauma-related acute lung injury (ALI) and adult respiratory distress syndrome (ARDS).

In 1974, Bryan was the first to suggest prone positioning to improve gas exchange in patients with severe ARDS [1]. Based on numerous studies indicating an improvement of gas exchange, the prone position has been increasingly used in the last decade. Prone positioning results in the recruitment of alveoli [2], a more uniform regional ventilation-perfusion relationship [3–5] and therefore an improvement of gas exchange [6–8] as a result of postural differences in chest-wall mechanics [9] and an eliminated compression of the lungs by the heart [10].

In a non-randomised study published recently, intermittent prone positioning improved pulmonary gas exchange significantly in multiple trauma patients with severe ARDS as well as in patients with moderate lung injury. However, the non-randomised study design did not provide conclusive evidence that intermittent prone positioning improves outcome [11]. The results of other studies were encouraging [12], but the findings needed to be confirmed by randomised controlled trials to determine whether intermittent prone positioning will improve outcome or shorten ventilatory support in patients with ALI or ARDS.

U. Lucangelo, P. Pelosi, W.A. Zin, A. Aliverti (eds.) *Respiratory System and Artificial Ventilation.* © Springer 2008

Gas Exchange and Mortality

A multicentre randomised trial was published recently by Gattinoni et al. [13]. Conventional treatment (in the supine position) of patients with ALI or ARDS was compared to a predefined strategy of placing patients in a prone position. The study confirmed that prone positioning improves oxygenation but no positive effects on outcome were demonstrated. The authors found that use of the prone position improved oxygenation in more than 70% of the instances in which it was used, with about 70% of the effect occurring during the first hour of pronation. However, the mortality rate did not differ significantly between the prone group and the supine group at the end of the 10-day study period (21.1 vs. 25.0%) and at the time of discharge from the intensive care unit (50.7 vs. 48.0%). However the study has been criticised because of inhomogeneous study population, the short period of ventilation in prone position and the relatively low PEEP-levels used.

In a randomised trial, we therefore assessed the effect of a predefined strategy of prone positioning on the duration of mechanical ventilation in multiple trauma patients with ALI or ARDS [14]. In this study involving a homogeneous series of 40 multiple-injured patients, intermittent prone positioning was not able to reduce the duration of mechanical ventilation. However, a significant improvement of pulmonary function in patients ventilated in the prone position was observed: (1) the PaO_2:FiO_2 ratio improved significantly over the first 4 days of treatment in the prone group; (2) the prevalence of ARDS and the number of days with ALI were reduced and (3) there was a lower incidence of pneumonia. These findings concerned the secondary endpoints. No differences between the two groups regarding various parameters of gas exchange were evident after 10 days. The lack of an associated reduction of ventilator time and mortality may reflect the small sample size in this study, and it is possible that with a larger group of patients significant reductions might be observed. Nonetheless, the improvement of gas exchange, reduction of days with ALI, and reduction of prevalence of ARDS following ALI demonstrates the potential benefit of prone positioning. These findings confirm the experimental results of the lung protective effects of the prone position [15,16]. Additionally in the worst-case analysis of all patients, a trend towards a reduction of the duration of ventilatory support was observed. A study on the influence of body position on the pulmonary surfactant system detected no effect of prone position on surfactant composition and surfactant function [17].

In the present study, the mortality of trauma patients was lower than that reported in other studies of prone positioning, including lung injury of various origins [13]. The mortality rate of 10% also compares favourably with other studies on prone positioning of trauma patients. Micheals et al. [18] and Fridrich et al. [8] reported a mortality rate of 14 and 10%, respectively. These low mortality rates in trauma-induced ARDS make it difficult to detect a reduction of mortality.

Based on the results of Gattinoni et al. [13] there might be some benefit of the prone position for patients with severe hypoxaemia. This is supported by the findings of Lee et al. [19] indicating that patients with larger shunts have a better oxygenation response. Therefore, mechanical ventilation in the prone position may be beneficial to outcome in patients with severe ARDS characterised by pronounced dorsal-lung densities, as shown in CT scans. Hence it may be speculated that further clinical studies on mechanical ventilation of patients in the prone position should focus on patients with severe ARDS, since they have a higher potential to benefit than patients with ALI.

Compared to the studies of Gattinoni and others [13,19,20], we found a remarkable low rate of non-responders (PaO_2:FiO_2 ratio <10% of baseline after a maximum of 24 h) at a mean duration of prone position of 11 h a day. Only one out of 21 patients did not respond to prone positioning. This result supports the observation that ventilation in the prone position for more prolonged periods may be required for optimal improvement [21].

In the randomised study of Mancebo et al., mortality in the intensive care unit was 58% (35/60) in patients ventilated supine and 43% (33/76) in patients ventilated prone (p=0.12) [22]. The latter group had a higher simplified acute physiology score II at inclusion. Multivariate analysis showed that the simplified acute physiology score II at inclusion (OR, 1.07; p<0.001), number of days elapsed between ARDS diagnosis and inclusion (OR, 2.83; p<0.001), and randomisation to the supine position (OR, 2.53; p=0.03) were independent risk factors for mortality. Prone position was applied for a mean of 17 h/day for a mean of 10 days.

Guerin et al. found an improved oxygenation by prone positioning but no reduction in mortality [23]. This result was obtained with lower VT, PEEP, and FIO_2 in the prone position group than in the supine group. Patients were randomly assigned to prone position placement (n=413), applied as early as possible for at least 8 h per day on standard beds, or to supine position placement (n=378). The 28-day mortality rate was 32.4% for the prone group and 31.5% for the supine group. The 90-day mortality for the prone group was 43.3 vs. 42.2% for the supine group. The mean duration of mechanical ventilation was 13.7 (7.8) days for the prone group vs. 14.1 (8.6) days for the supine group (p=0.93)

Reduction of Pneumonia

Immobility is an important risk factor for the development of atelectasis and nosocomial infections in critically ill patients requiring mechanical ventilation. Our study detected a reduction of the prevalence of nosocomial pneumonia in patients ventilated prone but the use of antibiotics was not different between the two groups [14]. This may be attributed to the enhanced mobilisation of secretions following alteration of the patients' position and the maintenance of airway patency [24–26], but we do not have data from the present investigation to support the assertion that prone positioning should be used to improve mucociliary clearance. In the study of Guerin et al., the incidence of ventilator-associated pneumonia was significantly lower in the prone group. The reported incidence of VAP in the prone and supine groups was 1.66 vs. 2.14 episodes per 100-patients days of intubation, respectively (p=0.045) [23].

As far as we know, other studies on intermittent prone positioning have not reported a reduction of pneumonia. However several randomised studies on continuous postural oscillation found a decreased prevalence of pneumonia but no difference in mortality [27,28]. All these data suggest that, although pneumonia and impaired gas exchange add to morbidity, they may not be the primary cause of mortality.

Kinetic Therapy

Kinetic therapy is defined by the Centers for Disease Control and Prevention as the use of a bed that turns continuously and slowly over >40° along its longitudinal axis. Clinical studies have shown advantages in using kinetic therapy to decrease atelectasis and pneumonia in trauma and surgical patients [28–30]. Additionally, the use of kinetic therapy significantly improved the PaO_2/FiO_2 ratio in mechanically ventilated patients with ALI or ARDS [31].

Nevertheless, no study to date has demonstrated a survival advantage with the use of kinetic therapy in trauma and surgical patients with ALI or ARDS. One prospective trial demonstrated no advantage to prone positioning over continuous lateral rotational therapy (roto-rest) in patients with ARDS [32]. A recent investigation in multiple trauma patients demonstrated improved oxygenation, PaO_2/FiO_2 ratio, and decreased FiO_2 requirement with continuous rotation in the prone position compared with continuous rotation in the supine position. That study demonstrated a significant reduction in mortality (overall and pulmonary related) with prone kinetic therapy. Additionally, patients who were prone had decreased duration of ventilatory support and length of stay. The use of a prone oscillating bed was advantageous in trauma and surgical patients with ALI or ARDS and was superior to supine kinetic therapy [33].

Neurotrauma

Neuro-intensivists are more hesitant to use prone positioning, considering the risk of intracranial hypertension caused by the turning procedure and prone posture itself. Positioning of the patient has a great effect on intracranial pressure (ICP). Supine 30° head-up posture is recommended to achieve the lowest ICP. However, in patients with severe respiratory insufficiency and hypoxaemia, the situation may be different. Theoretically, an improved gas exchange and arterial oxygenation result in lower ICP, because of a beneficial effect of improved oxygen transport to the damaged brain. In a pilot study [34], 11 out of 12 patients with reduced intracranial compliance who were placed in the prone position for 3 h had significantly improved PaO_2, SaO_2 and respiratory-system compliance without alterations in intracranial or circulatory parameters. Contrary to these results, Reinprecht et al. [35], in a retrospective investigation, found a significant increase in ICP and a significant decrease in cerebral perfusion pressure (CPP) in the prone position in patients suffering from subarachnoid haemorrhage (n=16). These patients were placed in the prone position for 14 h, which perhaps explains the differences in ICP and CPP results. Another study was undertaken to further explore whether the advantages of the prone position outweigh the risk of intracranial hypertension in patients with reduced intracranial compliance [36]. The principal finding was an improved oxygenation, a slightly increased ICP, and moderately increased mean arterial pressure (MAP) during treatment of patients in the prone position. As MAP increased to a greater extent than ICP, this resulted in an improved CPP in the prone position. However patients with high ICP were not included in the study.

Complications

Despite the encouraging results, prone ventilation has not been widely accepted in the management of ARDS. One reason for this reluctance is that prone positioning is viewed as a complex manoeuvre with potential life-threatening complications. Reports to date suggest that prone positioning is safe in critically ill patients; however, details have been lacking. The purpose of our study was to investigate the use of prone positioning in severely injured and critically ill postoperative patients with ARDS refractory to our standard management [14]. Particular attention was devoted to the complications of prone ventilation in this group of patients. Critically ill patients with ARDS frequently have multiple chest tubes, arterial and venous access catheters and endotracheal or tracheostomy tubes. Loss of any of these during turning may have devastating consequences. Other safety concerns include inability to perform cardiopulmonary resuscitation in the event of cardiac arrest, development of peripheral nerve injuries or skin necrosis and damage to the eyes. While most reports have suggested that prone positioning is safe, the associated complications have not been well-documented in the literature to date.

Comparison of the incidence of complications that were most likely related to positioning during the study period showed a tendency of an increased number of pressure sores in the prone group but a higher number of patients with swelling and oedema in the supine group. The number of pressure sores seemed to be high. This was explained by documenting all superficial skin lesions that could be attributed not only to positioning but also to trauma. Maximum standard bedside care was administered to all patients. Surprisingly, the number of patients with displacement of endotracheal tubes was similar in the two groups.

Since these events were expected to be more frequent in the prone group than in the supine group, our findings suggest that the use of appropriate nursing precautions may prevent them. However, in two patients of the prone group a transient decrease of minute ventilation and PaO_2 was observed immediately after posture change into the prone position. Furthermore, arrhythmias were observed more frequently in the prone group.

Offner et al. [37] noted significant complications in four of nine patients treated with prone positioning, including abdominal wound dehiscence, skin necrosis, and cardiac arrest. Facial and periorbital oedema was present in all patients and was not considered a complication.

In a multicentre trial, complications related to prone positioning per se were few and clinically mild [22]. Oedema (facial, limbs, thorax) was observed in 14 of the 80 patients, but rapidly improved when patients were turned supine. Conjunctival haemorrhage and pressure sores were observed in two patients each, and one patient exhibited a vascular catheter malfunction during continuous veno-venous haemofiltration. Complications directly attributable to the turning procedures were as follows: the inadvertent dislodging of a Swan-Ganz catheter during the turn was accompanied by cardiac arrest in one patient, but resuscitation was successful; in two other patients, lines were accidentally displaced (a urinary bladder catheter and a nasogastric feeding tube); and kinking occurred in the endotracheal tube of one patient and the thoracic drain of another. All together, a total of 28 complications were noted.

The risk of complications may be minimised with anticipation and attention to detail during implementation of the prone position. Several recommendations for prone ventilation are worth emphasising. An institutional protocol to standardise the process of prone positioning in critically ill trauma patients should be developed. Problems with the patient's airway, vascular access, and other invasive devices should be anticipated. During the turning process, an adequate number of personnel should be present. We use two intensive care unit nurses, one staff physician and a respiratory therapist who is responsible for ensuring a secure airway throughout the process. After the turn, all tubes and lines should be rechecked and secured. In addition, ventilator parameters should be reassessed because occasional changes in compliance can lead to changes in airway pressure or tidal volume. Pulmonary secretions may increase and necessitate more frequent suctioning. Care during prone positioning should include elevation of the head of the bed by 10–15° to minimise facial oedema. Moreover, particular attention should be given to protecting the eyes. Careful padding of pressure points and use of appropriate specialty beds may help reduce skin breakdown. Finally, the neck and extremities, especially if external fixators have been for fracture stabilisation, should be placed in appropriate physiologic positions to avoid compression neuropathy.

Conclusions

The present results confirm the role of prone positioning in our critical care armamentarium. The potential utility of this intervention regarding oxygenation and reduction of pneumonia is supported by data from recent studies. However, despite the enthusiasm related to improvement of gas exchange, there still is little encouragement in the conversion of physiologic improvement to clinical outcome benefit in adults. Using prone ventilation for prolonged periods of time is both feasible and safe, and it may reduce mortality in ARDS patients. To date, none of the four trials (Table 1) designed to evaluate the effect of prone ventilation on mortality in adult patients with ARDS have been sufficiently powered to confirm a benefit or the lack thereof. An appropriately powered trial is needed to re-evaluate whether prone ventilation reduces mortality in patients with ARDS.

Table 1 Randomised controlled trials evaluating ventilation in the prone position for the treatment of patients with ARDS

Study	Patients (*N*)	Intervention	Mortality	*p*
Gattinoni et al. [13]	304	Prone position 6 h/d for 10 days	63 vs. 59%	0.65
Guerin et al. [23]	791	Prone position 8 h/day	32 vs. 32%	0.77
Mancebo et al. [22]	136	Prone position 20 h/day	50 vs. 62%	0.22
Voggenreiter et al. [14]	41	Prone position 11 h/day	5 vs. 16%	0.27

References

1. Bryan AC (1975) Comments of a devil's advocate. Am Rev Respir Dis 110(Suppl):143–144
2. Guerin C, Badet M, Roselli S et al (1999) Effects of prone position on alveolar recruitment and oxygenation in acute lung injury. Intensive Care Med 25:1222–1230
3. Wiener CM, Kirk W, Albert RK (1990) Prone position reverses gravitational distribution of perfusion in dog lungs with oleic acid-induced injury. J Appl Physiol 68:1386–92
4. Pappert D, Rossaint R, Slama K et al (1994) Influence of positioning on ventilation-perfusion relationships in severe adult respiratory distress syndrome. Chest 106:1511–1516
5. Lamm WJ, Graham MM, Albert RK (1994) Mechanism by which the prone position improves oxygenation in acute lung injury. Am J Respir Crit Care Med 150:184–193
6. Blanch L, Mancebo J, Perez M et al (1997) Short-term effects of prone position in critically ill patients with acute respiratory distress syndrome. Intensive Care Med 23:1033–1039
7. Stocker R, Neff T, Stein S et al (1997) Prone postioning and low-volume pressure-limited ventilation improve survival in patients with severe ARDS. Chest 11:1008–1017
8. Fridrich P, Krafft P, Hochleuthner H, Mauritz W (1996) The effects of long-term prone positioning in patients with trauma-induced adult respiratory distress syndrome. Anesth Analg 83:1206–1211

9. Pelosi P, Tubiolo D, Mascheroni D et al (1998) Effects of the prone position on respiratory mechanics and gas exchange during acute lung injury. Am J Respir Crit Care Med 157:387–393
10. Albert R, Hubmayr R (2000) The prone position eliminates compression of the lungs by the heart. Am J Respir Crit Care Med 161:1660–1665
11. Voggenreiter G, Neudeck F, Aufmkolk M et al (1999) Intermittent prone positioning in the treatment of severe and moderate posttraumatic lung injury. Crit Care Med 27:2375–2382
12. Erhard J, Waydhas C, Ruchholz S et al (1998) Einfluss der kinetischen Therapie auf den Behandlungsverlauf bei Patienten mit posttraumatischem Lungenversagen. Unfallchirurg 101:928–934
13. Gattinoni L, Tognoni G, Pesenti A et al (2001) Effect of prone positioning on the survival of patients with acute respiratory failure. New Engl J Med 345:568–573
14. Voggenreiter G, Aufmkolk M, Stiletto RJ et al (2005) Prone positioning improves oxygenation in post-traumatic lung injury—a prospective randomized trial. J Trauma 59:333–343
15. Broccard A, Shapiro R, Schmitz L et al (2000) Prone positioning attenuates and redistributes ventilator-induced lung injury in dogs. Crit Care Med 28:295–303
16. Broccard AF, Shapiro RS, Schmitz LL et al (1997) Influence of prone position on the extent and distribution of lung injury in a high tidal volume oleic acid model of acute respiratory distress syndrome. Crit Care Med 25:16–27
17. Aufmkolk M, Voggenreiter G, Mattern T et al (2005) Effect of prone position on lung surfactant composition and function in multiple trauma patients with respiratory dysfunction. Eur J Trauma 31:33–38
18. Michaels A, Wanek S, Dreifuss B et al (2002) A protocolized approach to pulmonary failure and the role of intermittent prone positioning. J Trauma 52:1037–1047
19. Lee D, Chiang H, Lin S et al (2002) Prone-position ventilation induces sustained improvement in oxigenation in patients with acute respiratory distress syndrome who have a large shunt. Crit Care Med 30:1446–1452
20. Jolliet P, Bulpa P, Chevrolet JC (1998) Effects of the prone position on gas exchange and hemodynamics in severe acute respiratory distress syndrome. Crit Care Med 26:1977–1985
21. McAuley D, Giles S, Fichter H, Gao F (2002) What is the optimal duration of ventilation in the prone position in acute lung injury and acute respiratory distress syndrome. Intensive Care Med 28:414–418
22. Mancebo J, Fernandez R, Blanch L et al (2006) A multicenter trial of prolonged prone ventilation in severe acute respiratory distress syndrome. Am J Respir Crit Care Med 173:1233–1239
23. Guerin C, Gaillard S, Lemasson S et al (2004) Effects of systematic prone positioning in hypoxemic acute respiratory failure: a randomized controlled trial. JAMA 292:2379–2387
24. Blake J (1975) On the movement of mucus in the lung J Biomech 8:179–190
25. Douglas W, Rehder K, Beynen F et al (1977) Improved oxygenation in patients with acute respiratory failure: the prone position. Am J Respir Crit Care 115:559–566
26. Kaneko K, Milic-Emili J, Dolovich M et al (1966) Regional distribution of ventilation and perfusion as a function of body position. J Appl Physiol 21:767–777
27. Kirschenbaum L, Azzi E, Sfeir T et al (2002) Effect of continuous lateral rotational therapy on the prevalence of ventilator-associated pneumonia in patients requiring long-term ventilatory care. Crit Care Med 30:1983–1986
28. Fink M, Helsmoortel C, Stein K et al (1990) The efficacy of an oscillating bed in the prevention of lower respiratory tract infection in critically ill victims of blunt trauma. A prospective study. Chest 97:132–137
29. Gentillelo L, Thompson DA, Tonnesen AS et al (1988) Effect of a rotating bed on the incidence of pulmonary complications in critically ill patients. Crit Care Med 16:783–786
30. Choi SC, Nelson LD (1992) Kinetic therapy in critically ill patients: combined results on meta-analysis. J Crit Care 7:57–62
31. Raoof S, Chowdhery N, Raoof S et al (1999) Effect of combined kinetic therapy and percussion therapy on the resolution of atelectasis in critically ill patients. Chest 115:1658–1666

32. Staudinger T, Koffler J, Mullner M et al (2001) Comparison of prone positioning and continuous rotation of patients with adult respiratory distress syndrome: results of a pilot study. Crit Care Med 29:51–56
33. Davies JW, Lemaster DM, Moore EC et al (2007) Prone ventilation in trauma or surgical patients with acute lung injury and adult respiratory distress syndrome: is it beneficial? J Trauma 62:1201–1206
34. Thelandersson A, Cider A, Nellgard B (2006) Prone position in mechanically ventilated patients with reduced intracranial compliance. Acta Anaesthesiol Scand 50:937–941
35. Reinprecht A, Greher M, Wolfsberger S et al (2003) Prone position in subarachnoid hemorrhage patients with acute respiratory distress syndrome: effects on cerebral tissue oxygenation and intracranial pressure. Crit Care Med 31:1831–1838
36. Nekludov M, Bellander BM, Mure M (2006) Oxygenation and cerebral perfusion pressure improved in the prone position. Acta Anaesthesiol Scand 50:932–936
37. Offner PJ, Haenel JB, Moore EE et al (2000) Complications of prone ventilation in patients with multisystem trauma with fulminant acute respiratory distress syndrome. J Trauma 49:224–228

Old and New Artificial Ventilation Techniques

Advanced Modalities in Negative-Pressure Ventilation

V. Antonaglia, S. Pascotto, F. Piller

Introduction

Several devices that ensure oxygenation and correct chest-wall motion can support the ventilation of patients with acute respiratory failure (ARF). Ventilation is performed either by the introduction of a flow, and therefore a positive inspiratory pressure into the airways, or by the creation of a negative inspiratory pressure around the thorax and abdomen, which allows the airflow to enter the airways. This latter approach is referred to as external negative-pressure ventilation (NPV).

Positive-pressure ventilation (PPV) may be invasive (IPPV), when given through an endotracheal tube or a tracheostomy cannula, or non-invasive (NIPPV), when devices such as a nasal mask, face mask, or helmet are used.

Negative-pressure body ventilators were the first devices used to assist ventilatory function. The first tank ventilator, the Spirophone, was conceived of in 1876, but it was introduced into clinical practise only in 1928 [1]. These ventilators were frequently used for patients with neuromuscular disorders in acute respiratory failure, e.g. during the poliomyelitis epidemics of the 1930s and 1940s, or for acute respiratory failure due to congestive heart failure and pneumonia [2].

Introduction of the endotracheal tube, which ensures optimal control of the airways, led to the rapid development of invasive ventilation, which surpassed the use of negative ventilation. However, over the years, several complications associated with IPPV have been observed [3,4], and physicians have become more prudent in its use and more likely to use non-invasive ventilatory techniques whenever possible.

The availability of a new generation of negative-pressure ventilators capable of providing different types of NPV could widen the field of application of non-invasive mechanical ventilation to include patients in whom NIPPV has failed, either for clinical reason (such as excessive airway secretion) or patient intolerance (such as difficulty in wearing the mask). This would further reduce the need for endotracheal intubation [5,6].

In this chapter, the devices, physiological effects and possible clinical uses of NPV are considered.

U. Lucangelo, P. Pelosi, W.A. Zin, A. Aliverti (eds.) *Respiratory System and Artificial Ventilation.* © Springer 2008

Ventilators Around the Body

Several negative-pressure ventilators are currently available. All are characterised by either a pump that generates a sub-atmospheric pressure on the surface of the patient's thorax via an applicator or a chamber. From the shape and size of the applicator, three types of ventilators can be distinguished: tank ventilators (the 'iron lung'), chest-shell style ventilators (cuirass) and wrap-shell style ventilators (jacket ventilators or body suit). In the case of tank ventilators, the pump is incorporated into the structure of the ventilator [7–10]. Another kind of external ventilatory-assistance device is the body ventilator which applies a positive expiratory pressure around the abdomen (IAPV, intermittent abdominal positive ventilation) [10].

Tank Ventilator or Iron Lung

The iron lung is a stiff metal chamber completely enclosing the patient's body, with an airtight seal around the neck. The patient rests on his back on a thin mattress while his head lies outside on a rest; side portholes allow access to the patient.

A modified version of the iron lung (Portalung) is constructed of fibreglass, is much smaller and lighter (45 vs. >300 kg), and fits on a standard bed.

The modern models (such as NEV-100, 33-CR, Maxivent and others) are constructed of aluminium and plastic and are provided with windows for patient observation, portholes for catheters and monitoring passages. In some, the patient's head can be raised to prevent bronchoaspiration of secretions.

Since the tank applies negative pressure to the patient's entire body, it is very efficient and reliable. The principal disadvantage is the immobility of the patient inside.

Cuirass

The cuirass is a stiff plastic shell covering the anterior surface of the thorax and the upper abdomen. The edges are padded with airtight material and the device is attached to the patient with a back strap. A negative-pressure pump is fitted via a wide-bore hose inlet in the centre of the shell.

The cuirass applies a negative pressure over a small surface area and is therefore much less efficient than the iron lung.

The advantages of this ventilator are that it is easy to wear, light, suitable for home use and durable. However, pressures areas may develop at the point of contact between the cuirass and the patient, and pressure sores are common. In addition, musculoskeletal, back and chest pain may develop. Custom-made shapes ensure an adequate fit, which is particularly important for patients with severe skeletal deformities.

Today, these devices are used predominantly for nocturnal ventilatory assistance, while for daytime use NIPPV or IAPV methods are more practical.

Body Suits or Jacket Ventilators

Wrap ventilators are similar in principle and function to the cuirass and were developed after those devices. They consist of an airtight jacket with seals around the neck and extremities; the jacket covers an inner stiff framework that encloses the thorax and the abdomen of the patient and ensures negative pressure in the same way as the cuirass.

The prototype was the Tunnicliffe breathing jacket, described in 1955. Subsequently, several models were produced: Pulmo-wrap and Pneumo-wrap, which completely seal the extremities; Poncho Wrap (or Red Poncho), Pneumosuit, NuMo Suit and Zip-Suit, which separately seal each extremity and have a long anterior zipper-closure. Jacket ventilators are easy to wear and light, so they can be used for home care. However, they are not suitable for long-term management and are somewhat less efficient than the iron lung.

Intermittent Abdominal Positive Ventilation

Intermittent abdominal positive ventilation is provided by a body ventilator, such as the Pneumobelt and the Exsufflation Belt, which applies a positive expiratory pressure around the patient's abdomen. It consists of a cloth corset containing an elastic inflatable bladder, which is worn beneath the patient's clothing and over the abdomen. The bladder is inflated intermittently by a positive-pressure ventilator. This pushes the abdominal contents inward, displacing the diaphragm upward and assisting exhalation. Deflation of the bladder allows passive downward motion of the diaphragm. Since this requires gravitational forces, it functions only when the patient is sitting at an angle >30°, optimally at 75°.

This ventilator is not very efficient and requires synchronisation of the patient's breathing pattern; however, it is simple to use, portable and it can be useful for daytime ventilatory assistance in patients with less severe degrees of ventilatory insufficiency.

How the Negative Ventilator Works

The power unit consists of a pump that intermittently creates subatmospheric pressure around the thorax and abdomen, expanding the chest wall and inflating the lungs. Exhalation occurs by passive contraction of the lungs due to elastic recoil. This mechanism is very similar to that of normal respiration, with the work of the pump carried out by the inspiratory muscles [8,11].

The pump is pressure-cycled; that is, the ventilator continues to generate negative pressure during inspiration until a predetermined level is reached (between -50 and -100 cmH_2O in the adult, -20 cmH_2O in children), resulting in the expansion of the lungs and the drawing in of air. In some models, expiration can be supported by positive expiratory pressure (up to +80 cmH_2O in the adult; +6 cmH_2O in children), which may prevent the small increase in functional residual capacity (FRC) that otherwise occurs. All current models can provide a continuous negative extra-thoracic pressure. A control unit ensures that ventilatory variables are correctly set.

The delivery modes are the following:

- Cyclical negative pressure or intermittent negative pressure (INPV): a subatmospheric pressure is generated in inspiration and expiration is passive.
- Continuously negative extra-thoracic pressure (CNEP): subatmospheric pressure surrounds the patient throughout the respiratory cycle. The patient breathes spontaneously; a constant negative pressure throughout the respiratory cycle increases the patient's FRC and acts similarly to CPAP mode.
- Negative/positive pressure: negative pressure during inspiration and positive pressure during expiration.
- Negative pressure/CNEP: intermittent swings of negative pressure are generated upon a background of constant negative expiratory pressure. In this way, at the end of expiration the negative pressure (negative end-expiratory pressure, NEEP) is equivalent to the positive end-expiratory pressure (PEEP) produced inside the airway. NEEP added to NPV improves the patient/ventilator interaction, reducing both the effort of the diaphragm in the pre-trigger phase and non-triggering inspiratory efforts [12].

Most ventilators have controls to set inspiratory and expiratory times and end-inspiratory pauses. The ventilator may provide a control, assist or assist-control mode. The assist-control mode is effective in the relief of dyspnoea and influences the control of breathing to minimise respiratory discomfort [13]. The assist mode usually has a pressure trigger, which is the pressure generated at the nares of the patient; in some cases, there is a thermistor trigger, which is activated by a change in temperature due to the onset of inspiratory airflow [14]. Gorini et al. demonstrated that a microprocessor thermistor trigger performs assist NPV with a marked reduction in diaphragm effort and a low rate of non-triggering inspiratory effort, both in normal subjects and in patients with acute exacerbations of chronic obstructive pulmonary disease (COPD) [12].

Most modern ventilators are able to respond rapidly to changing gas leaks and to maintain the desired pressure; the pattern of the pressure wave may be a square wave, half-sine wave or intermediate wave, depending on the pump model. It has been argued that if the pressure of a pump producing a half-sine wave is made more negative to compensate for and produce an equivalent tidal volume, the patients is more likely to suffer upper airway obstruction. A square wave of pressure produces a tidal volume up to 30% greater than that generated by the half-sine wave [15].

Physiological Effects

Respiratory Effects

During NPV, tidal volume (V_T) and minute ventilation (V_E) are related to the peak inspiratory negative pressure [16]. In normal awake subjects, Glérant observed [17] that NPV can significantly increase V_T and V_E, leading to a decrease in end-tidal CO_2 pressure ($P_{ET}CO_2$), in spite of a large increase in inspiratory resistance. This is concomitant with an inhibition of the muscle activity of the diaphragm and a rest of the respiratory muscles.

In patients with stable COPD and chronic respiratory failure, NPV ensures increases in alveolar ventilation (V_A) and V_E, a reduction in respiratory frequency (RF), improvement of arterial blood gas exchange [18,19] and partial rest of the respiratory muscles [20]. The strength of the respiratory muscles is improved and the ventilatory response to hypoxia and hypercapnia is increased. This has been observed also in patients with severe airflow limitations in whom NPV was administered for 6–8 h/day for two consecutive days [21].

It also appears that NEEP added to NPV reduces dynamic intrinsic end-expiratory pressure (PEEPi) and non-triggering inspiratory efforts, thus improving the patient-ventilator interaction [19]. However, NPV is less effective than nasal PPV in stimulating ventilatory changes and in reducing diaphragmatic activity [22].

Upper-Airway Obstruction

During spontaneous breathing, pharyngeal and laryngeal muscles contract earlier than the inspiratory muscles, resulting in stiffening of the upper airway. When subatmospheric pressure is generated in the upper airway, the abductor muscles may be inhibited. This result is favoured by inhibition of the respiratory centres, especially during sleep or relaxation, and leads to the collapse of the upper airway, sleep apnoeas and impairment of the quality of sleep [23]. This phenomenon is particularly evident in patients with advanced COPD [24], restrictive ventilatory dysfunction and neuromuscular disorders [25], in whom recurrent episodes of sleep apnoea and hypopnoea may develop.

Series and colleagues observed that continuous negative airway pressure (CNAP) causes a decrease in lung volume, which increases upper airway resistance [26] and collapsibility [27]. The obstruction occurs at the glottic or supraglottic level and is reduced by activation of the upper airway muscles [28], which stabilises the upper airways [29]. For this reason, assist-mode ventilation is often very useful in preventing this series of events.

Another method to obviate this problem, at least in restrictive pulmonary disease, is the use of nasal continuous positive airway pressure (CPAP) or protriptyline [30]; the latter is a tryciclic antidepressant drug that appears to elicit selective activation of upper airway muscles.

Experimental studies have evidenced a reflex abduction of the vocal cords during the application of negative pressure to the upper airway, which seemed to counterbalance the tendency of the glottis to narrow in healthy subjects [31].

Cardiovascular Effects

When negative pressure is generated around the chest wall, as with the cuirass or jacket ventilators, intrathoracic pressure decreases. A more negative intrathoracic pressure enhances the gradient of venous return, which tends to increase cardiac output; at the same time, the transmural pressure in the left ventricle also rises, increasing left ventricular afterload and decreasing cardiac output. Consequently, there is some evidence for no effect [32] on cardiac output, even if it seems that NPV does not decrease cardiac output. With the iron lung, these effects are not observed, because intrathoracic pressure is increased relative to body-surface pressure, thereby reducing the gradient of venous return [33].

In an experimental model, Lockhat et al. [34] observed higher cardiac output during NPV and NEEP applied with the Pneumowrap ventilator than with an iron lung administering NPV and PEEP. Also, in mechanically ventilated patients with and without lung damage, CNEP may increase cardiac output to a greater extent than accomplished with zero end-expiratory pressure (ZEEP) and PEEP [35]. In patients with non-cardiogenic pulmonary oedema, NPV with NEEP offers a comparable improvement in gas exchange with the advantages of less cardiac depression [36].

Borelli et al. [37] compared the effects of CNEP and PEEP in patients with acute lung injury (ALI). A CNEP of -20 cmH_2O achieved a transpulmonary pressure and a lung function similar to those resulting from a PEEP of 15 cmH_2O, but venous return and the preload of the heart were increased, and the cardiac index was better.

Clinical Side-Effects and Contraindications

The most common side-effects that occur during NPV are poor compliance (with Pneumowrap) and upper airway obstruction (with iron lung and Pneumowrap), both in long-term administration at home and in critical care setting [38,39]. Also, musculoskeletal pain is rather frequent with Pneumowrap used for home ventilation [39]. Other less common side-effects with Pneumowap are oesophagitis, rib fractures and pneumothorax, impaired sleep quality, fatigue and depression [18].

Contraindications to NPV are gastrointestinal bleeding, rib fractures, recent abdominal surgery, uncooperative patients, sleep apnoea syndrome and neurological disorders with bulbar dysfunction [11].

Clinical Uses

Acute Respiratory Failure in COPD

Intermittent NPV has been successfully used in the treatment of COPD patients in ARF. A significant improvement in arterial oxygen tension (PaO_2) and arterial CO_2 tension ($PaCO_2$), associated with a significant increase in maximal inspiratory and expiratory pressure have been reported [40]; particular improvement was achieved by patients with a good tolerance of the procedure [38] in whom outcome also was good [41].

Corrado et al. [42] treated 150 COPD patients in hypoxic-hypercapnic coma with the iron lung; the success rate was 70%.

Compared with conventional mechanical ventilation, NPV has the same efficacy while avoiding the need for intubation. It also resulted in a similar length of hospital stay [43].

The only study that compared the iron lung with mask ventilation in COPD patients with ARF was a retrospective study which concluded that the two techniques are equally effective; however, prospective trials are needed to confirm these results [44].

Long-Term Application in Stable COPD

Patients with severe stable COPD have chronic ventilatory muscle fatigue [45], in which the force and the endurance of the inspiratory muscle are reduced. In such patients, NPV may be useful to obtain intermittent ventilatory muscle rest (VMR). NPV with a tank ventilator virtually eliminates electrical activity of the diaphragm and assumes the work of breathing [46], whereas more compliant devices, such as wrap ventilators, may be less effective in suppressing inspiratory muscle work.

There is some evidence that NPV improves blood gases, inspiratory muscle strength (measured by maximal inspiratory pressure, MIP), endurance and the clinical condition of patients with chronic airflow limitation and chronic hypercapnia, probably because of the correction with chronic inspiratory muscle fatigue [47,48]. However, the relationship between VMR and clinical improvement is not well-established and those studies did not report control groups. In contrast, the results of controlled studies on daily intermittent ventilation with the Poncho-wrap or Pulmowrap failed to show an improvement in pulmonary function, inspiratory muscle strength, arterial blood gas or endurance time [18,39,49,50]. Moreover, wrap ventilation was found to be poorly tolerated by patients with stable COPD [18].

Neuromuscular Disorders and Chest-Wall Diseases

Negative-pressure ventilation has been used successfully for long-term home care ventilation in patients with neuromuscular disorders (muscular dystrophies, myotonic dystrophy, amyotrophic lateral sclerosis or after poliomyelitis) and chest-wall diseases (scoliosis, kyphosis, following a thoracoplasty) [51–54].

Controlled studies on NPV and NIPPV administered to patients with neuromuscular disorders are still lacking; however, it has been observed that NIPPV is associated with a better outcome, lower hospital admission rate and higher patient tolerability of the device [55]. Non-invasive methods are considered by neuromuscular patients to be more convenient and more comfortable for speech and appearance than external devices [56]. Thus, non-invasive ventilation using nasal or face masks is usually the first choice for patients with chest-wall disorders and in those with neuromuscular disorders without impairment of bulbar function. In of the presence of the latter, tracheostomy is necessary. Negative pressure remains an alternative, but patients' range of movement is thereby restricted [57].

Paediatric Diseases

A report dating from the 1950s described the treatment of neonatal respiratory distress syndrome with NPV [58]. A later study showed that continuous negative pressure improves the respiratory outcome of neonates with respiratory failure and may reduce the need for intubation, thus avoiding the complications of invasive ventilation [59]. In older children and in adults, NIPPV has become the preferred route for delivering ventilatory assistance in chronic respiratory failure, but in some cases it can be extremely difficult to introduce a young child to a nasal or face mask, making this method of ventilation unsuitable [60].

Klonin et al. [61] reported a case series of 4- to 16-month-old children with pneumonia, bronchopulmonary dysplasia and bronchiolitis obliterans who were successfully treated with chest cuirass. Moreover, either CNEP or INPV mode may facilitate weaning from PPV; when administered after extubation it can be particularly useful in preventing the need for re-intubation in a fragile child [60].

In some difficult cases of respiratory failure involving refractory hypoxaemia in which conventional ventilation fails, to avoid the use of extracorporeal membrane oxygenation, CNEP generated by an iron lung may be employed in conjunction with intermittent mandatory ventilation via en endotracheal tube [62,63]. In children with central hypoventilation syndrome, NPV may be effective if initiated before tracheostomy, improving the children's quality of life during the daytime. If upper airway obstruction is a problem in the first year of life, NPV may be combined with nasal mask CPAP [64,65].

Shekerdemian et al. [66] studied the haemodynamic effects of cuirass ventilation of children in the early postoperative period after cardiac surgery for persistent arterial duct or tetralogy of Fallot repair. In these patients, who often develop low cardiac output after the intervention, NPV with cuirass produced a marked increase in the pulmonary blood flow and, hence, cardiac output [67,68].

Other Reported Applications

A woman with respiratory distress syndrome who did not tolerate NIPPV was successfully treated with CNEP via an iron lung to avoid tracheal intubation [69]. Another patient with face-mask intolerance was described by Ambrosino et al. [70]; the patient had developed ARF due to *Staphylococcus aureus* pneumonia after heart-lung transplantation and was treated with a Ponchowrap ventilator.

CNEP delivered by a chest shell stabilised persistent flail chest deformities in a man after sternotomy and allowed him to be removed from mechanical ventilation [71].

A few cases have involved pregnant patients with kyphoscoliosis, who developed cardiorespiratory complications. They were treated with tank ventilation, during or immediately after pregnancy, without any effect on foetal development [72].

Simonds et al. successfully administered NPV to eight of ten patients with severe pulmonary disease who were being weaned from mechanical ventilation [73].

A case of a patient with tracheal injury was managed with iron lung: NPV reduced air leak and allowed removal of an endotracheal tube [74].

Advanced Modalities in Negative-Pressure Ventilation

External High-Frequency Oscillation

This type of external ventilation is provided by the Hayek oscillator [75], a ventilator that was developed from the traditional cuirass: its chest shell is a light, flexible cuirass with soft closures to form a tight seal. Two pumps make up the power unit: a diaphragmatic pump that provides alternating positive-negative pressure cycles or oscillations with pressures from +70 to -70 cmH_2O, and a vacuum pump that enables the oscillations to be superimposed on a negative-pressure baseline [76].

The inspiratory negative pressure causes the chest wall to expand, whereas the expiratory pressure may be positive, atmospheric or negative, allowing ventilation to be above, at or below the patient's FRC. Alterations in the magnitude of the baseline pressure allow the control of lung volume, which reduces the occurrence of lung collapse. A control unit establishes the inspiratory chamber pressure (defined as the trough of the intrachamber pressure wave), peak expiratory pressure (the peak of the intrachamber pressure wave), frequency (8–999 cycles/min) and inspiratory/expiratory ratio (1:6 to 6:1).

A wide range of frequencies (up to 160 Hz) may be delivered, enabling oxygenation largely by diffusion. The delivery modes are: mandatory chest oscillation, upon which the patient can impose spontaneous breaths; continuous negative pressure and oscillation around a negative baseline followed by an artificial 'cough' (secretion clearance).

Clinical Applications of External High-Frequency Oscillation

Currently, the Hayek oscillator is the most versatile negative pressure ventilator. Its applications are increasing, even if there are still no clear guidelines on how best to adjust the device to achieve optimum ventilation. The Hayek oscillator can provide effective assisted ventilation for short periods in healthy conscious subjects with no adverse side effects on blood pressure [77,78]. Moreover, it can be effectively used in severe COPD and respiratory failure for assisting ventilation [79]. Al-Saady et al. [80] observed, in patients with respiratory failure, that the improvement in PaO_2 and a decrease in $PaCO_2$ were higher during external high-frequency oscillation (EHFO) than during IPPV, with greater haemodynamic stability as well; the most effective frequencies were 1–3 Hz. Maximal changes in gas exchange and a significant reduction in the spontaneous respiratory rate are seen when a combination of lower frequencies (30 and 60 oscillations/min) and higher pressure spans were used [78].

This ventilator achieves ventilatory support with less negative pressure than conventional external ventilators, but it is not yet clear whether it is associated with a decrease in obstructive sleep apnoeas [81].

EHFO also increases cardiac index and improves tissue perfusion; the increased pumping of the heart is probably caused by changes in intracardiac pressure–volume relationship [82].

Shiga et al. studied the haemodynamic effects of Hayek oscillator with trans-oesophageal echocardiography [83]. The external high-frequency oscillation induces an increase in the left ventricular end-diastolic area, without any changes in the velocity of pulmonary artery flow, suggesting an increased transmural pressure rather than an increased preload; different frequencies do not modify the haemodynamic effects.

Cuirass NPV using the Hayek oscillator has been reported as a important alternative over existing tubeless methods of anaesthesia for airway surgery, including laser procedures, with satisfactory gas exchange and cardiovascular parameters [84,85]. Some cases of anaesthesia management with the Hayek oscillator also have been reported; for example, when endotracheal intubation was not possible in a patient with severe extensive tracheal stenosis [86] and a failed fibre optic intubation [87].

External NPV appears to be a suitable choice during rigid bronchoscopy: both EHFO and INPV ensure effective ventilation and comfortable surgical conditions. Compared with INPV, EHFO requires a higher fraction of inspired oxygen [88].

Another field of application is the combination of EHFO with PPV: as a method of ventilation for patients with acute respiratory failure, EHFO combined with pressure support ventilation may have advantages over conventional mechanical ventilation when the drainage of secretions is facilitated [89].

RTX Respirator

The RTX respirator is an external bi-phasic negative-positive ventilator that can be considered as a modified cuirass: the shell is attached by a flexible large-bore tube to a portable computerised power and control unit. This unit generates a cyclic pressure change inside the cuirass (positive inspiratory pressure and negative expiratory pressure). Several delivery modes can be provided by the RTX: controlled/assisted ventilation, synchronised ventilation, EHFO, CNEP (in spontaneous breathing) and ECG-triggered ventilation.

The respirator delivers low and high breathing frequencies (6–1200 breaths/min) and can be used to treat respiratory failure in neonates, children and adults. It is compact, can be used in hospitals, clinics, and homecare settings and has a unique feature that synchronises ventilation with ECG. Thus, during exhalation/systole the heart is compressed, which provides 'cardiac assist'. During inhalation/diastole (sub-ambient phase), ventricle pre-load is improved. This is in contrast to PPV, which may reduce cardiac output. The device can be set to trigger a respiration cycle at every cardiac cycle or at other ratios [90]. Even if further studies are necessary to assess its fields of application, the RTX Respirator has been successfully used in infants with acute or chronic respiratory failure due to spinal muscular atrophy type 1 [91,92].

Conclusions

Recent advances in NPV have demonstrated that a new era of non-invasive mechanical ventilation with negative pressure has begun. Further studies will assess the feasibility of the new devices for NPV administered intra-hospitally and at home. Patient-tailored ventilation, with integration of negative and positive non-invasive ventilation strategies, may be expected.

References

1. Drinker P, Shore LA (1929) An apparatus for the prolonged administration of artificial respiration. J Clin Invest 7:229
2. Miller FL, Zerbi-Ortiz A, Elkins JT (1960) Use of the tank respirator in overwhelming bacterial pneumonia. N Engl J Med 262:1264–1266
3. Torres A, Aznar R, Gatell JM et al (1990) Incidence, risk, and prognosis factors of nosocomial pneumonia in mechanically ventilated patients. Am Rev Respir Dis 142(3):523–528
4. Slutsky AS, Ranieri VM (2000) Mechanical ventilation: lessons from the ARDSNet trial. Respir Res 1(2):73–77

5. Corrado A, Gorini M (2002) Negative-pressure ventilation: is there still a role? Eur Respir J 20:187–197
6. Wisocki M (1998) Being more positive about negative pressure ventilation. Eur Respir J 12:515–516
7. Schiavina M, Fabiani A, Gunella G (1994) External negative pressure ventilations techniques. Monaldi Arch Chest Dis 49(6):516–521
8. Levine S, Henderson D (1994) Negative pressure ventilation. In: Tobin MJ (ed) Principles and practice of mechanical ventilation. McGraw-Hill, New York, pp 393–411
9. Bach JR (1994) Update and perspectives on noninvasive respiratory muscle aids. Part 1: the inspiratory aid. Chest 105:1230–1240
10. Hill NS (1986) Clinical application of body ventilators. Chest 90(6):897–905
11. Corrado A, Gorini M, Villella G et al (1996) Negative pressure ventilation in the treatment of acute respiratory failure: an old noninvasive technique reconsidered. Eur Respir J 9:1531–1544
12. Gorini M, Villella G, Ginanni R et al (2002) Effect of assist negative pressure ventilation by microprocessor based iron lung on breathing effort. Thorax 57:258–262
13. Nishino T, Sino S, Ide T (1998) Effects of negative pressure assisted ventilation on dyspnoeic sensation and breathing pattern. Eur Respir J 12:1278–1283
14. Shepard FM (1970) A negative-pressure tank-type respirator for the neonate. Anesth Analg 49:413–419
15. Smith IE, King MA, Shneerson JM (1995) Choosing a negative pressure ventilation pump: are there any important differences? Eur Respir J 8(10):1792–1795
16. Drinker PA, McKhann CF (1986) The iron lung: first practical means of respiratory support. JAMA 255:1476–1480
17. Glérant JC, Jounieaux V, Parriera VF et al (2002) Effects of intermittent negative pressure ventilation on effective ventilation in normal awake subjects. Chest 122:99–107
18. Zibrak JD, Hill NS, Federman EC et al (1988) Evaluation of intermittent long-term negative-pressure ventilation in patients with severe chronic obstructive pulmonary disease. Am Rev Respir Dis 138(6):1515–1518
19. Gorini M, Corrado A, Villella G et al (2001) Physiologic effects of negative pressure ventilation in acute exacerbation of chronic obstructive pulmonary disease. Am J Respir Crit Care Med 163(7):1614–1618
20. Nava S, Ambrosino N, Zocchi L et al (1990) Diaphragmatic rest during negative pressure ventilation by pneumowrap: assessment in normal and COPD patients. Chest 98:857–865
21. Fernandez E, Weiner P, Meltzer E et al (1991) Sustained improvement in gas exchange after negative pressure ventilation for 8 hours per day on 2 successive days in chronic airflow limitation. Am Rev Respir Dis 144(2):390–394
22. Belman MJ, Soo Hoo GW, Kuei JH, Shadmehr R (1990) Efficacy of positive vs. negative pressure ventilation in unloading the respiratory muscles. Chest 98(4):850–856
23. Levy RD, Bradley TD, Newman SL et al (1989) Negative pressure ventilation. Effects on ventilation during sleep in normal subjects. Chest 95(1):95–99
24. Levy RD, Cosio MG, Gibbons L et al (1992) Induction of sleep apnoea with negative pressure ventilation in patients with chronic obstructive lung disease. Thorax 47(8):612–615
25. Bach JR, Penek J (1991) Obstructive sleep apnoea complicating negative-pressure ventilatory support in patients with chronic paralytic/restrictive ventilatory dysfunction. Chest 99(6):1386–1393
26. Series F, Marc I (1994) Influence of lung volume dependence of upper airway resistance during continuous negative airway pressure. J Appl Physiol 77(2):840–844
27. Series F, Marc I (1993) Effects of continuous negative airway pressure-related lung deflation on upper airway collapsibility. J Appl Physiol 75(3):1222–1225
28. Sanna A, Veriter C, Stanescu D (1993) Upper airway obstruction induced by negative-pressure ventilation in awake healthy subjects. J Appl Physiol 75:546–552
29. Sanna A, Veriter C, Kurtansky A, Stanescu D (1994) Contraction and relaxation of upper airway muscles during expiratory application of negative pressure at the mouth. Sleep

17(3):220–225

30. Goldstein RS, Molotiu N, Skrastins R et al (1987) Reversal of sleep-induced hypoventilation and chronic respiratory failure by nocturnal negative pressure ventilation in patients with restrictive ventilatory impairment. Am Rev Respir Dis 135(5):1049–1055
31. Van Lunteren E, Van de Graaff WB, Parker DM et al (1984) Nasal and laryngeal reflex responses to negative upper airway pressure. J Appl Physiol 56(3):746–752
32. Kinnear W, Petch M, Taylor G et al (1988) Assisted ventilation using cuirass respirators. Eur Respir J 1:198–203
33. Corrado A, Gorini M (2002) Long-term negative pressure ventilation. Respir Care Clin 8:545–557
34. Lockhat D, Langleben D, Zidulka A (1992) Hemodynamic differences between continual positive and two type of negative pressure ventilation. Am Rev Respir Dis 146:677–680
35. Torelli L, Zoccali G, Dalla Zuanna F et al (1995) Comparative evaluation of the haemodynamic effects of continuous negative external pressure (CNEP) and positive end-expiratory pressure (PEEP) in mechanically ventilated trauma patients. Intensive Care Med 21:67–70
36. Skaburskis M, Helal R, Zidulka A (1987) Hemodynamic effects of external continuous negative pressure ventilation compared with those of continuous positive pressure ventilation in dogs with acute lung injury. Am Rev Respir Dis 136(4):886–891
37. Borelli M, Benini A, Denkewitz T et al (1998) Effects of continuous negative extrathoracic pressure versus positive end-expiratory pressure in acute lung injury patients. Crit Care Med 26(6):1025–1031
38. Montserrat JM, Martos JA, Alarcon A et al (1991) Effect of negative pressure ventilation on arterial blood gas pressures and inspiratory muscle strength during an exacerbation of chronic obstructive lung disease. Thorax 46(1):6–8
39. Shapiro SH, Ernst P, Gray-Donald K et al (1992) Effect of negative pressure ventilation in severe chronic obstructive pulmonary disease. Lancet 340(8833):1425–1429
40. Corrado A, Gorini M, De Paola E et al (1994) Iron lung treatment for acute on chronic respiratory failure: 16 years of experience. Monaldi Arch Chest Dis 49(6):552–555
41. Corrado A, Bruscoli G, Messori A et al (1992) Iron lung treatment of subjects with COPD in acute respiratory failure. Evaluation of short and long-term prognosis. Chest 101:692–696
42. Corrado A, De Paola E, Gorini M et al (1996) Intermittent negative pressure ventilation in the treatment of hypoxic hypercapnic coma in chronic respiratory insufficiency. Thorax 51:1077–1082
43. Corrado A, Gorini M, Ginanni R et al (1998) Negative pressure ventilation versus conventional mechanical ventilation in the treatment of acute respiratory failure in COPD patients. Eur Respir J 12:519–525
44. Corrado A, Confalonieri M, Marchese S et al (2002) Iron lung vs. mask ventilation in the treatment of acute on chronic respiratory failure in COPD patients. Chest 121:189–195
45. Bellemare F, Grassino A (1983) Force reserve of the diaphragm in patients with chronic obstructive pulmonary disease. J Appl Physiol 55:8–15
46. Rochester DF, Braun NMT, Arora NS (1979) Respiratory muscle strength in chronic obstructive pulmonary disease. Am Rev Respir Dis 119:151–154
47. Gutierrez M, Beroiza T, Contreras G et al (1988) Weekly cuirass ventilation improves blood gases and inspiratory muscle strength in patients with chronic air-flow limitation and hypercarbia. Am Rev Respir Dis 138(3):617–623
48. Cropp A, DiMarco AF (1987) Effects of intermittent negative pressure ventilation on respiratory muscle function in patients with severe chronic obstructive pulmonary disease. Am Rev Respir Dis 135(5):1056–1061
49. Celli B, Lee H, Criner B et al (1989) Controlled trial of external negative pressure ventilation in patients with severe chronic airflow obstruction. Am Rev Respir Dis 140:1251–1256
50. Levine S, Levy SF, Henson DJ (1992) Effect of negative pressure ventilation on ventilatory muscle endurance in patients with severe chronic obstructive pulmonary disease. Am Rev Respir Dis 146:722–729
51. Garay SM, Turino GM, Goldring RM (1981) Sustained reversal of chronic hypercapnia in

patients with alveolar hypoventilation syndromes. Long-term maintenance with noninvasive nocturnal mechanical ventilation. Am J Med 70(2):269–274
52. Schiavina M, Fabiani A (1993) Intermittent negative pressure ventilation in patients with restrictive respiratory failure. Monaldi Arch Chest Dis 48(2):169–175
53. Jackson M, Kinnear W, King M et al (1993) The effects of five years of nocturnal cuirass-assisted ventilation in chest wall disease. Eur Respir J 6(5):630–635
54. Frederick C (1994) Noninvasive mechanical ventilation with the iron lung. Crit Care Nurs Clin North Am 6(4):831-840
55. Baydur A, Layne E, Aral H (2000) Long term non-invasive ventilation in the community for patients with musculoskeletal disorders: 46 year experience and review. Thorax 55:4–11
56. Bach JR (1993) A comparison of long-term ventilatory support alternatives from the perspective of the patient and care giver. Chest 104(6):1702–1706
57. Shneerson JM, Simonds AK (2002) Noninvasive ventilation for chest wall and neuromuscular disorders. Eur Respir J 20(2):480–487
58. Donald I, Lord J (1953) Augmented respiration. Studies in atelectasis neonatorum. Lancet 1:9–16
59. Samuels MP, Raine J, Wright T et al (1996) Continuous negative extrathoracic pressure in neonatal respiratory failure. Pediatrics 98(6 Pt 1):1154–1160
60. Thomson A (1997) The role of negative pressure ventilation. Arch Dis Child 77:454–458
61. Klonin H, Bowman B, Peters M et al (2000) Negative pressure ventilation via chest cuirass to decrease ventilator-associated complications in infants with acute respiratory failure: a case series. Respir Care 45(5):486–490
62. Sills JH, Cvetnic WG, Pietz J (1989) Continuous negative pressure in the treatment of infants with pulmonary hypertension and respiratory failure. J Perinatol 9(1):43–48
63. Cvetnic WG, Shoptaugh M, Sills JH (1992) Intermittent mandatory ventilation with continuous negative pressure compared with positive end-expiratory pressure for neonatal hypoxemia. J Perinatol 12(4):316–324
64. Hartmann H, Jawad MH, Noyes J et al (1994) Negative extrathoracic pressure ventilation in central hypoventilation syndrome. Arch Dis Child 70(5):418–423
65. Russell-Jones DL, Treacher DF, Lenicker HM et al (1989) Central hypoventilation in a seven year old child following pertussis treated with negative pressure ventilation. Postgrad Med J 65:768–770
66. Shekerdemian LS, Bush A, Lincoln C et al (1997) Cardiopulmonary interaction in healthy children and children after simple cardiac surgery: the effects of positive and negative pressure ventilation. Heart 78(6):587–593
67. Shekerdemian LS, Bush A, Shore DF et al (1997) Cardiopulmonary interactions after fontan operations. Augmentation of cardiac output using negative pressure ventilation. Circulation 96:3934–3942
68. Shekerdemian LS, Bush A, Shore DF et al (1999) Cardiorespiratory responses to negative pressure ventilation after tetralogy of Fallot repair: a hemodynamic tool for patients with low-output state. J Am Coll Cardiol 33(2):549–555
69. Morris AH, Elliott CG (1985) Adult respiratory distress syndrome: successful support with continuous negative extrathoracic pressure. Crit Care Med 13(11):989–990
70. Ambrosino N, Rubini F, Callegari G et al (1994) Noninvasive mechanical ventilation in the treatment of acute respiratory failure due to infectious complications of lung transplantation. Monaldi Arch Chest Dis 49(4):311–314
71. Hartke RH Jr, Block AJ (1992) External stabilisation of flail chest using continuous negative extrathoracic pressure. Chest 102(4):1283–1285
72. Sawicka EH, Spencer GT, Branthwaite MA (1986) Management of respiratory failure complicating pregnancy in severe kyphoscoliosis: a new use for an old technique? Br J Dis Chest 80(2):191–196
73. Simonds AK, Sawicka EH, Carroll N et al (1988) Use of negative pressure ventilation to facilitate the return of spontaneous ventilation. Anaesthesia 43(3):216–219
74. Chen JC, Brenner M, Milliken J et al (1997) Successful management of a complex tracheal

injury with the iron lung. J Trauma 43(2):362–364
75. Hayek Z, Sohar E (1993) External high frequency oscillation. Concept and practice. Intensive Care World 10:36–40
76. Fink JB, Mahlmeister MJ (2002) High-frequency oscillation of the airway and chest wall. Respir Care 47(7):797–807
77. Dolmage TE, DeRosie JA, Avendano MA et al (1995) Effect of external chest wall oscillation on gas exchange in healthy subjects. Chest 107:433–439
78. Hardinge FM, Davies RJ, Stradling JR (1995) Effects of short term high frequency negative pressure ventilation on gas exchange using the Hayek oscillator in normal subjects. Thorax 50(1):44–49
79. Spitzer SA, Fink G, Mittelman M (1993) External high-frequency ventilation in severe chronic obstructive pulmonary disease. Chest 104:1698–1701
80. Al-Saady NM, Fernando SS, Petros AJ et al (1995) External high frequency oscillation in normal subjects and in patients with acute respiratory failure. Anaesthesia 50(12):1031–1035
81. Dolmage TE, Heisenberg HA, Davis LL et al (1996) Chest wall oscillation at 1 Hz reduces spontaneous ventilation in healthy subjects during sleep. Chest 110:128–135
82. Sideno B, Vaage J (1997) Ventilation by external high-frequency oscillations improves cardiac function after coronary artery bypass grafting. Eur J Cardiothorac Surg 11(2):248–257
83. Shiga T, Takeda S, Nakanishi K et al (1998) Transesophageal echocardiograph evaluation during negative-pressure ventilation using the Hayek oscillator. J Cardiothorac Vasc Anesth 12(5):527–532
84. Dilkes MG, McNeill JM, Hill AC et al (1993)The Hayek oscillator: a new method of ventilation in microlaryngeal surgery. Ann Otol Rhinol Laryngol 102:455–458
85. Monks PS, Broomhead CJ, Dilkes MG et al (1995) The use of the Hayek Oscillator during microlaryngeal surgery. Anaesthesia 50(10):865–869
86. Sutcliffe N, Remington SA, Ramsay TM et al (1995) Severe tracheal stenosis and operative delivery. Anaesthesia 50(1):26–29
87. Broomhead CJ, Dilkes MG, Monks PS (1995) Use of the Hayek oscillator in a case of failed fibreoptic intubation. Br J Anaesth 74:720–721
88. Natalini G, Cavaliere S, Seramondi V et al (2000) Negative pressure ventilation vs. external high-frequency oscillation during rigid bronchoscopy. A controlled randomised trial. Chest 118:18–23
89. Takeda S, Nakanishi K, Takano T et al (1997) The combination of external high-frequency oscillation and pressure support ventilation in acute respiratory failure. Acta Anaesthesiol Scand 41(6):670–674
90. Plein S, Bulugahapitiya S, Jones TR et al (2003) Cardiac RM imaging with external respirator: sinchronizing cardiac and respiratory motion. Radiology 227:877–882
91. Marraro GA (2003) Innovative practices of ventilatory support with pediatric patients. Pediatr Crit Care Med 4:8
92. Marraro GA, Lucchetti M, Cereda G et al (2003) Non-invasive ventilation of acute respiratory failure in infants with spinal muscular atrophy (SMA) tipe 1. PCCM J, Abstracts' Book

High-Frequency Percussive Ventilation

U. Lucangelo, S. Gramaticopolo, L. Fontanesi

Introduction

High-frequency ventilation (HFV) techniques have been studied and applied for more than 40 years. Nonetheless, they are still largely unpopular in intensive care units (ICUs) and their use is limited to specialist applications in cases of acute respiratory failure refractory to conventional treatment. Results in clinical trials have been alternatively convincing or feebly positive in favour of HFV, and to most practitioners it is an unphysiological approach to the care of ICU patients.

In this chapter we discuss the physiological characteristics of high-frequency percussive ventilation (HFPV), explain why it is different from other forms of HFV, and why it is successful in managing patients with acute lung injury (ALI) or acute respiratory distress syndrome (ARDS). Moreover, HFV is not limited to intensive care use but can also be implemented in the operating room for better management of surgery involving the lower airways.

The Equation of Motion and HFV

High-frequency ventilation implies a ventilation frequency ranging from 60 to 3000 cycles per minute, tidal volumes smaller than dead space, lower peak airway pressures and a more efficient gas exchange than provided by conventional ventilation. The mechanisms by which HFV establishes alveolar ventilation is uncertain and differs according to the technique employed: gas distribution is governed by diffusion, convection and a combination of both. All forms of HFV are characterised by peak airway pressures that are lower than those of conventional ventilation, lower transpulmonary pressures and more efficient gas exchange than obtained with conventional ventilation [1].

HFV eliminates the phasic variations of chest volume during normal respiratory rhythm and is effective in the setting of bronchopleural fistulas that are

U. Lucangelo, P. Pelosi, W.A. Zin, A. Aliverti (eds.) *Respiratory System and Artificial Ventilation*. © Springer 2008

refractory to closure, in part because of lower peak airway pressures. Fistulas also tend to draw less flow at higher frequencies because the inertia of the fistulous pathway is greater than that of alternative routes [2].

As explained by the equation of motion:

$$\text{Prs} = (\dot{V} \times Rrs) + (V \times Ers) + (\ddot{V} \times Irs) \qquad \text{(Eq. 1)}$$

the pressure applied (Prs) is the sum of resistive, elastic and inertial pressure drops of the respiratory system. ($\dot{V} \times Rrs$) is the pressure that must be applied to balance frictional forces and is due chiefly to the resistance (*Rrs*) offered to flow ($\dot{V}$). ($V \times Ers$) is the pressure that must be applied to balance elastic forces and it depends on the volume (V) and on the elastance of the respiratory system (*Ers*). Lastly, the product ($\ddot{V} \times Irs$) is the pressure loss needed to overcome the system's inertia. This effect is referred to as the inertia of the respiratory system (*Irs*) and it depends on the acceleration ($\ddot{V}$).

During conventional mechanical ventilation, *Irs* is negligible and *Rrs* is the main determinant of flow distribution. In contrast, during HFV, *Irs* becomes relevant and the high acceleration of pulsatile flow in HFV renders flow distribution less dependent on very low resistance values, as may happen in main bronchial discontinuity (traumatic or surgical). As a result, notwithstanding leakage in the main bronchial tree, delivery of volume is guaranteed to the distal airways.

What Is High-Frequency Percussive Ventilation?

High-frequency percussive ventilation (HFPV) is a time-cycled pressure-limited mode of ventilation that delivers subphysiological tidal volumes at rates that range from 200 to 900 cycles/min. It can be described as a hybrid mode of mechanical ventilation that superimposes a conventional pressure-cycled breath on small pulsatile volumes delivered at high frequency (Fig. 1). High-frequency pulses of gas are delivered to the patient through a sliding Venturi connected to the endotracheal tube [3].

HFPV was introduced more than 20 years ago to overcome the drawbacks of other HFV modes (e.g. high-frequency oscillation, high-frequency jet ventilation). The only system that delivers HFPV is the VDR4 (volumetric diffusive respirator; Percussionaire, Sandpoint, ID, USA). This is a time-cycled pressure-controlled ventilator equipped with a high-frequency flow generator connected to a device (the phasitron) that provides the interface between the patient and the machine. The phasitron produces mini-bursts of subtidal volumes that generate intrapulmonary percussive waves, hence the denomination 'percussive ventilation.' The VDR4 is equipped with a system for the humidification and heating of the delivered gases; in addition, aerosolised topically active medications can be continuously or periodically delivered [4].

HFPV combines the positive aspects of conventional mechanical ventilation with those of HFV. The phasitron is driven by a high-pressure gas supply at a high-frequency rate of 200–900 beats/min superimposed on a conventional inspiratory/expiratory pressure-controlled cycle that is set at a rate of 10–15 breaths/min. During inspiration, lung volumes are progressively increased in a controlled, stepwise fashion by repetitively diminishing subtidal volume deliveries. Depending on the elastance of the respiratory system during inspiration, an oscillatory plateau can be reached and maintained (Fig. 1). As shown in Fig.

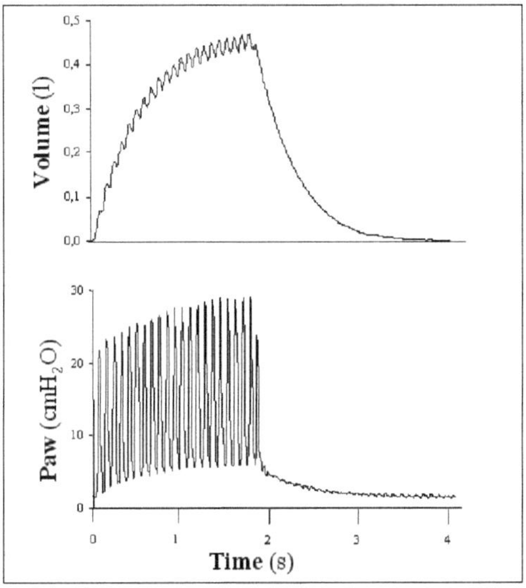

Fig. 1 Volume and pressure tracings during high-frequency pressure ventilation (HFPV)

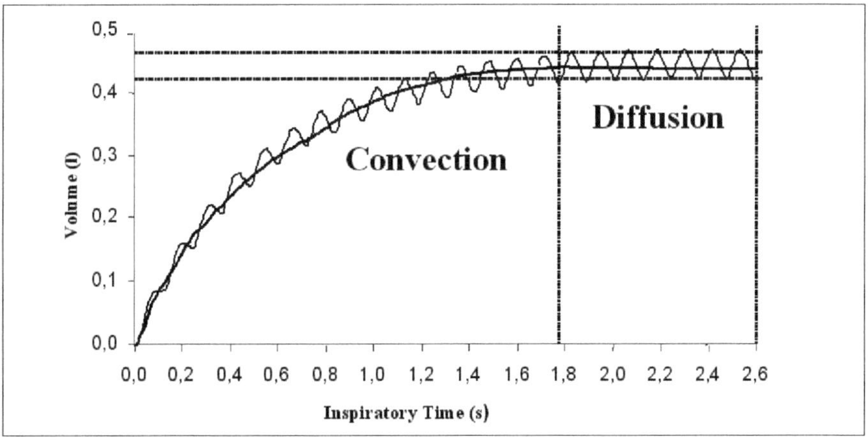

Fig. 2 Inspiratory phase of a typical HFPV cycle: the ranking part of the curve is responsible for the convection of gas delivery, while the plateau phase favours the diffusion of gases

2, where the inspiratory phase of a typical HFPV cycle is depicted, while the ranking part of the curve is mainly responsible for the convection of gas delivery, the plateau phase is mainly responsible for the diffusion of gases, thus allowing for a better gas exchange and favouring the removal of secretions.

HFPV in Acute Lung Injury and Acute Respiratory Distress Syndrome

Like other HFV techniques, HFPV offers an advantage over conventional ventilation (CV) in that it provides adequate oxygenation at lower airway pressure and tidal volume, thus diminishing the risk of volutrauma and barotrauma in acute lung injury/acute respiratory distress syndrome (ALI/ARDS) patients. Several trials comparing HFPV efficacy to CV demonstrated that HFPV improves oxygenation and promotes CO_2 removal at lower peak inspiratory pressure, with negligible effects on central haemodynamics [5–8].

In a bench-study, HFPV was applied to a single-compartment mechanical lung simulator in which resistance and elastance values were modified (simulating the augmented resistance of the airways or parenchymal stiffness) while the same ventilatory setting of the VDR4 was maintained. In that model, as the endobronchial inflation pressure increased against the respiratory system impedance, it was reflected into the Venturi device, causing its entrainment ratio to vary from a maximum of 5 to a minimum of zero. The response to transient intrapulmonary pressure changed in less than 3 ms, demonstrating that the Venturi serves as a fluidic clutch, with the rise in peak pressure governed by the selected pressure drop across the Venturi orifice. Thus, physiological/physical feedback serves to avoid a potentially hazardous rise in intrapulmonary pressure [9,10].

Drainage and recruitment of atelectatic lung areas are possible for three reasons. First, the application of PEEP allows areas of atelectatic lung recruited by the high-frequency percussive mechanism of the VDR4 that have been opened to be maintained in an open state. Second, aerosol is delivered at high flow; coupled with percussion, this produces an effective therapy and adequate humidification of the airway. Third, subtidal volume percussions and elevated flow mobilise mucosal plugs; acting together with the elastic force of the alveoli, this results in the transport of secretions into the upper airways.

The mobilisation of mucus is, in turn, due to: (1) successive pressure peaks, which provoke a vibratory effect on bronchial mucosa and on secretions; (2) variations in percussion frequency, which generate turbulence in the airways and (3) the elevated flow, which, combined with percussion, enhances mucociliary clearance [11].

HFPV has proved its unique efficacy in the treatment of ARDS in cases in which the response to CV was limited. Notwithstanding these results, no clinical trial has shown an improved survival or ICU length of stay in HFPV patients, demonstrating once again that improving oxygenation is only one aspect of a multi-facet approach to ARDS.

HFPV Applications in Major Conducting-Airway Lesions

When the tracheobronchial tree is normal, HFPV is set to allow time cycling between the inspiratory and expiratory phases. The inspiratory/expiratory ratio ranges from physiological values of 1:2 to 1:1, depending on the desired value of mean airway pressure.

The expiratory phase may be passive or pulsatile, as required by the target of gas exchange and the patient's haemodynamic response. Carbon dioxide monitoring is also possible if a proper pressure gap is achieved between inspiratory and expiratory phase.

When the tracheobronchial tree is interrupted, inspiratory phase must be prolonged to increase the diffusive phase and a short passive expiratory phase has been suggested to enhance CO_2 washout by convection.

High Frequency Percussive Ventilation During Surgical Bronchial Repair

High-frequency percussive ventilation has been employed mainly in intensive care settings, in burn patients and as rescue therapy in adult patients with refractory respiratory failure. As a form of high-frequency ventilation, HFPV can be employed during surgery on the major conducting airways, to guarantee an adequate gas exchange and to minimise shifting of the surgical field while ventilation is maintained in both the dependent and the independent lung.

Bronchial repair is a challenging procedure for the surgeon and for the anaesthetist, as ventilation must be guaranteed while isolating part of the conducting airway and at the same time allowing for ventilation of dependent parenchyma. This can be achieved by employing double-lumen tubes or bronchial blockage through single-lumen tubes. HFV has been used in thoracic surgery, where its main role is the delivery of small rapid tidal volumes through small-airway tubes. Thus, if a major conducting airway (trachea, carinal area, main-stem bronchus) has to be divided, the transit of a small-airway tube through the surgical field causes much less surgical interference than would occur with the passage of a large standard or double-lumen endotracheal tube. Small-airway catheters present the surgeon with a relatively accessible circumference of trachea and bronchus, so that the ends of a divided airway can be properly aligned for the construction of an unstressed and airtight anastomosis. However, with all types of HFV for airway surgery, the logistics of small-catheter placement and securement are formidable, and suctioning of the airway and distal lung may be problematic [12–15].

In employing HFPV during surgical repair of the major conducting airways, we have used a standard single-lumen tube in most cases and have obtained satisfactory gas exchange throughout surgery.

Standard management for surgery in which there is discontinuity in the main conducting airways (prior to or during surgery) starts with tracheal intubation with a standard single-lumen tube and HFPV set at about 500 cycles min^{-1}, with inspiratory and expiratory times of 2 s (15 bpm). Initially, the expiratory phase is passive in order to allow CO_2 monitoring during a pressure gap between inspiration and expiration. Peak airway pressure and the inspiratory oxygen fraction (FiO_2) are set to obtain sPO_2>90%. After thoracotomy and pleural opening, the inspiratory time is prolonged to obtain at least two pressure gaps per minute. Hyperinflation is avoided by allowing for two expiratory phases per minute, resetting the peak pressure and because gas delivery during HFPV is based on Venturi logic. The ability of HFPV to maintain acceptable blood gas levels in the face of leaky ruptured bronchial stems is a product of its ability to generate very high pulsatile flows, as the ventilator gas output is servo-adjusted to the output impedance. Interestingly, the VDR4 itself operates with an open-air circuit that is intended to prevent lung hyperinflation. The surgeon can manually deflate the lung when necessary; this manoeuvre will result in an acceptable immobilisation of the surgical field and a positive pressure inside the lung, similar to the application of continuous positive airway pressure (CPAP).

VDR4 settings can be modified to obtain CO_2 washout by decreasing the number of cycles per minute (to 300 cycles per minute). In contrast, oxygenation is improved at the highest number of cycles per minute (700–800 cycles per minute). Blood-gas analysis will guide the choice of the optimal number of cycles for each patient [16].

PV and Surgical Bronchial Repair in a One-Lung Patient

High-frequency percussive ventilation was successfully employed in the surgical repair of a tracheobronchial rupture in a one-lung patient. In this patient, who suffered iatrogenic bronchial rupture after right pneumonectomy, surgical repair was managed with a starting ventilation of 500 cyles min^{-1}, infinite inspiratory time, and a steady-state mean airway pressure. The retention of CO_2 ensued and the oscillation frequency was reduced from 500 to 300 cycles min^{-1}, thus reducing mean airway pressure. However this manoeuvre had no result: reduction of the oscillation frequency maintained the PaO_2/FiO_2 ratio and the $PaCO_2$ was unchanged, despite the fact that mean airway pressure was reduced by 3 cm H_2O (from 22 to 19 cmH_2O). Although at this stage the patient's gas exchange could be considered acceptable, CO_2 removal was enhanced by exploiting the bi-level ventilation mode. The VDR4 allows the use of a low-frequency (about 4 bpm) bi-level mean airway pressure (23 and 16 cmH_2O during inspiratory and expiratory phases, respectively), which led to a decrease in the $PaCO_2$ of 0.67 kPa 20 min after changing from the previous ventilatory strategy. However, it was considered that a larger gap in bi-level mean airway pressure would further improve CO_2 removal; indeed, when the mean expiratory airway pressure was 12 cm H_2O, the $PaCO_2$ dropped to 7.2 kPa. During bi-level ventilation, the calculated mean airway pressure was 22 cmH_2O and the percussion frequency was switched back to 500 cycles min^{-1}. This was done to highlight the fact that CO_2

washout depended mainly on the pressure gap created by the bi-level ventilation model [16].

HFPV During Sleeve Resection

A sleeve resection is an anatomical pulmonary resection (segmentectomy, lobectomy or pneumonectomy) that is combined with the excision of a bronchial segment, and the anastomosis between the airway proximal and distal to it. This technique allows a certain number of centrally located tumours to be completely resected with sufficient margins of healthy tissue.

We have employed HFPV during sleeve resection to simplify airway management and lung ventilation. The same principles described for bronchial rupture applied in this case. Moreover, we noted, particularly during carinal resection, that during HFPV, as long as the surgeon kept the distal bronchus aligned with the trachea in the surgical field, the distal lung, despite the airway interruption, was successfully inflated.

This is an extreme application of the equation of motion, in which airways resistance becomes almost negligible and distal ventilation is guaranteed only by the high value of the third term of the equation.

References

1. Branson RD (1995) High frequency ventilators. In: Branson RD, Hess DR, Chatburn, RL (eds) Respiratory care equipment. Lippincott, Philadelphia, pp 458–469
2. Turnbull AD, Carlon G, Howland WS et al (1981) High-frequency jet ventilation in major airway or pulmonary destruction. Ann Thorac Surg 32:468–474
3. Salim A, Martin M (2005) High-frequency percussive ventilation. Crit Care Med 33:S241-S245
4. Anonymous (1996) A manual on volumetric diffusive respiration (VDR). Product information. Percussionaire Corporation, Sandpoint, ID
5. Gallagher TJ, Boysen PG, Davidson DD et al (1989) High-frequency percussive ventilation compared with conventional mechanical ventilation. Crit Care Med 17:364–366
6. Velmahos GC, Chan LS, Tatevossian R et al (1999) High-frequency percussive ventilation improves oxygenation in patients with ARDS. Chest 116:440–446
7. Paulsen SM, Kyllyon GW, Barillo DJ (2002) High-frequency percussive ventilation as a salvage modality in adult respiratory distress syndrome: a preliminary study. Am Surg 10:854–856
8. Salim A, miller K, Dangleben D et al (2004) High-frequency percussive ventilation: an alternative mode of ventilation for head injured patients with adult respiratory distress syndrome. J Trauma 57:542–546
9. Lucangelo U, Antonaglia V, Zin WA et al (2006) Mechanical loads modulate tidal volume and lung washout during high-frequency percussive ventilation. Respir Physiol Neurobiol 150(1):44–51
10. Lucangelo U, Antonaglia V, Zin WA et al (2004) Effects of mechanical load on flow, volume and pressure delivered by high-frequency percussive ventilation. Respir Physiol Neurobiol 142(1):81–91

11. Lucangelo U, Fontantesi L, Antonaglia V et al (2003). High frequency percussive ventilation (HFPV). Principles and techniques. Minerva anestesiol 69:841–851
12. Brodsky JB, Fitzmaurice B (2001) Modern anesthetic techniques for thoracic operations. World J Surg 25:162–166
13. McGlade DP, Slinger PD (2003) The elective combined use of a double-lumen tube and endobronchial blocker to provide selective lobar isolation for lung resection following contralateral lobectomy. Anesthesiology 99:1021–1022
14. Perera ER, Vidic DM, Zivot J (1993) Carinal resection with two high-frequency jet ventilation delivery systems. Can J Anaesth 40:59–63
15. Ratzenhofer-Komenda B, Prause G, Offner A et al (1996) Intraoperative application of high frequency ventilation in thoracic surgery. Acta Anaesthesiol Scan 109(S):149–153
16. Lucangelo U, Zin WA, Antonaglia V et al (2006) High-frequency percussive ventilation during surgical bronchial repair in a patient with one lung. Br J Anaesth 96(4):533–536

Non-invasive Ventilation

Non-invasive Ventilation in Patients with Acute Respiratory Failure and COPD or ARDS

G. Hilbert, F. Vargas, D. Gruson

Introduction

A major driving force behind the increasing use of non-invasive ventilation (NIV) has been the desire to avoid the complications of invasive ventilation. Although invasive mechanical ventilation is highly effective and reliable in supporting alveolar ventilation, endotracheal intubation is associated with numerous risks of complications. These include upper-airway injuries, tracheal stenosis, tracheomalacia, sinusitis, and ventilator-associated pneumonia [1]. Torres et al. considered the correlation between several risk factors and the development of nosocomial pneumonia: the presence of chronic obstructive pulmonary disease (COPD) and invasive ventilation for more than 3 days were significantly associated with an increased risk [2]. This complication of invasive ventilation is associated with a longer stay in the intensive care unit (ICU), increased costs and a worse outcome [2]. Furthermore, weaning difficulties are frequent in COPD patients [3], and the management of difficult-to-wean patients is a major clinical challenge that constitutes a large portion of the workload in an ICU [4].

In NIV, a tight-fitting face mask is used as an alternative interface between the patient and the ventilator to avoid these complications. In contrast to invasive ventilation, NIV leaves the upper airway intact, preserves airway defence mechanisms and allows patients to eat, drink, verbalise and expectorate secretions. The development of improved masks and ventilator technology has made this mode of ventilation acceptable.

In the early 1980s, continuous positive airway pressure (CPAP) delivered through a nasal mask was described in the treatment of obstructive sleep apnoea [5]. With the realisation that patients could tolerate positive pressure delivered through such masks during sleep, NIV was developed for the management of chronic nocturnal hypoventilation in patients with chronic respiratory failure caused by a variety of neuromuscular diseases and chest wall deformities [6–8]. The combination of non-invasive positive-pressure ventilation and long-term oxygen therapy may be more effective than treatment with long-term oxygen in

U. Lucangelo, P. Pelosi, W.A. Zin, A. Aliverti (eds.) *Respiratory System and Artificial Ventilation*. © Springer 2008

COPD patients [9]. However, the efficacy of NIV in patients with stable COPD is still debated [10,11].

Thus, NIV was applied first to patients with chronic pulmonary disease but is now being used to support those with acute respiratory failure (ARF). In these patients, the role of NIV in the management of patients with ARF and two very different pathologies, i.e., COPD and acute respiratory distress syndrome (ARDS), must be considered. The goals of NIV differ according to the clinical context. During acute exacerbations of COPD, the goal is to reduce CO_2 by unloading the respiratory muscles and augmenting alveolar ventilation, thereby stabilising arterial pH until the underlying problem can be reversed. When NIV is employed during episodes of hypoxaemic ARF, the goal is to ensure an adequate PaO_2 until the underlying problem can be reversed.

Furthermore, several controlled studies have clearly demonstrated the benefits of NIV in acute exacerbations of COPD and, as stated in the conclusions of the recent international consensus conference considering the role of NIV in ARF, patients hospitalised for exacerbations of COPD with rapid clinical deterioration should be considered for NIV to prevent further deterioration in gas exchange, respiratory workload and the need for endotracheal intubation [12]. The situation is very different for patients with ARDS. Based on the good results obtained in patients with acute exacerbations of COPD, NIV is now being used to support those with hypoxaemic ARF, some of them with acute lung injury (ALI) or ARDS. Nevertheless, in contrast to COPD patients with acute exacerbation, who constitute a relatively homogeneous group of patients, those with hypoxaemic ARF make up a much more heterogeneous group. Overall, in patients with hypoxaemic ARF, the clinical experience with NIV is less extensive than in COPD patients. The consensus conference concluded that larger, controlled studies are required to determine the potential benefit of adding NIV to standard medical treatment in the avoidance of endotracheal intubation in hypoxaemic ARF [12]. While it seems logical to propose NIV in patients with ARDS, the approach remains to be validated in this pathology. Thus, in this review, NIV in COPD patients and in patients with ARDS is discussed separately.

NIV in COPD Patients with Acute Respiratory Failure

Mechanisms of Improvement of NIV in COPD Patients

Failure of conventional treatment in patients with acute or chronic respiratory failure is characterised by the development of a rapid and shallow pattern of breathing, acute hypercapnia, and respiratory acidosis [13]. Thus, during acute exacerbations of COPD, the goal is to reduce CO_2 by unloading the respiratory muscles and augmenting alveolar ventilation, thereby stabilising arterial pH until the underlying problem can be reversed.

Meduri et al. have shown that assisted ventilation may be delivered non-invasively via a full face mask with the same immediate efficacy obtained through an endotracheal tube. Their study consisted of seven patients who had post-extubation hypercapnic respiratory distress [14]. In a physiologic study in 11 patients with acute exacerbation of COPD, Brochard et al. showed that 45 min of NIV with pressure support (PS) mode induced a rise in pH from 7.31±0.08 to 7.38±0.07, a drop in mean $PaCO_2$ from 68±17 to 55±15 mmHg, while PaO_2 was increased from 52±12 to 69±16 mmHg [15]. Bott et al. randomised 60 patients with acute exacerbations of COPD to receive nasal NIV or conventional treatment. Within the first hour of therapy, mean $PaCO_2$ fell from 65 to 55 mmHg, and dyspnoea scores improved among treated patients, whereas no significant changes occurred among control subjects [16]. Subsequent controlled studies comparing NIV and conventional therapy have confirmed that the use of NIV in acute exacerbations of COPD is associated with prompt improvement in acid–base balance and pulmonary gas exchange, as determined by arterial blood gases obtained within the first few hours [17–20].

Several theories have been proposed to explain why NIV is effective in the treatment of acute exacerbations of COPD. Numerous studies have examined the effects of NIV on breathing pattern and indices of work of breathing in these patients. In successfully treated patients, the respiratory rate invariably falls as tidal volume is augmented; NIV reduces the work of breathing and improves alveolar ventilation during acute exacerbations with hypercapnic respiratory failure [15,21,22]. As detailed elsewhere in this volume, the former can be further alleviated by addition of a moderate amount of positive end expiratory pressure (PEEP) to counterbalance intrinsic PEEP (PEEPi) [23]. Accordingly, NIV can correct the causes of increased work of breathing, i.e. the combination of PS and PEEP can offset the PEEPi level, reduce this inspiratory additional load and decrease the amount of work of breathing that the inspiratory muscle must generate to produce the tidal volume. When appropriate levels of PS and PEEP are used, the tidal volume increases and the respiratory rate decreases; then, NIV is able to rapidly increase PaO_2, reduce $PaCO_2$ and increase pH.

Diaz et al. demonstrated that improvement in respiratory blood gases during NIV was essentially due to higher alveolar ventilation and not to improvement in pulmonary ventilation–perfusion relationships [24]. Indeed, in their study, both the increase of PaO_2 and the decrease of $PaCO_2$ during NIV appeared to be related to the development of greater alveolar ventilation due to reduced respiratory frequency and increased tidal volume. In contrast, implementation of NIV did not result in recruitment of non-ventilated and/or of poorly ventilated alveolar units, in that there were no changes in the extent of blood-perfusing areas with shunt and very low ventilation–perfusion ratio [24].

The favourable effects of NIV in patients with ARF are thought to be at least partly related to a reduction in inspiratory muscle work, improvement in respiratory muscle function and avoidance of respiratory muscle fatigue. Ventilatory failure in patients with COPD is associated with inspiratory muscle fatigue and dysfunction. Brochard et al. demonstrated that PS ventilation via a face mask reduced the transdiaphragmatic pressure and electromyographic activity of the diaphragm in patients with acute exacerbations of COPD [15]. An improvement in oxygenation increases the flow of oxygen to the diaphragm and is also associated with the improvement observed with NIV.

The early demonstration that NIV reduces oesophageal pressure swings, diaphragmatic electromyographic activity and respiratory muscle work in patients with respiratory disease led investigators to hypothesise that NIV would be useful for supporting ventilation in patients with ARF who were at risk for respiratory muscle fatigue.

Equipment and Techniques

Interface

Non-invasive ventilation can be administered to COPD patients through different types of interfaces: face masks that cover the nose and mouth, nasal masks and 'nasal pillows' that fit into the nostrils. The patient interface most commonly employed is a full-face or nasal mask secured firmly, but not tightly, with a head-strap [12]. The full-face mask delivers higher ventilation pressures with fewer leaks, requires less patient cooperation and permits mouth breathing. However, it is less comfortable, increases dead space, impedes communication and limits oral intake. The nasal mask needs patent nasal passages and requires mouth closure to minimise air leaks. Leaks through the mouth decrease alveolar ventilation and may decrease the efficacy of NIV to reduce the work of breathing [21]. Furthermore, high flows of gas passing through the nose in case of mouth leaks can markedly increase nasal resistance and thus further reduce the efficacy of nasal NIV [25].

The standard masks exert pressure over the bridge of the nose in order to achieve an adequate air seal, often causing skin irritation and redness, and occasionally ulceration. Various modifications are available to minimise this complication, such as use of forehead spacers or the addition of a thin plastic flap that permits air sealing with less mask pressure on the nose. Straps that hold the mask in place are also important for patient comfort, and many types of strap assemblies are available. Most manufacturers provide straps that are designed for use with a particular mask. More points of attachment add to stability, and strap systems with Velcro fasteners are useful.

The efficacy of nasal and full-face masks was recently compared in a controlled trial of 26 patients with stable hypercapnia caused by COPD or restrictive thoracic disease. The nasal mask was better-tolerated than either nasal pillow or an oro-nasal mask but was less effective at lowering $PaCO_2$ [26]. However, to our knowledge, there are no studies comparing the effects of nasal and face masks on the efficacy of NIV in patients with acute respiratory distress. A selection of different sizes of nasal masks and full-face masks should be available for NIV. The different types of interfaces used in several controlled studies carried out in patients with acute exacerbations of COPD are reported in Table 1.

Table 1 Controlled studies examining the efficacy of non-invasive ventilation (*NIV*) in patients with acute exacerbations of chronic obstructive pulmonary disease (COPD)

Authors	Number of patients	pH at inclusion	Mask	Ventilatory mode	Hours of NIV/day	Duration of NIV (days)	Intubation rate (NIV/standard[b])
Brochard (1990) [15]	26	7.31	Facial	PS	7.6	3	8/85
Bott (1993) [16][a]	60	7.35	Nasal	ACV	7.6	6	Not compared
Vitacca (1993) [27]	60	7.27	Facial	PS-PEEP/ACV	CM	3	18/46
Brochard (1995) [17][a]	85	7.27	Facial	PS	7.6	4	26/74
Confalonieri (1996) [28]	48	7.29	Nasal	PS-PEEP	CM	10	8/38
Hilbert (1997) [18]	84	7.29	Facial, nasal	PS-PEEP	7	6	26/71
Celikel (1998) [19][a]	30	7.27	Facial	PS-PEEP	CM	1	7/40
Plant (2000) [20][a]	236	7.32	Facial, nasal	PS-PEEP	8	3	15/27

PS, Pressure support; *PEEP*, positive end-expiratory pressure, *ACV*, assisted control ventilation, *CM*, continuous mode

[a]Prospective, randomised controlled studies

[b]Standard medical treatment

Ventilators

Many different types of ventilator have been used successfully to provide NIV to patients with acute exacerbations of COPD. NIV can be administered by a volume ventilator, a pressure-controlled ventilator, a bilevel positive airway pressure (BiPAP) ventilator or a CPAP device. Ventilators employed in NIV range from ICU ventilators with full monitoring and alarm systems normally employed in the intubated patient, to lightweight, free-standing devices with limited alarm systems specifically designed for non-invasive respiratory support.

Life-support ICU ventilators separate inspiratory and expiratory gas mixtures. This prevents re-breathing and allows monitoring of inspiratory pressure and exhaled minute ventilation, on which monitoring and alarm limits are based.

Devices that use a common inspiratory and expiratory line can cause re-breathing of exhaled gas and persistent hypercapnia. Re-breathing has been shown to occur with low expiratory pressure settings and the standard exhalation device during BiPAP [29,30]. The use of an alternative exhalation device or expiratory pressures of at least 6 cmH_2O reduces re-breathing of carbon dioxide. In our practice, we never use an expiratory pressure <6 cmH_2O, with BiPAP ventilators, in COPD patients. Some BiPAP ventilators offer not only a spontaneously triggered PS mode but also pressure-limited, time-cycled and assist modes. Some also offer adjustable trigger sensitivities, time required to reach peak pressure and inspiratory duration, all features that may enhance patient-ventilator synchrony and comfort. Recently, new versions of BiPAP ventilators have been introduced that have more sophisticated alarm and monitoring capabilities, graphic displays and oxygen blenders; these are quite suitable for use in the acute care setting. Further, the performance characteristics of these ventilators compare favourably with those of critical care ventilators [31].

Pennock et al. were the first to demonstrate BiPAP as an effective method for treatment of acute respiratory episodes [32]. The degree of hypercapnia and acidosis were moderate in this initial study (at inclusion, mean $PaCO_2$ = 50 mmHg, mean pH = 7.38). Hilbert et al. demonstrated that BiPAP may also be used in the management of patients with severe acute exacerbations of COPD (at inclusion, mean $PaCO_2$ = 74 mmHg, mean pH = 7.29) [18].

Ventilatory Modes

During *volume-cycled* ventilation, the ventilator delivers a set tidal volume for each breath and inflation pressures may vary. The *assist-control* mode ensures that tidal breaths are triggered or imposed depending on the presence and magnitude of inspiratory efforts. Volume-cycled NIV can improve outcomes in ARF [33,34]. However, patient tolerance of this therapy is often poor [33,35], in part because the inspiratory pressure may be elevated, which can be uncomfortable and cause leaks [36].

During *pressure-support* ventilation, the ventilator is triggered by the patient, delivers a set pressure for each breath (commonly given with standard ventilators that use PS or with BiPAP ventilators) and cycles to expiration either when it senses a fall in inspiratory flow rate below a threshold value, or at a preset time. Non-invasive PS ventilation offers the potential of excellent patient-ventilator synchrony, reduced diaphragmatic work and improved patient comfort. However, it may also contribute to patient-ventilator asynchrony, particularly in patients with COPD. High levels of PS and the resulting large tidal volumes may contribute to inadequate inspiratory efforts on subsequent breaths, leading to failure to trigger. Also, brief rapid inspiration, as is often observed in patients with acute exacerbations of COPD, may not permit adequate time for the PS ventilation mode to cycle into expiration, so that the patient's expiratory effort begins while the ventilator is still delivering inspiratory pressure [37]. The patient must exert expiratory force to cycle the ventilator, and this may contribute to breathing discomfort. These forms of asynchrony are exacerbated in the presence of air leaks during NIV [38].

Intrinsic PEEP is often present in patients with COPD and can require great respiratory effort to trigger the ventilator. This can be alleviated by the addition of external PEEP [23]. Appendini et al. assessed the physiologic effects of PEEP during non-invasive PS ventilation in seven patients with acute exacerbation of COPD. PS ventilation increased minute ventilation, improved gas exchange and decreased diaphragmatic effort. PEEP added to PS ventilation further significantly decreased the diaphragmatic work by counterbalancing PEEPi, which was reduced from 5.4±4.0 to 3.1±2.3 cmH_2O [23].

At a recent consensus conference, NIV was defined as any form of ventilatory support applied without the use of an endotracheal tube and was considered to include CPAP, with or without inspiratory PS [12]. By counterbalancing the PEEPi imposed by the inspiratory threshold load, CPAP may reduce the work of breathing in patients with COPD. A few uncontrolled trials have observed improved vital signs and gas exchange in patients with acute exacerbations of COPD treated with CPAP alone, suggesting that this modality is beneficial to these patients [39–41]. Nevertheless, CPAP alone is less effective than PS to improve respiratory blood gases, because the technique does not directly increase tidal volume [41,42].

The ventilatory modes used in several controlled studies of patients with acute exacerbations of COPD are reported in Table 1. Volume-cycled and PS modes have both been shown to be effective in COPD, but few comparative studies have been reported. Vitacca et al. found no difference in outcome whether volume or pressure ventilators were used [27]. Girault et al. found greater respiratory muscle rest with volume assist, but at the cost of greater patient discomfort compared with PS [43].

Clinical Studies in Patients with Acute Exacerbations of COPD

Patients with acute exacerbations of COPD constitute the largest single diagnostic category among reported recipients of NIV. In one of the first studies dedicated to NIV in ARF, Meduri et al. reported positive results in a small sample of COPD patients; their results suggested the possibility of avoiding endotracheal intubation with use of this technique. Among the numerous subsequent uncontrolled studies, success rates in avoiding intubation have ranged from 58 to 93%. However, despite these encouraging results, uncontrolled studies are unable to provide evidence.

Controlled studies performed in patients with acute exacerbations of COPD are cited in Table 1. Studies using historical controls [15,18,27,28] and overall prospective, randomised studies [16,17,19,20,44] strongly support the use of noninvasive mechanical ventilation in patients with severe exacerbations of COPD.

In an early study using historically matched control subjects, Brochard et al. reported that only one of 13 patients with acute exacerbations of COPD treated with face-mask NIV required endotracheal intubation, compared with 11 of 13 control subjects [15]. In addition, patients treated with NIV were weaned from the ventilator faster and spent less time in the ICU than did the control subjects.

A larger, more recent, historically controlled trial yielded similar results; indeed, 11 of the 42 patients (26%) in the NIV group needed tracheal intubation compared with 30 of the 42 control patients (71%) [18]. Furthermore, this study evidenced that a simple device, such as BiPAP, initially designed for home NIV, may also be used in the management of severe ARF. One of the originalities of this trial is that NIV was used in a sequential, discontinuous mode with some specificity, i.e. predetermination of the duration of the ventilation sessions and of the time between NIV sessions.

In the first prospective, randomised study, Bott et al. randomised 60 patients with acute exacerbations of COPD to receive nasal NIV or conventional therapy [16]. Mortality fell from 30% among control patients to 10% among NIV-treated patients, although this reduction became statistically significant only after the exclusion of four patients randomised to the NIV group but who never actually received it.

Kramer et al. randomised 31 patients with various aetiologies for respiratory failure, 21 of whom had COPD, to receive BiPAP ventilation through a nasal mask or conventional therapy [44]. Among patients with COPD, the need for intubation was reduced from 67% among control patients to 9% among those given NIV.

Subsequently, a multicentre randomised study found significant benefits of NIV (PS of 20 cmH_2O, and PEEP of 0 cmH_2O) delivered by face mask as compared with standard treatment among 85 COPD patients [17]. The NIV group had significantly lower rates of complications (including nosocomial pneumonia, 16 vs. 48%), a reduced need for endotracheal intubation (26 vs. 74%), shorter hospital lengths of stays (23 vs. 35 days) and lower mortality (9 vs. 29%) than those receiving standard treatment. It is important to note that 69% of the total group of patients with COPD who had acute or chronic respiratory failure were excluded from the study: that is, the patients were highly selected. It is therefore clear that careful patient selection is important to the success of NIV.

Among the controlled studies examining the efficacy of NIV in ARF due to

COPD, only one obtained negative results [45]. Nevertheless, in this study comprising only 24 patients, the lack of difference between the two groups was not surprising as, given the modest level of acidosis at presentation, the majority were likely to improve with standard treatment.

NIV is the only therapeutic measure to produce a survival advantage for individuals with severe exacerbations of COPD. This advantage, previously established in ICUs, has now been shown by Plant et al. to be obtainable also on general medical or respiratory wards [20]. Plant et al. carried out the most recent and largest randomised controlled trial on 236 patients with COPD exacerbations and pH values between 7.25 and 7.35 who were treated on general respiratory wards. After staff training, NIV was applied by the usual ward staff according to a simple protocol. The need for intubation was reduced from 27 to 15% by NIV ($p<0.05$). Subgroup analysis suggested that the outcome in patients with pH<7.30 after initial treatment was inferior to that in studies performed in the ICU. Thus, the authors suggested that these patients are probably best managed in a higher-dependency setting with individually tailored ventilation.

In summary, the addition of NIV to standard medical treatment may prevent endotracheal intubation, and reduce the rate of complications and mortality, in patients with severe exacerbations of COPD. Thus, the recent international consensus conference recommended: 'patients hospitalized for exacerbations of COPD with rapid clinical deterioration should be considered for NIV to prevent further deterioration in gas exchange, respiratory workload, and the need for endotracheal intubation' [12].

Use of NIV for Weaning and To Avoid Re-intubation

As noted above, Torres et al. found that several risk factors were correlated with the development of nosocomial pneumonia. Their findings, that the presence of COPD and intubation and mechanical ventilation for more than 3 days were significantly associated with an increase risk of nosocomial pneumonia, support the need to shorten the duration of intubation as an attractive strategy to reduce hospital stay and decrease morbidity and mortality [2].

Nava et al. compared weaning using NIV or continued invasive ventilation in 50 COPD patients who had been intubated and ventilated either from the outset or following a failed trial of NIV [46]. After 48 h, patients on invasive ventilation were subjected to a 2-h T-piece trial; those who failed were randomised to receive either a standard weaning process with invasive PS ventilation or to be extubated and receive NIV. There was a clear advantage for the non-invasive approach in the percentage of patients successfully weaned, duration of need for assisted ventilation, ICU stay, survival, and incidence of ventilator-associated pneumonia. This suggests a role for NIV in patients who initially have had to be ventilated invasively.

Girault et al. compared NIV with continued invasive ventilation in another randomised study of 33 patients who failed a T-piece trial [47]. Patients who received NIV could be extubated earlier, but there was no difference in the number who could be weaned, the length of ICU stay, or survival at 3 months. In 43 mechanically ventilated patients with persistent weaning failure, the NIV group, when compared with the conventional-weaning group, had increased ICU and 90-day survival [48]. The conventional-weaning approach was an independent risk factor of decreased ICU and 90-day survival [48].

The failure of extubation and re-intubation are not infrequent clinical problems in the ICU setting and represents a risk factor for the development of nosocomial pneumonia. In a prospective randomised study, comparing four methods of weaning patients from mechanical ventilation, the incidence of extubation failure was 24% in COPD patients [49]. Epstein et al. reported that the incidence of post-extubation failure is relatively high and that the prognosis of these patients is poor, since their hospital mortality exceeds 40–50%, with the cause of extubation failure and the time to re-intubation being independent predictors of outcome [50,51].

A prospective case-controlled study using historical controls seemed to confirm the utility of NPPV in the setting of hypercapnic respiratory failure occurring within 72 h post-extubation [52]. In that study, respiratory distress was defined as the combination of a respiratory rate >25 breaths/min, an increase in $PaCO_2$ of at least 20% as compared to the value measured after extubation, and pH<7.35. The use of NIV significantly reduced the need for endotracheal intubation (20 vs. 67%, $p<0.001$). In-hospital mortality was not significantly different between the two groups, but the mean duration of ventilatory assistance for the treatment of the post-extubation distress, and the length of ICU stay related to this event, were both significantly shortened by NIV.

The factors related to higher rates of pneumonia and mortality in the population of patients needing to be re-intubated remain unidentified, but instability between extubation and reintubation may be responsible. If this period is prolonged, the probability of complications and death increases. Bearing in mind the importance of these issues, the early institution of NIV in this population is theoretically attractive. A simple and precocious measurement of occlusion pressure at 0.1 s after extubation could help to indicate the need for NIV in COPD patients [53].

To assess a new and very attractive application of NIV, a prospective randomised controlled trial was conducted in 162 mechanically ventilated patients who tolerated a spontaneous breathing trial after recovery from the acute episode but had increased risk for respiratory failure after extubation [54]. Patients were randomly allocated after extubation to receive NIV for 24 h or conventional management with oxygen therapy. In the NIV group, respiratory failure after extubation was less frequent. However, NIV improved ICU mortality and 90-day survival in hypercapnic patients ($PaCO_2$>45 mmHg during the spontaneous breathing trial) only; these patients had chronic respiratory disorders [54]. Further studies are needed to valid this novel indication of NIV in COPD patients, i.e. as an alternative to conventional weaning, and its role in the prevention of post-extubation respiratory distress.

Side Effects, Limits and Factors Predictive of NIV Outcome

Some authors have emphasised that NIV is not easily accepted by ARF patients [35,55]. This explains, at least partly, why in numerous studies the objectives of either continuous ventilation or prolonged periods of ventilation have not been achieved. In the study of Foglio et al., patients were submitted to an average of only 4 h of NIV [35]. In the study of Bott et al., patients were encouraged to use NIV up to 16 h a day and finally received 7.6 h of ventilation per day [16]. The difficulties of acceptance on behalf of the patients, and most NIV failures, are due to technical problems. When NIV is applied, patients must be watched for signs of mask intolerance, claustrophobia, ventilator-patient asynchrony, serious air leaks, gastric distention, drying of the eyes, and facial-skin breakdown.

Gastric distention is very unlikely with PS levels <25 cmH_2O. Eye irritation or conjunctivitis has been reported in up to 18% of patients. The most serious problems concern air leaks and facial-skin breakdown, especially at the bridge of the nose.

Gas Leaks

Gas leaks around the mask or from the mouth limit the efficacy of the device, make monitoring of tidal volume difficult, may prevent adequate ventilatory assistance in patients who require high inspiratory airway pressures and represent a cause of failure. Carrey et al. showed that significant reduction of the diaphragmatic electromyographic signal, related to partial unloading of inspiratory muscles, with the use of nasal NIV was observed only during periods when the patient's mouth was closed [21]. This supports the commonly held belief that in the acute setting full-face masks are preferable to nasal masks, because dyspnoeic and poorly cooperative patients are unable to close their mouth, predisposing to greater air leakage and reduced effectiveness during nasal mask ventilation.

In the case of leaks at end-inspiration, PS ventilation may fail to synchronise with termination of the patient's inspiratory effort; then, the end-inspiration off-switch mechanism may not be detected by the ventilator, which may result in a prolonged insufflation time with major dyssynchrony [38].

Facial-Skin Breakdown

Both nasal and full-face masks can lead to pressure necrosis of the skin over the nasal bridge. Facial-skin necrosis has been reported in up to 18% of patients [44]. Avoiding this complication requires the selection of different sizes of nasal and full-face masks, careful attention, the use of cushioning materials and 'rest' periods. Thus, discontinuous administration of NIV, by the inclusion of rest periods during which oxygen is conventionally delivered, together with the alternation between different types of interface according to patient's needs, cooperation and tolerance may be an interesting approach to reduce the side effects of

NIV and improve its performance. In our experience, the sequential mode, which is a discontinuous mode with some specificity, is well tolerated by COPD patients [18,52,56,57]. Ventilatory support should also be introduced gradually, starting with low levels of PS and PEEP and increasing the pressure levels as required. The process should be controlled by an experienced attendant working with the patient and observing his or her response and comfort level. A manual mask should be applied at first to minimise the patient's sense of claustrophobia.

The fact that most NIV failures are due to technical problems justifies the recent studies evaluating new interfaces. In a recent multicentre randomised study, Gregoretti et al. evaluated patient comfort, skin breakdown and eye irritation in a comparison of conventional face masks and a prototype face mask to administer NIV [58]. This prototype was specifically designed for NIV to allow a more comfortable patient-mask interface where the mask is in contact with the nasal bridge and to reduce air leaks. The new mask significantly reduced skin breakdown and improved patient comfort compared to the conventional face mask.

Influence of NIV on the Workload of ICU Nurses

An early work suggested that NIV created an excessive workload for ICU nurses: Chevrolet et al., in a study of six patients, three of whom had COPD, showed that, in the case of COPD patients, the nursing time spent with the patient was close to the ventilatory time [55]. However, it is necessary to point out that these results were based solely on three patients whose respiratory insufficiency was very severe and in whom NIV had failed; thus experience with this method is limited. As Pennock et al. [59] and Meduri et al. [60] demonstrated, it is likely that training of personnel is necessary before optimal routine daily use of NIV can be expected.

Other studies have shown that while extra time is required to set up NIV compared to that needed for routine care, maintenance of the patient on NIV does not require a large amount of extra nursing and/or physiotherapy time [44,61]. When invasive ventilation and NIV were compared, no differences were found in the time doctors, nurses, or therapists spent at the bedside during the initial 6 h of ventilatory support [62]. In the subsequent 42 h, less nursing time was required to monitor patients receiving NIV. However, these studies were performed in respiratory ICUs, i.e. with specialised activity, and where patient/staff ratios are generally lower than in general ICUs [44,61,62].

Thus, we conducted a trial to prospectively study, in a medical ICU, the assistance time spent by nurses in relation to ventilatory time when NIV was used in COPD patients with either acute exacerbations or post-extubation hypercapnic respiratory insufficiency [56]. The nurse time consumed per session was 25% of the ventilatory time during the first 24 h after enrolment and dropped significantly to 15% of the ventilatory time after the first 24 h of the protocol. The study seemed to favour a very low assistance time spent by nurses in relation to ventilatory time when NIV is used in COPD patients with respiratory distress. As in other studies by our team that have dealt with NIV in COPD patients, NIV was used in a sequential, discontinuous mode. Accordingly, the reported results could be compared with those of other studies with some specificity regarding predetermination of the duration of the ventilation sessions and of the time between NIV sessions. For example, in our first study on NIV in patients with acute exacerbations of COPD, BiPAP was used for at least 30 min every 3 h [18]. The nurse and physiotherapist were asked to perform periods of ventilation for as long as possible, mainly in the beginning of the protocol, taking into account the patient's tolerance and always trying to encourage a minimal duration of ventilation of 30 min. Between periods of ventilation, patients received a minimal oxygen flow adjusted to blood gas analysis data, with continuous monitoring of the haemodynamic state, respiratory rate and pulse oxygen saturation (SaO_2). Patients were systematically returned to BiPAP when SaO_2 was <0.85 or when dyspnoea worsened (respiratory rate >30 breaths/min). After the first 24 h of the protocol, if the patient improved, the interval between ventilation sessions could be increased. One of the potential advantages of the sequential approach is a harmonious distribution of NIV sessions, better acceptance and tolerance by patients, and better management by the nursing staff. The protocol of sequential ventilation is appreciated by our staff and has contributed to the standardisation of NIV techniques in our ICU. It was not necessary to modify the organisation of our unit due to the introduction of these new techniques.

A recent study confirmed that the workload of nurses should not be overestimated [20]. This study showed that, in acute exacerbations of COPD, the use of NIV on general respiratory wards (with a median nurse/patient ratio of 1/11) was both feasible and clinically effective, and led to a modest 26 min increase in nursing workload in the first 8 h of admission. No difference in workload was identified after 8 h between patients treated with NIV and those who received standard treatment. However, these results were only obtained by ensuring that the staff within the participating wards was trained to provide NIV and that these skills were maintained over time. The mean amount of formal training given in the first 3 months of opening a ward by the research doctor and nurse was 7.6 h. Thereafter, each centre received 0.9 h training per month to maintain skills.

An educational and supervision program is essential to successfully implement and develop NIV methods. In our ICU, the personnel have benefited from the training they have received in the techniques of ventilation, which is performed by medical doctors, respiratory therapists, and the most experienced nurses.

Factors Predictive of NIV Outcome

During acute exacerbations of COPD, the goal is to reduce CO_2 by unloading the respiratory muscles and augmenting alveolar ventilation, thereby stabilising arterial pH until the underlying problem can be reversed. A number of studies have shown that rapid (1–4 h) improvement in blood pH is crucial for successful NIV.

Soo Hoo et al., in a small study (14 episodes in 12 patients) in which NIV was successful in 50% of patients, found that there were no differences in age, prior pulmonary function, baseline arterial blood gas tensions, admission arterial blood gas tensions, or respiratory rate between patients successfully treated and those who failed NIV [36]. Unsuccessfully treated patients had more severe illness than successfully treated patients, as indicated by a higher Acute Physiology and Chronic Health Evaluation II score, and had pneumonia or excess secretions. In addition, they were edentulous and had pursed lip breathing, both of which are factors that prevent adequate mouth seal and contribute to greater mouth leaks than in successfully treated patients. Successfully treated patients were those who were able to adapt more rapidly to the nasal mask and ventilator, with greater and more rapid reduction in $PaCO_2$, correction of pH, and reduction in respiratory rate.

Ambrosino et al., in a larger study of 59 episodes in 47 patients of whom 78% were successfully treated with NIV, found that success was more likely in patients with less severely abnormal baseline clinical and functional parameters and with less severe levels of acidosis [63]. Pneumonia was associated with a worse outcome.

At the beginning of the protocol of Hilbert's et al. study, patients benefited from a first session of BiPAP of 30 min, then, after blood gas analysis, a second session of 45 min of ventilation with optimisation of ventilator adjustments [18]. Two initial closely following sessions of a total of 75 min may be sufficient to halt the worsening of respiratory failure and significantly correct acidosis, this being considered the main cause of persistent respiratory muscle fatigue. In patients successfully ventilated with NIV, correction of pH, measured after 45 min of support with optimal settings, was greater than in those in whom NIV had failed (7.38 vs. 7.28).

A recent prospective study examined COPD patients with and without home ventilatory support and compared those patients who were successfully ventilated with NIV and those who failed with NIV for treatment of acute exacerbations of lung disease [57]. A greater correction of pH, after 45 min of NIV with optimal settings, was recorded in the group of successful patients than in the group of failure patients: in those receiving home NIV, 7.34 ± 0.04 vs. 7.31 ± 0.04 ($p=0.06$) and in the group without home NIV, 7.34 ± 0.04 vs. 7.30 ± 0.04 ($p=0.001$).

The study by Plant et al., on 118 COPD patients treated with NIV, adds data that support monitoring the change in pH and shows that changes in respiratory rate can also be informative, i.e. after 4 h of treatment, an improvement in acidosis (OR 0.89 per nmol/l, 95% CI 0.82–0.97, $p<0.01$) and a fall in respiratory rate (OR 0.92 per breaths/min, 95% CI 0.84–0.99, $p=0.04$) were associated with success [64].

Taken together, these data suggest that NIV is more likely to be successful in patients with a less severe physiological derangement at baseline, in whom a rapid improvement in respiratory rate and in pH can be expected.

Future Developments

Patient comfort and therapeutic compliance are critical to the success of NIV; thus, newer modes of ventilation that closely mirror the patient's desired breathing pattern are of great interest. One such new ventilator mode is *proportional assist ventilation* (PAV), which targets patient effort rather than pressure or volume [65]. By instantaneously tracking patient inspiratory flow and its integral (volume) using an in-line pneumotachograph, PAV has the capability of responding rapidly to the patient's ventilatory effort. Since the gain on the flow and volume signals is adjustable, the operator is able to select the proportion of breathing work that is to be assisted. In seven COPD patients with hypercapnic ARF, NIV-PAV improved arterial blood gases while unloading inspiratory muscles, and was well-tolerated by the patients compared to CPAP [66]. In a recent study, the short-term administration of NIV-PAV and NIV with PS ventilation was compared in 12 COPD patients with hypercapnic ARF [67]. Breathing pattern, arterial pH and $PaCO_2$ were similarly improved and indices of inspiratory muscle effort were similarly reduced with the two modalities, but patients found NIV-PAV to be more comfortable than NIV-PS ventilation, perhaps related to the more variable tidal volume obtained with PAV. Nevertheless, in a prospective randomised controlled trial, even though PAV was better-tolerated, intubation and mortality rates were similar between NIV-PAV and NIV-PS modes [68].

The decrease in the resistance to gas flow achieved by a gas of low density, such as helium, might facilitate wider use of NIV. The administration of helium-oxygen (He/O_2) was tested in combination with NIV in ten patients with acute exacerbation of COPD. Results of NIV-HeO_2 were compared with those obtained with standard NIV ($AirO_2$) at two levels of PS ventilation [69]. The low-density gas mixture conferred significant reductions in inspiratory effort, work of breathing and $PaCO_2$, and no change in breathing pattern or oxygenation. Nevertheless, in a prospective randomised controlled trial, NIV with HeO_2 did not significantly reduce intubation rate when compared with $AirO_2$ [70]. If the problems of infrastructure and the high cost of the He/O_2 mixture and of the equipment needed to deliver He/O_2 are considered, this well-conducted clinical study offers few arguments to persuade physicians to modify their approach in the treatment of acute exacerbations of COPD [71].

NIV in Patients with ARDS

The mainstay of supportive care of ALI and ARDS is mechanical ventilation. By stabilising respiration, mechanical ventilation allows time for treatment of the underlying cause of these conditions, i.e. infection, and for the evolution of natural healing processes. Improved understanding of the pathogenesis of ALI/ARDS has led to important advances in the treatment of ALI/ARDS, particularly in the area of ventilator-associated lung injury. Standard supportive care for ALI/ARDS should now include a protective ventilatory strategy with low tidal volume ventilation, such as outlined in the protocol developed by the National Institutes of Health ARDS Network [72]. The decrease in ALI/ARDS mortality reported since the early 1990s is attributable to improvements in many aspects of care, such as ventilator management, diagnosis and treatment of infections [73]. However, mortality is still high, and survivors may suffer from the various sequelae for months after recovery from critical illness [74,75]. Thus, further improvements in treatment are needed. Mortality from ARDS has long been associated with the development of multiple organ failure rather than death from hypoxaemic ARF per se. If intubation could be avoided in such patients, the risk from ventilator-associated lung injury and/or nosocomial pneumonia and sepsis might be substantially reduced. In this way, NIV could have its place in the therapeutic armamentarium of physicians dealing with patients with ALI or ARDS. Based on the good results obtained in patients with acute exacerbations of COPD, NIV is now being used to support those with hypoxaemic ARF, including some with ALI or ARDS.

Mechanisms of Improvement Following NIV in Patients with ARDS

In many ALI/ARDS patients, intrapulmonary shunt and ventilation-perfusion imbalances cause life-threatening hypoxaemia. Moreover, the high work of breathing from increased alveolar dead space and reduced respiratory system compliance may cause ventilatory failure with hypercapnia and respiratory acidosis. When employed during episodes of hypoxaemic ARF, the goal of NIV is to ensure an adequate PaO_2 until the underlying problem can be reversed.

Numerous case series and reports have shown that CPAP improves oxygenation, reduces respiratory rate and lessens dyspnoea in hypoxaemic ARF patients [76–82]. Kesten et al. applied 10 cmH_2O of nasal CPAP in nine subjects with *Pneumocystis carinii* pneumonia and AIDS, all of whom had presented with bilateral pulmonary infiltrates and hypoxaemia [79]. Twenty minutes of nasal CPAP without supplemental oxygen increased mean PaO_2 from 56 to 68 mmHg and decreased the calculated alveolar-arterial oxygen gradient from 48 to 34 mmHg.

In a trial that specifically included patients with ALI or ARDS, baseline PaO_2/FiO_2 was <120 on 11 of 12 occasions [83]. In response to NIV, 2–6 h after administration, PaO_2/FiO_2 was measured in ten patients; it remained <200 in seven, but improved by >25% in nine patients, and was unchanged in one.

Antonelli et al. conducted a prospective, randomised trial in which NIV was compared with endotracheal intubation with conventional mechanical ventilation in 64 patients with hypoxaemic ARF who required mechanical ventilation [84]. Seven (22%) of 32 patients randomised to NIV had ARDS of varied aetiology. Patients in the two groups had similar initial changes in PaO_2/FiO_2: within the first hour of ventilation, 20 patients (62%) in the NIV group and 15 (47%)

in the conventional ventilation group showed improvement in PaO_2/FiO_2. Their PaO_2/FiO_2 ratios increased significantly from 116±24 to 230±76 mmHg with NIV and from 124±25 to 211±68 mmHg with conventional ventilation.

Numerous prospective controlled studies comparing NIV with standard medical treatment showed that the use of NIV in hypoxaemic ARF is associated with prompt improvement in pulmonary gas exchange, as determined by arterial blood gases obtained within the first few hours [85–87]. In a study comparing NIV with standard treatment using supplemental oxygen administration in recipients of solid-organ transplants who developed hypoxaemic ARF, seven (22%) of 32 patients randomised to NIV had ARDS of varied aetiology [85]. Within the first hour of treatment, 14 patients (70%) in the NIV group but only five patients (25%) in the standard treatment group had an improved PaO_2/FiO_2. In another randomised controlled trial, the physiologic effects of CPAP vs. standard oxygen therapy were compared in 123 patients with hypoxaemic ARF and $PaO_2/FiO_2 \leq 300$ due to bilateral pulmonary oedema, 102 of them with ALI [86]. After one hour of treatment, median PaO_2/FiO_2 was greater with CPAP (203 vs. 151, $p=0.02$). In a prospective, randomised trial of NIV compared with standard medical treatment with supplemental oxygen in immunosuppressed patients with hypoxaemic ARF, initial improvement in PaO_2/FiO_2 was observed in 46% of patients in the NIV group and in 15% in the standard group ($p=0.02$) [87]. Even though NIV was used intermittently and in a sequential mode, the improvement in gas-exchange abnormalities achieved with the NIV protocol was significantly higher than that in patients who received standard treatment [87]. Reducing the work of breathing during NIV sessions may also allow respiratory muscles to be more efficient during non-assisted breaths.

NIV can improve the pathophysiology of hypoxaemic respiratory failure. Mechanisms of improvement can include the beneficial effects of PEEP on the distribution of extravascular lung water and on alveolar recruitment of under-ventilated alveoli by increasing lung volume at end expiration, and in the early treatment of atelectasis. In addition, ventilation/perfusion ratios or even shunt undoubtedly improve in patients with ARDS, in whom the application of expiratory pressure should have an effect similar to that of PEEP in invasively ventilated patients. By lowering left ventricular transmural pressure, CPAP may reduce afterload and increase cardiac output, making it an attractive modality for therapy of acute pulmonary oedema. Even if CPAP alone is able to improve lung mechanics in patients with ARF and decrease work of breathing compared with unsupported ventilation [88], the addition of PS has a positive effect in reducing the work of breathing and maintaining a tidal volume compatible with adequate alveolar ventilation [89].

Equipment and Techniques in the NIV of ARDS Patients

There is no evidence to support the use of a particular patient interface device in patients with hypoxaemic ARF. Nevertheless, clinical experience suggests that full-face masks improve efficacy by reducing leaks and are more appropriate for use in the setting of severe hypoxaemic ARF, including ALI and ARDS. As shown in Table 2, a face mask was used preferentially in controlled studies examining the efficacy of NIV in hypoxaemic ARF.

One of the main differences between COPD patients and patients with hypoxaemic ARF is the place of CPAP in the therapeutic armamentarium of physicians treating the latter. Pressures commonly used to deliver CPAP to those patients range from 5 to 15 cmH_2O. Pressure can be applied using a wide variety of devices, including CPAP valves connected to a compressed gas source, small portable units used for home therapy of obstructive sleep apnoea and ventilators designed for use in the ICU. Depending on the critical care ventilator selected, CPAP may be administered using 'demand,' 'flow-by,' or 'continuous flow' techniques, with the imposed work differing slightly between them [90]. CPAP is widely used in the belief that it may reduce the need for intubation and mechanical ventilation in patients with acute hypoxaemic respiratory insufficiency. Nevertheless, to our knowledge, although several studies have shown the ability of the method to improve hypoxaemia, only one randomised study has demonstrated that the use of CPAP reduces the need for endotracheal intubation in patients with severe hypercapnic cardiogenic pulmonary oedema [91]. A recent study showed that, compared with standard oxygen therapy, CPAP neither reduced the need for intubation nor improved outcomes in patients with hypoxaemic ARF [86]. In contrast, positive results have been reported in randomised controlled studies (discussed in the next chapter) in which PS + PEEP was used.

The choice of NIV with PS and PEEP, rather than CPAP, a technique previously systematically used in treating hypoxaemic ARF in our ICU [82], has undoubtedly contributed to the good results recently reported in immunosuppressed patients [87]. In our practice, after the mask is secured, the level of PS is progressively increased and adjusted such that the patient obtains an expired tidal volume of 7–10 ml per kg body weight and a respiratory rate of <25 breaths per minute. PEEP is repeatedly increased by 2 cmH_2O, up to a level of 10 cmH_2O, until the FiO_2 requirement is 70% or less. The FiO_2 is adjusted to maintain SaO_2 above 90%. Ventilator settings are adjusted on the basis of continuous monitoring of SaO_2, clinical data and measurements of arterial-blood gases.

Studies comparing the impact on clinical outcome of CPAP and PS + PEEP in patients with hypoxaemic ARF should be useful. For the moment, and looking forward to the results of further studies, PS ventilation + PEEP could be the ventilatory mode recommended for treatment with NIV of hypoxaemic ARF, including ALI/ARDS.

Main Clinical Studies

CPAP has been used successfully for years to correct severe hypoxaemia in patients with hypoxaemic ARF [76–82]. For instance, Gregg et al. studied the efficacy of CPAP in ten AIDS patients with pneumonia; in seven of them intu-

Table 2 Controlled studies examining the efficacy of non-invasive ventilation (*NIV*) in hypoxaemic acute respiratory failure

Author	Number of patients	Comments	Mask	Ventilatory mode	Intubation rate (NIV/standard[a])
Wysocki (1995) [92]	41	Variety of causes of acute respiratory failure	Facial	PS-PEEP	62/70
Antonelli (1998) [84]	64	Criteria for intubation	Facial	PS-PEEP	31[b]
Confalonieri (1999) [61]	56	Community-acquired pneumonia $PaO_2/FiO_2 \leq 250$	Facial	PS-PEEP	21/50
Martin (2000) [93]		Variety of causes of acute respiratory failure	Nasal/facial	PS-PEEP	7/23
Delclaux (2000) [86]	123	$PaO_2/FiO_2 \leq 300$	Facial	CPAP	34/39
Antonelli (2000) [85]	40	Solid-organ transplantation	Facial	PS-PEEP	20/70
Hilbert (2001) [87]	52	Immunosuppressed patients$PaO_2/FiO_2 \leq 200$	Facial	PS-PEEP	46/77
Ferrer (2003) [94]	105	Variety of causes of acute respiratory failure	Facial	PS-PEEP	13/29

PS, Pressure support; *PEEP*, positive end-expiratory pressure; *CPAP* continuous positive airway pressure; *PAV*, proportional assist ventilation
[a]Standard medical treatment related to the aetiology of hypoxaemic acute respiratory failure with O_2 supplementation
[b]In this study NIV was compared to invasive ventilation and not to standard treatment

bation could be avoided [80]. Among 64 neutropaenic patients with febrile acute hypoxaemic normocapnic respiratory failure who were treated by CPAP in addition to standard therapy in the study by Hilbert et al., CPAP was efficient in only 25% of cases [82]. The enrolled patients were critically ill, with a high SAPS II and dysfunction of more than two organs, explaining, in part, the poor results obtained. Nevertheless, all the responders and only four non-responders survived their ICU stay. Recently, in a case report, Rabitsch et al. reported the successful management through high-flow CPAP of a neutropenic patient with ARDS [95].

In the large series of Meduri et al., 41 of 158 patients had hypoxaemic respiratory failure [60] arising from multiple causes, including ARDS. Despite an average initial PaO_2/FiO_2 of 110 mm Hg, these hypoxaemic patients, who were treated with NIV, required intubation in only 34% of cases. In a prospective study, variables predictive of NIV failure were investigated in 354 patients with hypoxaemic ARF [96]. NIV failed in 30%. Endotracheal intubation was required in 51% of the 86 patients with ARDS, in 54% of the 59 patients with ARDS of extrapulmonary aetiology and in 46% of the 27 patients with ARDS of pulmonary origin.

Only two trials enrolled exclusively patients with ALI/ARDS [83,97]. Rocker et al., in an uncontrolled study, reported the outcome of 12 episodes of ALI/ARDS in ten patients treated with NIV [83]. The overall success rate in the NIV trials was 50%. In detail, avoidance of intubation was achieved on six of the nine occasions (66%) when NIV was used as the initial mode of assisted ventilation; it failed after three episodes of planned (1) or self (2) extubation. In a prospective, multiple-centre cohort study, NIV applied as first-line intervention in ARDS led to the avoidance of intubation in 54% of treated patients [97]. These encouraging results showed that NIV should be considered as a treatment option for patients in stable condition in the early phase of ALI/ARDS.

Table 2 lists reported the controlled studies that have examined the efficacy of NIV in hypoxaemic ARF. Numerous randomised trials tested the hypothesis that NIV prevents endotracheal intubation in patients with hypoxaemic ARF, compared with those that received medical treatment, with O_2 supplementation, according to related the aetiology of the ARF [61,85–87,92–94]. A trial of patients with a variety of causes for their ARF found no benefit of NIV over conventional therapy among all enrolled patients [95]. When patients with a $PaCO_2$ <45 mmHg (90% of whom required intubation) were excluded in a post hoc analysis, NIV significantly reduced intubation rate, length of ICU stay and ICU mortality among the remaining hypercapnic patients. The implication of these findings is that hypoxaemic ARF without CO_2 retention responds poorly to NIV. Confalonieri et al. randomised 56 patients with severe community-acquired pneumonia to receive NIV plus conventional therapy or conventional therapy alone. The intubation rates of patients treated with NIV were lower (21 vs. 50, $p<0.03$) and their duration of ICU stay was shorter (1.8 vs. 6 days, $p<0.04$) than was the case for control subjects, although hospital lengths of stay and hospital mortality rates were similar [61]. In addition, a subgroup analysis revealed that significant benefits were attributable only to patients with underlying COPD. However, more recent controlled studies suggested that some patients with hypoxaemic ARF, without COPD and/or CO_2 retention, may respond favourably to NIV. A randomised controlled trial of 61 patients with various forms of ARF found a significantly reduced intubation rate when patients with hypoxaemic ARF were treated with NIV as opposed to conventional therapy (7.5 vs. 22.6 intubations per 100 ICU days), although mortality rates were not significantly different [96].

Five randomised trials included patients with ALI/ARDS [84–87,94]. In the study by Antonelli et al. [84] described above, more patients in the conventional ventilation group had serious complications (66 vs. 38%, p=0.02) and pneumonia or sinusitis related to the endotracheal tube (31 vs. 3%, p=0.003). Among the survivors, patients in the NIV group had shorter periods of ventilation (p=0.006) and shorter stays in the ICU (p=0.002). Seven (22%) of 32 patients randomised to NIV had ARDS of varied aetiology. Four (58%) of them with ARDS avoided intubation and survived, while three (42%) required intubation and died. In a randomised controlled trial of CPAP in 123 patients with hypoxaemic ARF, including 102 with ALI, treatment with CPAP failed to reduce the endotracheal intubation rate, hospital mortality, or median ICU length of stay [86]. In that study, despite early physiologic improvement, CPAP neither reduced the need for intubation nor improved outcomes in patients with acute hypoxaemic, non-hypercapnic respiratory insufficiency primarily due in majority to ALI. In the most recent controlled study, NIV significantly decreased the need for intubation compared with oxygen therapy (13 vs. 29%) and ICU mortality, and increased cumulative 90-day survival [94]. Only seven patients in the NIV group and eight in the control group had criteria of ARDS. Six of the seven NIV patients and the eight control patients were intubated. However, it is important to underline that patients with very severe ARDSwere included since the mean ratio PaO2/FiO2 was 102, and certainly lower for ARDS. In addition, ARDS was not secondary to pneumonia and in some patients was of extra-pulmonary origin [94].

'Immunocompromised patients with ARF who require mechanical ventilation have notoriously poor prognoses, with mortality rates ranging from 60 to 100%. Traditionally, immunocompromised patients have undergone endotracheal intubation when their respiratory failure becomes severe. Too often, this intervention has been followed by further, ultimately fatal complications, including pneumonia and sepsis. New therapeutic approaches are clearly needed' [98], and avoiding intubation should be an important objective in the management of hypoxaemic ARF in immunosuppressed patients.

In a study comparing NIV with standard treatment consisting of supplemental oxygen administration in solid-organ transplant recipients who developed hypoxaemic ARF, NIV resulted in lower intubation rates (20 vs. 70%, p=0.002), fewer fatal complications (20 vs. 50%, p=0.05) and reduced ICU stay and mortality (20 vs. 50%, p=0.05) [85]. However, hospital mortality did not differ between the NIV and standard therapy groups. In a subgroup analysis, patients with ARDS randomised to NIV had an intubation rate of 38 vs. 86% in the standard treatment group (p=0.08).

We conducted a prospective, randomised trial comparing NIV with standard medical treatment of supplemental oxygen and no ventilatory support in 52 immunosuppressed patients (30 of them with haematological malignancies and neutropaenia) with pulmonary infiltrates and fever and hypoxaemic ARF [87]. A third of the enrolled patients, at least, had criteria of ALI/ARDS (subgroup analysis not published). Randomisation was made at an early stage of respiratory failure, well before intubation of the patients became a consideration. NIV was delivered discontinuously through a face mask, with a protocol resembling the one previously described for COPD patients. In the NIV group, compared with the standard-therapy group, fewer patients required endotracheal intubation (12 vs. 20, p=0.03) and there were fewer complications (13 vs. 21, p=0.02). Overall, with NIV, there were improvements in mortality in the ICU (10 vs. 18, p=0.03) and in total in-hospital mortality (13 vs. 21, p=0.02).

It is important to note that ventilator-associated pneumonia was associated with in-ICU death in 100% of cases in two randomised controlled studies dealing with immunosuppressed patients [85,87].

In summary, despite the limitations posed by the fact that only two uncontrolled trials have studied NIV specifically in ARDS patients, and the small size of the sample populations in the those and other published reports, the technique seems to prevent endotracheal intubation and reduce the rate of complications and mortality in selected patients with ALI or ARDS. A reduction in the incidence of nosocomial infection is a consistent and important advantage of NIV compared with invasive ventilation and is probably one of the major advantages of this strategy. For the moment, it seems suitable to limit NIV to haemodynamically stable ALI/ARDS patients who can be closely monitored and in units where intubation can be promptly performed. The studies published to date should provide the rationale for prospective randomised studies. Our own prospective involving randomised trial immunocompetent patients with ARDS compared NIV with standard medical treatment including supplemental oxygen and no ventilatory support. We obtained positive results, but to date the study has been published only in an abstract form.

NIV as a Means of Assisting Ventilation During Fibre-Optic Bronchoscopy

It is important to establish the specific causes of an immunosuppressed patient's pulmonary disease, so that specific therapy can be instituted. Furthermore, a correct diagnosis and well-adapted treatment could be the main determinants of improved outcome of immunosuppressed patients managed with NIV [87]. Consequently, fibre-optic bronchoscopy and bronchoalveolar lavage are major tools in diagnosing the diffuse infiltrates that often occur in association with fever and new onset of respiratory symptoms in this group of patients

[87,99,100]. Nevertheless, although there is no absolute contraindication to this procedure, severe hypoxaemia is an accepted contraindication to fibre-optic bronchoscopy in non-intubated patients. The American Thoracic Society recommends avoiding bronchoalveolar lavage in patients who are breathing spontaneously and who have hypercapnia and/or hypoxaemia that cannot be corrected to a PaO_2 of $\geq$75 mmHg with supplemental oxygen.

In a study of eight immunosuppressed patients with suspected pneumonia and $PaO_2/FiO_2 \leq 100$, Antonelli et al. assessed the feasibility and safety of fibre-optic bronchoscopy with NIV [101]. They found that NIV during bronchoscopy was well-tolerated, significantly improved the PaO_2/FiO_2 ratio, and successfully avoided the need for endotracheal intubation. Another recent study, consisting of 46 patients, suggested that the application of another non-invasive interface, i.e., the laryngeal airway mask, is also a safe and effective alternative to intubation for accomplishing bronchoscopy with bronchoalveolar lavage in immunosuppressed patients with suspected pneumonia and severe hypoxaemia ($PaO_2/FiO_2 \leq 125$) [102]. In a recent prospective randomised trial involving 26 patients, NIV was shown to be superior to conventional oxygen supplementation in preventing gas-exchange deterioration, and with better haemodynamic tolerance during fibre-optic bronchoscopy in patients with less severe forms of hypoxaemia ($PaO_2/FiO_2 < 200$) [103].

Side Effects and Factors Predictive of NIV Outcome

Gas Leaks

Gas leaks around the mask or from the mouth limit the efficacy of the device, make monitoring of tidal volume difficult, may prevent adequate ventilatory assistance in patients who require high inspiratory airway pressures and represent an important cause of failure. Leaks may also indicate low compliance or ventilation close to total lung capacity. Thus, particular attention should be paid to leaks during the administration of NIV in patients with ARDS. A study of six patients with ALI due to AIDS-related opportunistic pneumonia found that, in the presence of air leaks during NIV, a time-cycled expiratory trigger provided a better patient-machine interaction than a flow-cycled expiratory trigger [36].

Facial-Skin Breakdown

In a study consisting exclusively of patients with ALI/ARDS, none of the patients developed complications related to the use of NIV, such as skin necrosis, gastric distention, nosocomial pneumonia, or evidence of barotrauma (pneumothorax, pneumomediastinum, pneumoperitoneum or pulmonary interstitial emphysema) [83]. No patients vomited and/or aspirated after initiation of NIV.

Data from the literature and observations from our practice have suggested that the highest incidence of facial-skin breakdown and/or intolerance of the interface occur in patients with hypoxaemic ARF and haematological malignancies. Three patients were excluded from the study by Hilbert et al. because they refused to keep the face mask during the first CPAP session [82]. The reason was acute stress in one patient and major painful mucositis in two. Poor tolerance of CPAP was reported in five intubated patients enrolled in that study.

Mask intolerance because of pain, discomfort or claustrophobia may require the discontinuation of NIV and endotracheal intubation. The fact that most NIV failures are due to technical problems supports recent studies that evaluated new interface devices. In an attempt to improve patient tolerance of NIV, Antonelli et al. provided patients with a transparent *helmet* made from latex-free polyvinyl chloride that allows patients to see, read, and speak during NIV. A prospective trial, with a matched control group, was conducted in order to investigate the efficacy of NIV in hypoxaemic ARF patients wearing the helmet [104]. Six patients (18%) in the helmet group and nine (13%) in the facial-mask group had ARDS. Eight patients (24%) in the helmet group and 21 patients (32%) in the facial-mask group failed NIV and were intubated. No patients failed NIV because of intolerance of the technique in the helmet group, compared with eight patients (38%) in the mask group (p=0.047). Complications related to the technique (skin necrosis, gastric distension, and eye irritation) were fewer in the helmet group than in the standard mask group (no patients vs. 14 patients, 21%, p=0.002). The helmet allowed the continuous administration of NIV for a longer period of time (p=0.05). The authors concluded that NIV by helmet successfully treated hypoxaemic ARF, with better tolerance and fewer complications than occur with face mask NIV.

Factors Predictive of NIV Outcome

In their randomised study, Antonelli et al. reported that among patients in the NIV group, those requiring intubation were older (p=0.006), had a higher SAPS I (p=0.009) and were less likely to show improvement of PaO_2/FiO_2 (p=0.003) over time [84]. Nonetheless, initial improvement in PaO_2/FiO_2 (within 1 h after study entry) was not significantly different between success and failure patients in the NIV group.

In the randomised study of Hilbert et al., the effect on outcome of the presence or absence of a final diagnosis of the cause of pneumonitis with respiratory failure was studied [87]. In the NIV group, patients with a final diagnosis had significantly lower rates of intubation (p=0.03) and death in the ICU (p=0.04) or in the hospital (p=0.006). Thus, a positive diagnosis and a well-adapted treatment may be the main determinants of an improved outcome of immunosuppressed patients managed with NIV.

In a prospective study, variables predictive of NIV failure were investigated in 354 patients with hypoxaemic ARF, 86 of them with ARDS [93]. Multivariate analysis identified age >40 years (OR 1.72, 95% CI 0.92–3.23), SAPS II score ≥35 (OR 1.81, 95 % CI 1.07–3.06), the presence of ARDS or community-acquired pneumonia (OR 3.75, 95% CI 2.25–6.24), and a $PaO_2/FiO_2 \leq 146$ after 1 h of NIV (OR 2.51, 95% CI 1.45–4.35) as factors independently associated with the failure of NIV. In a recent cohort study in which NIV was applied as first-line intervention in ARDS, only SAPS II >34 and a $PaO2/FiO2 \leq 175$ after 1 h of NIV were independently associated with NIV failure and need for endotracheal intubation.[94]

In summary, it is difficult to apply these results to ARDS patients, and controlled studies that specifically include patients with ALI/ARDS are clearly needed.

Conclusions

Recent studies demonstrated that NIV is an effective treatment for selected patients with ARF, with lower rates of endotracheal intubation, fewer complications and improved survival. A reduction in the incidence of nosocomial infection is a consistent and important advantage of NIV compared with invasive ventilation and is probably one of the most important advantages of avoiding endotracheal intubation by using NIV.

Patients hospitalised for exacerbations of COPD with rapid clinical deterioration should be considered for NIV to prevent further deterioration in gas exchange, respiratory workload and the need for endotracheal intubation. Avoiding reintubation should also be an important objective in the management of respiratory failure in COPD patients, and NIV may help achieve that goal.

Based on the good results obtained in patients with acute exacerbations of COPD, NIV is now being used to support those with hypoxaemic ARF, including some patients with ALI or ARDS. Despite the limitations due to the fact that only two uncontrolled trials have studied NIV specifically in ARDS patients and that the sample populations in the published reports have been small, NIV seems able to prevent endotracheal intubation and to reduce the rate of complications and mortality in selected patients with ALI or ARDS.

Experience gradually acquired by the different care units, the regular training of personnel, further technological advances and future research will position NIV more accurately in the therapeutic armamentarium of physicians dealing with patients with ARF, and is likely to improve the conditions for performing NIV in the future.

References

1. Stauffer JL (1994) Complications of translaryngeal intubation. In: Tobin MJ (ed) Principles and practice of mechanical ventilation. McGraw-Hill, New York, pp 711–747
2. Torres A, Aznar R, Gatell JM et al (1990) Incidence, risk, and prognosis factors of nosocomial pneumonia in mechanically ventilated patients. Am Rev Respir Dis 142:523–528

3. Lemaire F (1993) Difficult weaning. Intensive Care Med 19:S69-S73
4. Tobin MJ (1994) Mechanical ventilation. N Engl J Med 330:1056–1061
5. Sullivan CE, Issa FG, Berthon-Jones M et al (1981) Reversal of obstructive sleep apnea by continuous positive airway pressure applied through the nares. Lancet 1:862–865
6. Rideau Y, Gatin G, Bach J et al (1983) Prolongation of life in Duchenne's muscular dystrophy. Acta Neurol Belg 5:118–124
7. Kerby GR, Mayer LS, Pingleton SK (1987) Nocturnal positive pressure ventilation via nasal mask. Am Rev Respir Dis 135:738–740
8. Ellis ER, Bye PT, Bruderer JW et al (1987) Treatment of respiratory failure during sleep in patients with neuromuscular disease: positive pressure ventilation through a nose mask. Am Rev Respir Dis 135:148–152
9. Meecham Jones DJ, Paul EA, Jones PW et al (1995) Nasal pressure support ventilation plus oxygen compared with oxygen therapy alone in hypercapnic COPD. Am J Respir Crit Care Med 152:538–544
10. Rossi A (2000) Noninvasive ventilation has not been shown to be ineffective in stable COPD. Am J Respir Crit Care Med 161:688–689
11. Hill NS (2000) Noninvasive ventilation has been shown to be ineffective in stable COPD. Am J Respir Crit Care Med 161:689–690
12. Evans TW (2001) International Consensus Conferences in Intensive Care Medicine: noninvasive positive pressure ventilation in acute Respiratory failure. Am J Respir Crit Care Med 163:283–291
13. Tobin MJ, Perez W, Guenther SM et al (1986) The pattern of breathing during successful and unsuccessful trials of weaning from mechanical ventilation. Am Rev Respir Dis 134:1111–1118
14. Meduri GU, Abou-Shala N, Fox RC et al (1991) Noninvasive face mask mechanical ventilation in patients with acute hypercapnic respiratory failure. Chest 100:445–454
15. Brochard L, Isabey D, Piquet J et al (1990) Reversal of acute exacerbations of chronic obstructive lung disease by inspiratory assistance with a face mask. N Engl J Med 323:1523–1530
16. Bott J, Caroll MP, Conway JH et al (1993) Randomized controlled trial of nasal ventilation in acute ventilatory failure due to chronic obstructive airways disease. Lancet 341:1555–1557
17. Brochard L, Mancebo J, Wysocki M et al (1995) Noninvasive ventilation for acute exacerbations of chronic obstructive pulmonary disease. N Engl J Med 333:817–822
18. Hilbert G, Gruson D, Gbikpi-Benissan G et al (1997) Sequential use of noninvasive pressure support ventilation for acute exacerbations of COPD. Intensive Care Med 23:955–961
19. Celikel T, Sungur M, Ceyhan B et al (1998) Comparison of noninvasive positive pressure ventilation with standard medical therapy in hypercapnic acute respiratory failure. Chest 114:1636–1642
20. Plant PK, Owen JL, Elliott MW (2000) A multicenter randomized controlled trial of the early use of non invasive ventilation for acute exacerbations of chronic obstructive pulmonary disease on general respiratory wards. Lancet 355:1931–1935
21. Carrey Z, Gottfried SB, Levy RD (1990) Ventilatory muscle support in respiratory failure with nasal positive pressure ventilation. Chest 97:150–158
22. Nava S, Ambrosino N, Rubini F et al (1993) Effect of nasal pressure support ventilation and external PEEP on diaphragmatic activity in patients with severe stable COPD. Chest 103:143–150.
23. Appendini L, Patessio A, Zanaboni S et al (1994) Physiologic effects of positive end-expiratory pressure and mask pressure support during exacerbations of chronic obstructive pulmonary disease. Am J Respir Crit Care Med 149:1069–1076
24. Diaz O, Iglesia R, Ferrer M et al (1997) Effects of noninvasive ventilation on pulmonary gas exchange and hemodynamics during acute hypercapnic exacerbations of chronic obstructive pulmonary disease. Am J Respir Crit Care Med 156:1840–1845
25. Richards GN, Cistulli PA, Ungar RG et al (1996) Mouth leak with nasal continuous positive

airway pressure increases nasal airway resistance. Am J Respir Crit Care Med 154:182–186
26. Navalesi P, Fanfulla F, Frigeiro P et al (2000) Physiologic evaluation of noninvasive mechanical ventilation delivered with three types of masks in patients with chronic hypercapnic respiratory failure. Chest 28:1785–1790
27. Vitacca M, Rubini F, Foglio K et al (1993) Non-invasive modalities of positive pressure ventilation improve the outcome of acute exacerbations in COLD patients. Intensive Care Med 19:450–455
28. Confalonieri M, Parigi P, Scartabellati A et al (1996) Noninvasive mechanical ventilation improves the immediate and long-term outcome of COPD patients with acute respiratory failure. Eur Respir J 9:422–430
29. Ferguson GT, Gilmartin M (1995) CO2 rebreathing during BiPAP ventilatory assistance. Am J Respir Crit Care Med 151:1126–1135
30. Lofaso F, Brochard L, Touchard D et al (1995) Evaluation of carbon dioxide rebreathing during pressure support ventilation with airway management system (BiPAP) devices. Chest 108:772–778
31. Bunburaphong T, Imaka H, Nishimura M et al (1997) Performance characteristics of bilevel pressure ventilators: a lung model study. Chest 11:1050–1060
32. Pennock BE, Kaplan PD, Carlin BW et al (1991) Pressure support ventilation with a simplified ventilatory support system administered with a nasal mask in patients with respiratory failure. Chest 100:1371–1376
33. Marino W (1991) Intermittent volume cycled mechanical ventilation via nasal mask in patients with respiratory failure due to COPD. Chest 99:681–684
34. Benhamou D, Girault C, Faure C et al (1992) Nasal mask ventilation in acute respiratory failure: experience in elderly patients. Chest 102:912–917
35. Foglio C, Vitacca M, Quadri A et al (1992) Acute exacerbations in severe COLD patients: treatment using positive pressure ventilation by nasal mask. Chest 101:1533–1538
36. Soo Hoo GW, Santiago S, Williams AJ (1994) Nasal mechanical ventilation for hypercapnic respiratory failure in chronic obstructive pulmonary disease: determinants of success and failure. Crit Care Med 22:1253–1261
37. Jubran A, Van de Graaff WB, Tobin MJ (1995) Variability of patient-ventilator interaction with pressure support ventilation in patients with chronic obstructive pulmonary disease. Am J Respir Crit Care Med 152:129–136
38. Calderini E, Confalonieri M, Puccio PG et al (1999) Patient-ventilator asynchrony during noninvasive ventilation: the role of expiratory trigger. Intensive Care Med 25:662–667
39. Goldberg P, Reissmann H, Maltais F et al (1995) Efficacy of noninvasive CPAP in COPD with acute respiratory failure. Eur Respir J 8:1894–1900
40. DeLucas P, Tarancon C, Puente L et al (1993) Nasal continuous positive airway pressure in patients with COPD in acute respiratory failure. Chest 104:1694–1697
41. Miro AM, Shivaram U, Hertig I (1993) Continuous positive airway pressure in COPD patients in acute hypercapnic respiratory failure. Chest 103:266–268
42. Petrof BJ, Legare M, Goldberg P et al (1990) Continuous positive airway pressure reduces work of breathing and dyspnea during weaning from mechanical ventilation in severe chronic obstuctive pulmonary disease. Am Rev Resp Dis 141:281–289
43. Girault C, Richard JC, Chevron V et al (1997) Comparative physiologic effects of noninvasive assist-control and pressure support ventilation in acute hypercapnic respiratory failure. Chest 111:1639–1648
44. Kramer N, Meyer TJ, Meharg J et al (1995) Randomized, prospective trial of noninvasive positive pressure ventilation in acute respiratory failure. Am J Respir Crit Care Med 151:1799–1806
45. Barbe F, Togores B, Rubi M et al (1996) Noninvasive ventilatory support does not facilitate recovery from acute respiratory failure in chronic obstructive pulmonary disease. Eur Respir J 9:1240–1245
46. Nava S, Ambrosino N, Clini E et al (1998) Noninvasive mechanical ventilation in the wean-

ing of patients with respiratory failure due to chronic obstructive pulmonary disease. A randomized, controlled trial. Ann Intern Med 128:721–728

47. Girault C, Daudenthun I, Chevron V et al (1999) Non-invasive ventilation as a systematic extubation and weaning technique in acute-on-chronic respiratory failure. Am J Respir Crit Care Med 160:86–92
48. Ferrer M, Esquinas A, Arancibia F et al (2003) Noninvasive ventilation during persistent weaning failure: a randomized controlled trial. Am J Respir Crit Care Med 168:70–76
49. Esteban A, Frutos F, Tobin MJ et al (1995) A comparison of four methods of weaning patients from mechanical ventilation. Spanish Lung Failure Collaborative Group. N Engl J Med 332:345–350
50. Epstein SK, Ciubotaru RL, Wong JB (1997) Effect of failed extubation on the outcome of mechanical ventilation. Chest 112:186–192
51. Epstein SK, Ciubotaru RL (1998) Independent effects of etiology of failure and time to reintubation on outcome for patients failing extubation. Am J Respir Crit Care Med 158:489–493
52. Hilbert, G, Gruson D, Portel L et al (1998) Non-invasive pressure support ventilation in COPD patients with postextubation hypercapnic respiratory insufficiency. Eur Respir J 11:1349–1353
53. Hilbert G, Gruson D, Portel L et al (1998) Airway occlusion pressure at 0.1 s (P0.1) after extubation: an early indicator of postextubation hypercapnic respiratory insufficiency. Intensive Care Med 24:1277–1282
54. Ferrer M, Valencia M, Nicolas JM et al (2006) Early noninvasive ventilation averts extubation failure in patients at risk: a randomized trial. Am J Respir Crit Care Med 173:164–170
55. Chevrolet JC, Jolliet P, Abajo B et al (1991) Nasal positive pressure ventilation in patients with acute respiratory failure: difficult and time consuming procedure for nurses. Chest 100:775–782
56. Hilbert G, Gruson D, Vargas F et al (2000) Noninvasive ventilation for acute respiratory failure: Quite low time consumption for nurses. Eur Respir J 16:710–716
57. Hilbert G, Vargas F, Valentino R et al (2002) Noninvasive ventilation in acute exacerbations of chronic obstructive pulmonary disease in patients with and without home noninvasive ventilation. Crit Care Med 30:1453–1458
58. Gregoretti C, Confalonieri M, Navalesi P et al (2002) Evaluation of patient skin breakdown and comfort with a new face mask for non-invasive ventilation: a multi-center study. Intensive Care Med 28:278–284
59. Pennock BE, Crawshaw L, Kaplan PD (1994) Noninvasive nasal mask ventilation for acute respiratory failure. Institution of a new therapeutic technology for routine use. Chest 105: 441–444
60. Meduri GU, Turner RE, Abou-Shala N et al (1996) Noninvasive positive pressure ventilation via face mask. First-line intervention in patients with acute hypercapnic and hypoxemic respiratory failure. Chest 109: 179–193
61. Confalonieri M, Potena A, Carbone G et al (1999) Acute respiratory failure in patients with severe community acquired pneumonia: a prospective randomized evaluation of noninvasive ventilation. Am J Respir Crit Care Med 160:1585–1591
62. Nava S, Evangelisti I, Rampulla C et al (1997) Human and financial costs of noninvasive mechanical ventilation in patients affected by COPD and acute respiratory failure. Chest 111:1631–1638
63. Ambrosino N, Foglio K, Rubini F et al (1995) Non-invasive mechanical ventilation in acute respiratory failure due to chronic obstructive airways disease: correlates for success. Thorax 50:755–757
64. Plant PK, Owen JL, Elliott MW. Non-invasive ventilation in acute exacerbations of chronic obstructive pulmonary disease: long term survival and predictors of in-hospital outcome. Thorax 56:708–712
65. Younes M, Puddy A, Roberts D et al (1992) Proportional assist ventilation: results of an initial clinical trial. Am Rev Respir Dis 145:121–129

66. Vitacca M, Clini E, Pagani M et al (2000) Physiologic effects of early administered mask proportional assist ventilation in patients with chronic obstructive pulmonary disease and acute respiratory failure. Crit Care Med 28:1791–1797
67. Wysocki M, Richard JC, Meshaka P (2002) Noninvasive proportional assist ventilation compared with noninvasive pressure support ventilation in hypercapnic acute respiratory failure. Crit Care Med 30:323–329
68. Gay PC, Hess DR, Hill NS (2001) Noninvasive proportional assist ventilation for acute respiratory insufficiency. Comparison with pressure support ventilation. Am J Respir Crit Care Med 164:1606–1611
69. Jaber S, Fodil R, Carlucci A et al (2000) Noninvasive ventilation with helium–oxygen in acute exacerbations of chronic obstructive pulmonary disease. Am J Respir Crit Care Med 161:1191–1200
70. Jolliet P, Tassaux D, Roeseler J et al (2003) Helium-oxygen versus air-oxygen noninvasive pressure support in decompensated chronic obstructive disease: a prospective, multicenter study. Crit Care Med 31:878–884
71. Hilbert G (2003) Noninvasive ventilation with helium-oxygen rather than air-oxygen in acute exacerbations of chronic obstructive disease? Crit Care Med 31:990–991
72. The Acute Respiratory Distress Syndrome Network (2000) Ventilation with lower tidal volumes as compared with traditional tidal volumes for acute lung injury and the acute respiratory distress syndrome. N Engl J Med 342:1301–1308
73. Brower RG, Ware LB, Berthiaume Y et al (2001) Treatment of ARDS. Chest 120:1347–1367
74. Weinert CR, Gross CR, Kangas JR et al (1997) Health-related quality of life after acute lung injury. Am J Respir Crit Care Med 156:1120–1128
75. Davidson TA, Caldwell ES, Curtis JR et al (1999) Reduced quality of life in survivors of acute respiratory distress syndrome compared with critically ill control patients. JAMA 281:354–360
76. Greenbaum DM, Millen JE, Eross B et al (1976) Continuous positive airway pressure without tracheal intubation in spontaneously breathing patients. Chest 69:615–621
77. Smith RA, Kirby RR, Gooding JM et al (1980) Continuous positive airway pressure (CPAP) by face mask. Crit Care Med 8:483–485
78. Covelli HD, Weled BJ, Beekam JF (1982) Efficacy of continuous positive airway pressure administered by face mask. Chest 81:147–150
79. Kesten S, Rebuck AS (1988) Nasal continuous positive airway pressure in Pneumocystis carinii pneumonia. Lancet 17:1414–1415
80. Gregg RW, Friedman BC, Williams JF et al (1990) Continuous positive airway pressure by face mask in Pneumocystis carinii pneumonia. Crit Care Med 18:21–24
81. Brett A, Sinclair DG (1993) Use of continuous positive airway pressure in the management of community acquired pneumonia. Thorax 48:1280–1281
82. Hilbert G, Gruson D, Vargas F et al (2000) Non-invasive continuous positive airway pressure in neutropenic patients with acute respiratory failure requiring intensive care unit admission. Crit Care Med 28:3185–3190
83. Rocker GM, Mackenzie MG, Williams B et al (1999) Noninvasive positive pressure ventilation: successful outcome in patients with acute lung injury/ARDS. Chest 115:173–177
84. Antonelli M, Conti G, Rocco M et al (1998) A comparison of noninvasive positive pressure ventilation and conventional mechanical ventilation in patients with acute respiratory failure. N Engl J Med 339:429–435
85. Antonelli M, Conti G, Bufi M et al (2000) Noninvasive ventilation for treatment of acute respiratory failure in patients undergoing solid organ transplantation. A randomized trial. JAMA 283:235–241
86. Delclaux C, L'Her E, Alberti C et al (2000) Treatment of acute hypoxemic nonhypercapnic respiratory insufficiency with continuous positive airway pressure delivered by a face mask: A randomized controlled trial. JAMA 284:2352–2360
87. Hilbert G, Gruson D, Vargas F et al (2001) Noninvasive ventilation for treatment of acute respiratory failure in immunosuppressed patients with pulmonary infiltrates and fever, a randomized trial. New Engl J Med 344:481–487

88. Katz JA, Marks JD (1985) Inspiratory work with and without continuous positive airway pressure in patients with acute respiratory failure. Anesthesiology 63:598–607
89. Appendini L, Patessio A, Zanaboni S et al (1994) Physiologic effects of positive end-expiratory pressure and mask pressure support during exacerbations of chronic obstructive pulmonary disease. Am J Respir Crit Care Med 149:1069–1076
90. Sassoon CSH, Lodia R, Rheeman CH et al (1992) Inspiratory muscle work of breathing during flow-by, demand-flow and continuous-flow systems in patients with chronic obstructive pulmonary disease. Am Rev Respir Dis 145:1219–1222
91. Bersten AD, Holt AW, Vedig AE et al (1991) Treatment of severe cardiogenic pulmonary edema with continuous positive airway pressure delivered by face mask. N Engl J Med 1991 325:1825–1830
92. Wysocki M, Tric L, Wolff MA et al (1995) Noninvasive pressure support ventilation in patients with acute respiratory failure. A randomized comparison with conventional therapy. Chest 107:761–768
93. Martin TJ, Hovis JD, Costantino JP et al (2000) A randomized prospective evaluation of noninvasive ventilation for acute respiratory failure. Am J Respir Crit Care Med 161:807–813
94. Ferrer M, Esquinas A, Leon M et al (2003) Noninvasive ventilation in severe hypoxemic respiratory failure: a randomized clinical trial. Am J Respir Crit Care Med 168:1438–1444
95. Rabitsch W, Staudinger T, Brugger SA et al (1998) Successful management of adult respiratory distress syndrome (ARDS) after high-dose chemotherapy and peripheral blood progenitor cell rescue by non-invasive ventilatory support. Bone Marrow Transpl 21:1067–1069
96. Antonelli M, Conti G, Moro ML et al (2001) Predictors of failure of noninvasive positive pressure ventilation in patients with acute hypoxemic respiratory failure: a multi-center study. Intensive Care Med 27:1718–1728
97. Antonelli M, Conti G, Esquinas A et al (2007) A multiple-center survey on the use in clinical practice of noninvasive ventilation as a first-line intervention for acute respiratory distress syndrome. Crit Care Med 35:18–25
98. Hill NS (2001) Noninvasive ventilation for immunocompromised patients. N Engl J Med 344:522–524
99. Stover DE, Zaman NB, Hadjou SI et al (1984) Bronchoalveolar lavage in the diagnosis of diffuse pulmonary infiltrates in the immunosuppressed host. Ann Intern Med 101:1–7
100. Levine SJ, Stover DE (1991) Bronchoscopy, and related techniques. In: Shelhamer J (ed) Respiratory disease in the immunosuppressed host. Lippincott, Philadelphia, pp 73–93
101. Antonelli M, Conti G, Rocco M et al (2002) Noninvasive positive-pressure ventilation vs. conventional oxygen supplementation in hypoxemic patients undergoing diagnostic bronchoscopy. Chest 121:1149–1154
102. Hilbert G, Gruson D, Vargas F et al (2001) Bronchoscopy with bronchoalveolar lavage via the laryngeal mask airway in high-risk hypoxemic immunosuppressed patients. Crit Care Med 29:249–255
103. Antonelli M, Conti G, Rocco M et al (2002) Noninvasive positive-pressure ventilation vs. conventional oxygen supplementation in hypoxemic patients undergoing diagnostic bronchoscopy. Chest 121:1149–1154
104. Antonelli M, Conti G, Pelosi P et al (2002) New treatment of acute hypoxemic respiratory failure: Noninvasive pressure support ventilation delivered by helmet—A pilot controlled trial. Crit Care Med 30:602–608

Non-invasive Respiratory Assistance in Paediatric Patients

G. Chidini, D. d'Onofrio, E. Calderini

Introduction

In the last decade, non-invasive ventilation (NIV) has been used to provide respiratory assistance in various groups of patients, mainly in those with COPD, cardiogenic pulmonary oedema and acute hypoxaemic respiratory failure. Most of the experience originates from studies carried out in adult patients. In contrast, data regarding the use of NIV in infants and children are scarce, and case series constitute the majority of knowledge in acute and in home settings. Moreover many of the published studies reported data derived from the treatment of mixed groups of children and diseases, making it more difficult to draw conclusions with respect to any specific population or disease.

In the past several years, surveys carried out in the USA, Europe and Canada have indicated that the use of home-care ventilation of children is rapidly increasing. Two recent surveys focused on the use of non-invasive and invasive respiratory support in the paediatric population. The first was that of the ADEPT (a French organisation that manages home mechanical ventilation), which reported that in 2002 515 children were being ventilated at home. A survey in the UK noted that, of the 141 children who required long-term ventilator assistance, 33 of them used tracheostomy invasive positive-pressure ventilation (IPPV), 103 nocturnal nasal IPPV, and nine negative-pressure body ventilators. Ninety-six children had primary ventilatory impairment, and some children used more than one mode of ventilatory support [1,2].

Two major factors that explain the important development in the use of NIV in this population are: first, hypoventilation is the main cause of respiratory failure and can be managed at home with non-invasive respiratory support, with great benefit regarding symptoms related to CO_2 retention; second, NIV can be applied on demand, resulting in much less morbidity, discomfort and disruption of social life and family than is the case with tracheostomy [3–5].

Following successful application of NIV in the home-care setting, in the past 10 years interest in the use of NIV in acute setting has rapidly increased, and

U. Lucangelo, P. Pelosi, W.A. Zin, A. Aliverti (eds.) *Respiratory System and Artificial Ventilation*. © Springer 2008

many studies on adults have been carried out. Unlike endotracheal intubation, NIV requires the patients to be alert and cooperative. Especially in the acute setting, the patient-ventilator interaction is crucial to successful respiratory support. However, non-invasive respiratory support is usually applied by nasal or face mask, and this interface may cause air leaking, discomfort, need of sedation and pain, all of which can lead to a discontinuation of ventilatory treatment [6]. Whereas adult patients play the major role in choosing an interface and in cooperating with medical staff, for infants, the success of NIV depends on the clinic's appropriate choice of interface, ventilator and mode of ventilation. Another problem is the choice of ventilatory mode, which should be based on the clinical experience of the staff. Ventilator setting should be adjusted to provide the lowest PEEP and positive end-inspiratory pressure (PIP) or the volumes needed to improve patients comfort (decrease in respiratory rate and muscle unloading) and to ameliorate gas exchange. Technically, NIV is more difficult to apply in infants and young children because of problems related to tolerance of the interface and technical aspects related to ventilator characteristics. A typical major problem with the ventilator is the triggering system. Autotriggering, development of intrinsic PEEP and the presence of unsupported inspiratory efforts could also increase the work of breathing and reduce the efficacy of the support. This is a major concern, because infants and children have greater difficulties with synchronisation with and triggering of the ventilator. There are also greater limitations in commercially available interfaces. In this chapter, the term 'non-invasive ventilation' refers to continuous positive airway pressure (CPAP) as well as to the combination of PEEP and positive inspiratory pressure (BiPAP, pressure support ventilation). Here, the focus is on non-invasive ventilator management of infants and children. The first section examines the physiology of the respiratory system in infants and children. The second section deals with the possible physiological effects of ventilatory assistance in children and the clinical application of NIV in this population. The third section focuses on special considerations for infants and children regarding ventilation techniques and equipment as well as their use.

Physiological Characteristics of the Respiratory System in Infants and Children

Major differences exist between the respiratory-system characteristics of preterm neonates, infants and very young children and those of adults [7]. With increasing age these differences tend to lessen and the basic characteristics of the respiratory systems become more similar. The respiratory system of the neonate is characterised by a relatively stiff lung and a very compliant chest wall. Thus, the lung tends to collapse such that in the absence of opposing forces the functional residual capacity (FRC) would only be 15–20% of total lung capacity. However, infants are able to maintain a FRC of at least 40% of total lung capacity by different physiological manoeuvres, such as laryngeal breaking [8], maintenance of post-inspiratory tone in the muscles of the chest wall [9] and through respiratory rates fast enough to allow the expiratory time to be less than the time constant of the respiratory system. The neonatal ability to generate adequate tidal volume is partially impeded by the compliant chest wall; thus, the work of breathing is increased by the wasting of muscle forces on chest-wall distortion instead of the production of effective alveolar ventilation. This contributes to muscle fatigue and is likely to negatively affect normal growth.

Other factors may contribute to hamper the neonatal respiratory system, such as high flow resistance of the nasal airway and small airways, increased propensity to hypertrophy of the adenoids and tonsils, a reduced zone of apposition of the diaphragm, horizontal ribs and, in the very young, the presence of immature muscles. In addition, metabolism is doubled that in adults, resulting in a dramatically higher alveolar ventilation/FRC ratio than in adults (5/1 vs. 1.5/1) [10]. In pre-term neonates, the surfactant deficiency, which manifests as a diminution of surface tension, leads to further collapse of alveolar segments [11].

The diaphragms of pre-term neonates have fewer high-oxidative fibres, such that fatigue of this muscle is probable [12]. Muller et al. [13] using EMGs recorded with surface electrodes demonstrated that the diaphragms of normal pre-term neonates and infants operate very close to the threshold of diaphragmatic fatigue.

The hypoxaemic response is also attenuated in the infant and apnoeas are more frequent than in the adult [14]. Thus, increased thoracic compliance combined with the surfactant deficiency, especially in pre-term neonates, leads to a loss of FRC; effectively, this means that the infant is attempting to achieve adequate gas exchange in a smaller compartment of ventilated lung. The ventilation of lungs below normal FRC can result in the cyclical opening and closing of lung units, and thereby injury [15]. This has been termed *low-volume injury* or atelectotrauma, and it causes inflammatory changes associated with severe alterations in the lung structure [16].

Thus, it appears that the respiratory systems of pre-term neonates, infants and children are extremely weak; thus, the presence of even a minimal abnormality can cause a rapid deterioration of respiratory function. The rationale for respiratory support is to increase and maintain FRC, prevent atelectasis (even by augmenting surfactant production in the case of pre-term neonates), support the easily fatigued ventilatory muscles and provide respiratory stimulation (against apnoea), and in doing so provide gaseous exchange of both oxygen and carbon dioxide.

Bronchopulmonary Dysplasia

Bronchopulmonary dysplasia (BPD), is characterised by early interstitial and alveolar oedema, which progresses to persistent inflammation and fibrosis. As the survival rates of pre-terms have improved over the years, the numbers of infants with BPD has increased [17]. Infants with BPD have a higher mortality and morbidity; they receive more ventilation, drugs, oxygen and intensive care and have higher hospital readmission rates in the first year of life than infants of similar gestational age who do not develop BPD [18]. The advent of antenatal steroids and surfactant has altered the definition of BPD, which was previously regarded as the stress patterns incurred by early ventilatory support of hyaline membrane disease, coupled with long exposure to ventilation and oxygen.

Several authors have proposed a new definition of BPD in extremely low-birth-weight infants [19]: in the first days to weeks of life, infants require only modest or no respiratory support, but it becomes necessary later. Thus, infants with chronic pulmonary insufficiency of prematurity (CPIP) form the current 'epidemic' of the new BPD.

Conventional mechanical ventilation via an endotracheal tube has undoubtedly led to improvements in neonatal survival in the last 30 years. However, prolonged use of an endotracheal tube and mechanical ventilation may cause upper airway damage, alter normal mucociliary flow, lead to infection and predispose the infant to BPD. Intubation can also cause fluctuations in oxygenation and blood pressure that may have potentially harmful consequences for the cerebrum.

Although multiple factors contribute to BPD, intubation and mechanical ventilation of pre-term infants is the single most important predictor of subsequent BPD [20]. Recognition of this has, in part, contributed to the general term of 'ventilator-induced lung injury' (VILI), which can be applied to both adults and children. The risk factors for VILI are very similar to those of BPD, namely volutrauma, barotrauma and atelectasis or end-expiratory alveolar collapse. These mechanical stresses are most likely transduced into a final common biological signal via the presence of toxic reactive-oxygen species and associated inflammation. Moreover, they are certainly not mutually exclusive, as the relationship between volume and pressure indicates.

Since the structural abnormalities of injured lungs cannot be easily reversed, preventative measures, like non-invasive respiratory support, aimed at minimising the incidence and severity of BPD are very attractive.

Hypoxaemic Respiratory Failure

Hypoxaemic respiratory failure consists primarily of hypoxaemia with low oxygenation and normal to low capnia, usually of acute onset. The predominant mechanism in hypoxaemic respiratory failure is uneven or mismatched ventilation and perfusion in regional lung units. In infants and children, this kind of respiratory failure mainly occurs in disorders characterised by airway obstruction, such as status asthmaticus and bronchiolitis. Furthermore, the presence of pneumonia due to different aetiological agents can lead to hypoxaemic respiratory failure. Bronchiolitis occurs mainly in children <2 years old. RSV is estimated to be the most frequent aetiological cause for over half of the cases of bronchiolitis [21]. Respiratory syncytial virus (RSV) bronchiolitis involves mainly the small airways but also the lung interstitium. Also, *Streptococcus pneumoniae* can be considered the most frequent agent of pneumonia, although other microorganisms can play a relevant role. Additional causes include non-infectious ones, such as of lobar atelectasis, mainly occurring in the postoperative period.

Hypercapnic Respiratory Failure

Hypercapnic chronic respiratory failure arises from the presence of alveolar hypoventilation associated with normal or reduced oxygenation. The predominant mechanism in this disorder is reduced ventilation caused by a depressed neuronal ventilatory drive (central hypoventilation disorders), acute or chronic upper airway obstruction (obstructive sleep apnoea), neuromuscular weakness (Duchenne muscular dystrophy and spinal muscular atrophy), rib-cage abnormalities, marked obesity and parenchymal conditions (advancing cystic fibrosis). Hypercapnic respiratory failure may be insidious in its onset and may develop when respiratory muscle fatigue occurs. Thus, it is more frequently associated with the chronic stages of respiratory failure.

Non-invasive Ventilation: Indications and Clinical Data

Indications for CPAP in Pre-term Neonates

Indications and physiological effects of CPAP are shown in Tables 1 and 2. CPAP is now used for a variety of neonatal conditions. It is effective in supporting recently extubated infants and for treating apnoea of prematurity [22,23].

Table 1 Physiologic benefits of continuous positive airway pressure (CPAP)

–	Produces a more regular breathing pattern
–	Establishes and maintains functional residual capacity
–	Decreases upper airway resistance
–	Results in progressive alveolar recruitment, inflates collapsed alveoli and reduces intrapulmonary shunting
–	Decreases upper airway collapsibility
–	Reduces obstructive apnoeas
–	Promotes the release and conservation of surfactant on the alveolar surface
–	Increases lung volume and lung weight in immature animals

Table 2 Clinical indications for continuous positive airway pressure (CPAP)

–	Respiratory support of the recently extubated infant
–	Management of apnoea of prematurity
–	Treatment of hyaline membrane disease
–	Hypoxaemic respiratory failure
–	Prevention and treatment of post-operative respiratory complications
–	Alternative to mechanical ventilation in resource-scarce areas?

Increasingly, CPAP is being seen as an alternative to intubation and ventilation in the treatment of hyaline membrane disease [24]. In a historical case series, a team at Columbia University consistently demonstrated a decreased prevalence of BPD compared to other neonatal ICUs (NICUs) [25]. This result was credited to a management strategy emphasising the early and routine use of CPAP for the treatment of HMD and the more limited use of intubation, surfactant and mechanical ventilation; but this conclusion has never been tested in a randomised controlled trial [26].

The conditions in which CPAP may not be useful include upper airway abnormalities (e.g. Pierre-Robin sequence), severe cardiovascular instability and intractable apnoeic episodes.

Upper airway obstruction due to congenital abnormalities of the larynx and trachea can cause severe respiratory distress in infancy. Laryngomalacia is the most frequent congenital abnormality of the larynx and the most common cause of stridor in newborns and infants. Non-invasive CPAP and positive-pressure ventilation [27,28]. The use of CPAP requires meticulous attention to the infant's airway. The correct prong size is essential and the infant's neck to be properly positioned to avoid excessive flexion or extension. The airway requires frequent suction to clear accumulated secretions (the optimal frequency of airway suction has yet to be determined), breathing patterns must be constantly observed and standardised and rigorous training of physicians, respiratory practitioners and/or nursing staff are of the utmost importance. CPAP should be administered early and judiciously, allowing both $PaCO_2$ (permissive hypercapnia) and the FiO_2 to rise. Apnoeic episodes should be tolerated and treated accordingly.

In the developing world, infants prone to higher mortality and morbidity are often denied access to neonatal intensive care because 'scarce' financial resources are directed towards more viable infants. In a prospective study from South Africa, Pieper et al. conducted a quasi-randomised control trial of CPAP for very-low-birth-weight infants denied access to the NICU compared to those receiving standard therapy of head-box oxygen [29]. Although CPAP was initially placed by respiratory therapists, ongoing care was continued by nursing staff with no intensive care or CPAP experience. Infants who received CPAP under these circumstances had a significantly improved short-term survival (<24 h), with trends towards improved long-term survival. None of the infants in the study received surfactant therapy. Further studies are warranted to define whether the routine early use of CPAP in areas of diminished neonatal resources offers an alternative to conventional mechanical ventilation and a reduction in costs and waste of resources.

Indications for Intermittent Positive-Pressure Ventilation in Neonates

In addition to CPAP, NICUs have adopted nasal intermittent positive pressure ventilation (NIPPV), via nasal prongs, with and without synchronisation as an alternative non-invasive strategy for respiratory support [30]. Nasal IPPV may improve patency of the upper airway by creating intermittently elevated pharyngeal pressures and, by intermittent inflation of the pharynx, i.e. activate respiratory drive. With respect to this second mechanism, Greenough demonstrated that lung inflation, by artificial ventilation, provokes an augmented inspiratory reflex, i.e. Head's paradoxical reflex, in certain pre-term infants. Moretti et al. demonstrated improved efficiency of the patient's breaths obtained by synchronised NIPPV compared to nasal continuous positive pressure ventilation, leading to larger tidal volumes (V_T) and minute volume. In response to the increase in V_T, the respiratory rate decreased by a statistically significant amount and $PaCO_2$ was reduced [31].

Physiologically synchronised NIPPV (sNIPPV) may offer advantages over nasal CPAP by improving tidal and minute volumes and by activating respiratory drive, which is poorly controlled in extremely low-birth-weight infants.

Bases on the three randomised control trials published, sNIPPV appears to provide superior respiratory support for recently extubated pre-term infants; the number needed to treat being three infants to prevent one extubation failure. A trend towards lower rates of BPD in infants randomised to sNIPPV was noted in the two trials reporting this outcome but did not reach statistical significance; and the trials were not powered for this outcome [32–34]. Moreover, these trials reported only short-term benefits of sNIPPV over nasal CPAP and were not powered to detect a benefit of sNIPPV for clinically relevant long-term outcomes such as BPD and death. Whether the short-term advantages of sNIPPV over CPAP following extubation lead to a real and meaningful clinical outcome in the longer term remains to be determined. Also, there are no studies describing the use of sNIPPV in the first-line management of hyaline membrane disease.

Indications for Nasal/Mask CPAP in Infants and Children

The experience of non-invasive CPAP in infants and children is scarce; so far, case series without any control group constitute the vast majority of the available knowledge, especially in the acute setting. Furthermore, many of the published case series reported results from the treatment of patients with acute respiratory failure of different aetiologies and severity, making it even more difficult to draw conclusions with respect to any specific disease. Finally, there are no generally accepted guidelines for NIV in infants and children.

Soong et al. investigated ten infants with an average age of 6 months and severe bronchiolitis who were treated with CPAP by nasal prongs. They found an improvement in respiratory rate and gas-exchange [35].

A recent study in infants and young children with a mean age of 10 months and chronic upper airway obstruction showed that CPAP and BiPAP delivered by nasal mask were associated with a significant and comparable decrease in respiratory effort but patient-ventilator asynchrony was more frequent during BiPAP ventilation [36].

Indications for NIPPV in Infants and Children

Data regarding the effect of positive pressure ventilation in infants and children in the acute setting are astonishingly scarce and mainly derive from case reports or small number of patients. In 1993, Akingbola et al. published a case report describing the effectiveness of NIPPV to prevent intubation after extubation in two paediatric patients with acute respiratory distress due to leukaemia [37]. Since that time, NIPPV has been applied in paediatric patients with a variety of respiratory disorders associated with acute hypoxaemic and chronic hypercapnic respiratory failure. Marino et al. reported the effectiveness of prolonged NIPPV to stabilise oxygenation and avoid intubation in one leukaemia patient with acute respiratory failure including lung infiltrates [38]. Fortenberry et al. reported an intubation rate lower than expected (11 vs. 42%) in a group of 28 patients with pneumonia and neurological disorders. Akingbola et al., in nine patients with pulmonary oedema, atelectasis and pneumonia, found an improvement in oxygenation but not ventilation [39,40]. Teague et al. evaluated 26 patients with status asthmaticus and reported improvement in oxygenation in 70% but a high rate of intubation (26%) [41].

NIPPV has been also found effective in improving ventilation and oxygenation in children with upper airway obstruction [42] and following corrective spinal repair [43].

NIPPV has been reported effective also in chronic disorders. Padman et al. improved dyspnoea scores and oxygen saturation in 43 patients with neuromuscular disease, obesity and encephalopathy, with an intubation rate of 9% [44]. In another study, Niranjan et al. combined the use of NIPPV with expiratory support (manual and assisted coughing) in ten children with neuromuscular disease. The authors pointed out that patient cooperation was critical for success [45]. Rosen et al. reported the effectiveness of NIPPV in five patients with obstructive apnoea post-tonsillectomy with no intubation [46]. Bimkrant et al., in 25 patients with spinal muscular atrophy, found that NIPPV allowed weaning from an invasive airway in 80% of the cases; similarly, Bach et al. reported that NIPPV was successful in 11 very young children with severe skeletal and bulbar weakness due to spinal muscular atrophy [47,48].

The possible use of NIPPV as a bridge to lung transplantation was reported by Padman et al. in seven patients with advanced cystic fibrosis [49]. However, another study showed that, in stable patients with advanced cystic fibrosis, NIPPV did improve respiratory gas exchange, but long-term acceptance of NIPPV in this population was poor [50]. NIPPV can also play a role in the early management of acute chest syndrome in children with sickle-cell anaemia, restoring lung volume and thereby preventing atelectasis [51].

However, in the majority of these studies, in premature neonates, infants and children, the overall rate of endotracheal intubation was relatively low due to the light to mild respiratory insufficiency of the majority of the patients included. Since control groups were not considered, it was not possible to conclude that the administration of NIV in infants and children with severe hypoxaemic respiratory failure can prevent endotracheal intubation.

Equipment

This section focuses on technical aspects regarding interfaces to deliver CPAP and NIV, equipment to deliver CPAP (flow generator and pressurisation system) and equipment to deliver NIV (ventilators, trigger system and modes of ventilation).

Interfaces To Deliver CPAP/NIV

A bewildering array of interfaces between the circuits and the infant's airway have been used: single prongs, binasal prongs, nasopharyngeal prongs, endotracheal tubes, head boxes, pressurised plastic bags, nasal cannulae and face masks and helmets (Figs. 1–3).

Currently, the most commonly used route is nasal CPAP, which was introduced in the early 1970s [51]. In pre-term neonates, a Cochrane Systematic Review suggested that short binasal prongs are more effective at preventing re-intubation than single nasal prongs. Nasal prongs are very easy to apply and comparatively non-invasive to the airways. The infant can still be nursed and handled with uninterrupted CPAP. The prongs can, however, cause nasal excoriation and scarring [52].

In neonates, the use of nasal cannulae has been shown to be effective in the treatment of apnoea of prematurity; however, there still may be associated nasal mucosal trauma and bleeding associated with their use [53,54].

The most common interfaces used in infants and children are nasal and face masks. The most important principle in guiding the selection of an interface is

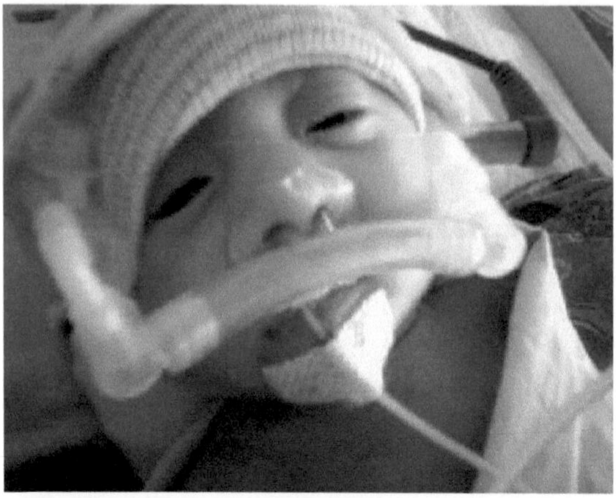

Fig. 1 Nasal prongs

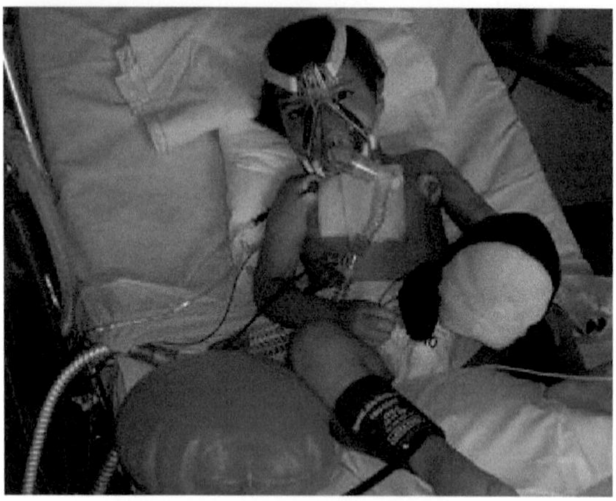

Fig. 2 Face mask

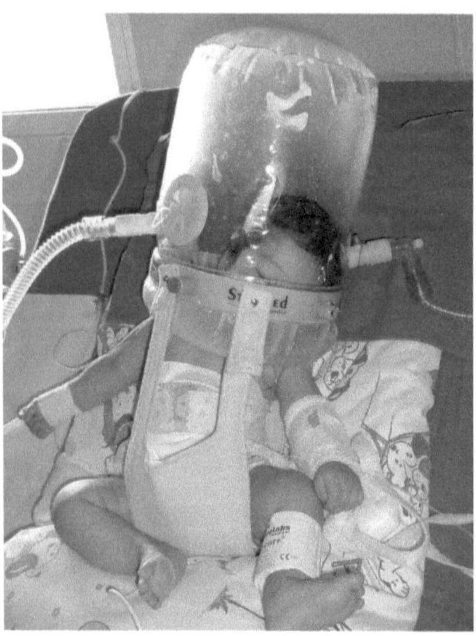

Fig. 3 The helmet

that it should fit comfortably. However, while nasal masks can leak gas when the infant opens its mouth, face masks can cause significant gastric distension and a tendency for infants to vomit, with the potential risk of aspirating gastric contents. The various complications, such as air leaks, skin irritation on the bridge of the nose and discomfort, that have been reported with nasal or face masks in children frequently lead to interruption of ventilatory treatment.

Masks (nasal or facial) can be divided into standard industrial masks, which are commonly available in different sizes, and moulded masks, moulded from an impression previously obtained from the patient.

It remains a matter of debate whether industrial masks or custom-made masks are preferable for use in neonates and infants. Masks should aim to exert the lowest amount of skin pressure compatible with ventilation and to obtain good efficiency in respiratory support and good CO_2 washout, because of their reduced dead space. If a nasal face mask is applied over the long term, then use of the mask should be monitored with respect to the effects of the interface on pressure marks, in particular on the maxillary bone, skull and eyes, in order to avoid the risk of cranial deformity in neonates.

The advantages of a nasal mask compared to a face mask are: less interference with speech, feeding or close contact with relatives, possible better comfort, reduced skin lesions and better removal of CO_2. Great priority should be given to using the smallest mask, which minimises dead space and facilitates triggering of the ventilator. CO_2 re-breathing in the mask depends on the type of interface, the interface's dead space, PEEP levels and flow through holes.

For nasal masks, transparent models are preferred as they readily allow inspection of infants' nostrils to ensure that they are not occluded by secretions or from dislocation of the mask. The smaller the child, the greater the risk of obstructed airways, even with small displacement of the interface. The long-term use of a face mask is correlated with adverse effects on the maxillary bone. Particular attention should be paid to the risk of narrowing the bony airway in the anterior-posterior plane. Monitoring with serial lateral X-ray of the skull is recommended.

In general nasal masks are effective interfaces for NIPPV in most paediatric patients even in the presence of a mouth leak; they also have the advantage of producing less anxiety in small children. Nasal oral masks eliminate significant oral gas leaks and should be considered in the acute setting when oral leaks appear to limit the effectiveness of NIPPV administered by nasal mask.

Nasal pillows or cushions are a third type of interface that may be effective in children who do not tolerate mask interfaces. They may be also used in the event of skin breakdown at the nasal bridge.

Recently, a new interface for infants was developed: its consist of a new type of helmet that offers several potential advantages over nasal or whole-face masks: (a) ease of use, (b) good tolerability, (c) less risk of disconnection from CPAP, (d) no air leakage when the infant opens its mouth, so pressure in the system remains stable, (e) a fixation system that avoids the risk of cutaneous lesions [55,56].

A rigid helmet was used to deliver CPAP in pre-term infants with apnoea and/or mild respiratory distress; the helmet improved gas exchange similar to the nasal mask but was tolerated better [57]. Piastra et al. used the helmet in four severely hypoxaemic children with acute leukaemia (mean age 14 years) who received positive-pressure NIV. The authors found an immediate improvement in oxygenation, with no complications. The helmet was also successful and better-tolerated than a face mask in the delivery of CPAP and positive pressure in adults with acute respiratory failure [58]. Squadrone et al. showed that CPAP delivered by a helmet successfully lowered the tracheal intubation rate and reduced clinical complications in postoperative adults [59].

Data regarding tolerability, safety and efficacy of the helmet compared to the different interfaces in the paediatric population are virtually absent in spite of the crucial role this device plays in obtaining successful NIV. There also limitations in commercially available interfaces. In contrast to adults, the children's nasal mask seems to be the preferred interface in both the chronic and the acute setting. The face mask is less well-tolerated than the nasal mask because of the risk of aspiration, technical difficulties in obtaining a good fit with children's facial contours, and the lack of cooperation. Previously, a helmet targeted for use as a paediatric interface was developed in an attempt to improve tolerability and to deliver prolonged respiratory support; these aspects are currently under evaluation.

Equipment To Deliver CPAP

Since its introduction [21] more than 30 years ago, CPAP has evolved with the development of a large number of different delivery systems and flow drivers. The physiological benefits of CPAP and its main clinical indications are shown in Tables 1 and 2. Fundamentally, CPAP delivery requires three components [60]: (1) a flow generator, (2) an airway interface (see above) and (3) a positive-pressure system.

Flow Generators

There are two major varieties of flow generators: constant flow and variable flow (demand). The flow generator should also warm and humidify the inhaled gases.

Constant flow is usually provided by an infant ventilator; this limits costs because of the dual use of a single piece of equipment. Most often, the amount of flow is set by the clinical team. Alternatively, variable-flow devices use a dedicated flow generator. Here, the 'expiratory' limb of the circuit is open to the atmosphere and the infant can draw extra gas from it to support inspiratory efforts. This device has gained widespread acceptance in Europe and North America. However, despite the theoretical advantages of the variable flow device, there are no consistent data showing clinically meaningful benefits over constant-flow devices [20].

Positive-Pressure System

At its simplest, expiratory pressure is provided by a fluid column (bubble CPAP), but more frequently by resistance at the expiratory valve of the ventilator. In the Benveniste device, pressure is generated at the nasal level or by generating CPAP in the immediate vicinity of the nasal airway through the conversion of kinetic energy from a jet of fresh gas [54]. The aim is to achieve constant distending pressure throughout the respiratory cycle to maintain FRC.

Bubble CPAP is a form of oscillatory pressure delivery in which mechanical vibrations are transmitted into the chest secondary to the non-uniform flow of gas bubbles across a downstream underwater seal. Its proponents point to the generation of waveforms similar to those produced by high-frequency ventilation, as recorded by a transducer at the airway. In pre-term lambs, bubble CPAP resulted in lower indicators of acute lung injury (neutrophils and hydrogen peroxide) than obtained with mechanical ventilation in the first 2 h of life. Bubble CPAP has the advantage of being simple and inexpensive [61].

Studies are required to identify the most effective pressure source for supplying continuous distending pressure.

There are no compelling data identifying the optimal pressure for CPAP in infants [62]. Traditionally, pressures of 4–6 cm H_2O have been used. Some investigators have claimed that higher pressures should be used, and some studies have involved pressures as high as 10 cmH_2O. We suggest a tailoring of the pressure to the infants' needs, i.e. increasing oxygen requirements, low-volume lung fields on chest radiograph and an increase in apnoeic episodes should prompt a judicious increase in the distending pressure by 1-cmH_2O increments to a maximum of 10 cmH_2O. There are few clinical studies on this approach, although it is consistent with the results of older physiologic studies.

Positive-pressure systems can be used to deliver positive-pressure ventilation. Most bilevel ventilators available for commercial use are remarkably adept at delivering CPAP, but problems arise when positive-pressure ventilation is used.

A significant barrier to effective CPAP in young or very small patients is the inability to achieve sufficient inspiratory flow to trigger the inspiratory pressure support feature. This problem can be solved by replacing the connector circuit between the mask interface and ventilator, consisting of standard tubing supplied by the manufacturer, to a connector tube that it is shorter and less compliant. However, this is a departure from the standard procedure and it is not recommended by the manufacturer.

Equipment To Deliver NIPPV

The application of NIPPV is facilitated by the cyclical application of positive pressure to the child's airway. Previous studies reported the use of volume-targeted ventilators, but pressure-targeted ventilators have also been employed.

In pressometric mode (pressure support ventilation, BiPAP), the, tidal volume delivered depends on the mechanical characteristics of the infant's respiratory system. Thus, any change in compliance, resistance or intrinsic PEEP reflects on the delivered tidal volume. Tidal volume can be enhanced during partial ventilatory support by increasing inspiratory effort.

The volume-targeted mode of ventilation delivers a pre-set tidal volume at timed intervals and specific frequency or in response to an inspiratory effort [63,64].

Independent variables are volume and flow while airway pressure depends on respiratory impedance. During assisted partial ventilation, the patient triggers a pre-set inspiratory volume, flow and time cycled breath, and cannot generate a tidal volume greater than that pre-set by the ventilator.

The major problem with NIPP is the effect of significant air leaks around the interface. In the presence of a significant leak, the inspiratory pressure target is never achieved, resulting in a very long insufflation time as the unit delivers massive amounts of inspiratory flow in an attempt to attain the pre-set inspiratory pressure. Some modern ventilators have an adjustable inflation time that can be set to limit this problem. The clinical impact of these ventilator differences vary between patients, with a significant impact on respiratory effort shown in some patients but not in others. These discrepancies may be explained by the different devices tested but also by the patients' diseases. A bench study showed that the performance of a home bilevel ventilator decreased as the respiratory effort increased [28]. Furthermore, leaks can also affect the quality of the trigger increasing the inspiratory trigger delays by slowing the decline in mask pressure [64].

A crucial role is also represented by the pressurisation rate, which can have marked, individual effects on the work of breathing and dyspnoea. This rate has been shown to differ greatly among the different ventilators [65,66].

It must be underlined that these studies were either bench studies or clinical studies performed in adult patients. However, the respiratory effort of those patients was not as great as the effort measured in the infants in the present study. Moreover, the breathing pattern of the infants also differed, with a higher respiratory rate and a smaller tidal volume, which could promote patient ventilator asynchrony.

Often, the inspiratory effort of infants may not be sufficient to generate pressure or flows and to trigger the ventilator. The majority of positive-pressure ventilators used in paediatric patients have fixed inspiratory and expiratory flow triggers, and both bench and clinical studies have shown significant differences in the trigger sensitivity and performance of the various bilevel pressure devices [67]. Expiratory triggers play a major role in achieving efficient NIPPV. They also detect the end of inspiration phase during pressure support ventilation by measuring inspiratory flow, thus allowing inspiratory/expiratory cycling.

The expiratory trigger can be activated by an inspiratory flow drop below a threshold value, by pre-set inspiratory flow termination criteria and by an algorithm-generated sequence.

The expiratory trigger depends on the reduction in expiratory flow and is time related; in cases of leaks, inspiration may continue when the infant has ceased to inspire, thus impeding expiration and adding to the work of breathing. Autotriggering of the ventilator is a common problem in infants who are non-invasively supported. Major causes of autotriggering are: air leaks, noise (excessive humidification, heart beat), low respiratory rate and low respiratory drive [68]. Another problem is the generation of an inspiratory effort in the absence of consisted pressurisation of the airway. This phenomenon can be generated by the presence of major air leaks, low inspiratory flow, heat and moisture exchange in the circuit, a ventilation time that is longer than the neurally activated one.

In order to allow better interaction between infants and the machine during NIV, a new system to deliver respiratory support, the Bipulse Machine, is currently under evaluation (Fig. 4). It consists of a mechanical PEEP valve positioned on the expiratory limb during high continuous flow (80–100 l/min) CPAP. The Bipulse machine is mechanically regulated, and alternates between low and high PEEP levels. Preliminary data indicate that with this approach respiratory function is supported without the need of a ventilator.

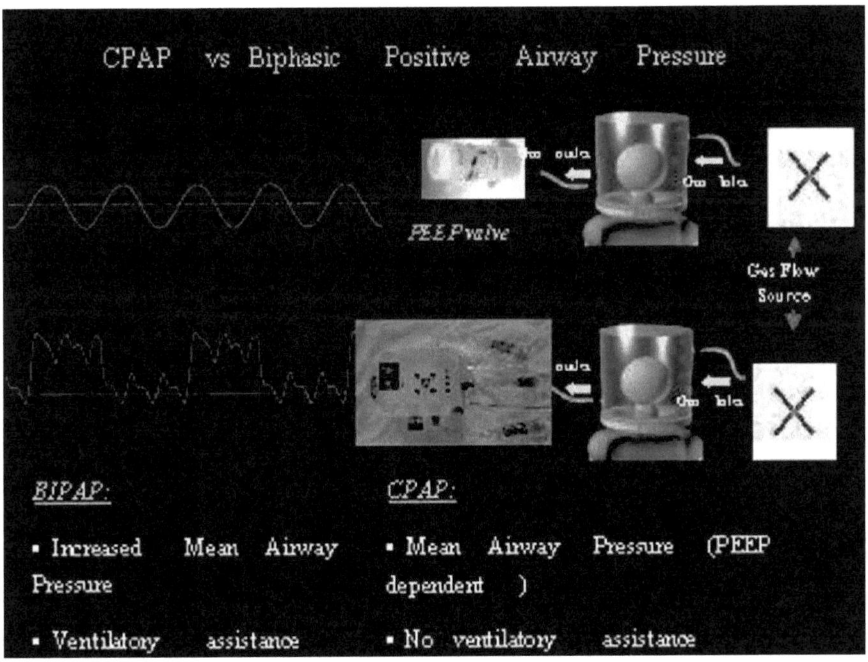

Fig. 4 Bipulse machine

Conclusions

For more than 10 years, NIV has been widely employed in the home setting to treat children with chronic respiratory failure, but the use of this technique in the paediatric ICU is expanding. However, physiological studies on the effects of NIV in children are lacking such that this approach has been employed on an empirical basis, with a considerable gap between the expanding use of paediatric NIV and the lack of knowledge of its physiological effects. This makes it difficult to establish both the appropriate timing of initiation of NIV and the most pertinent therapeutic goals. Moreover, technical problems related to interface and ventilator performances remain major obstacles to adequately supported respiratory function in acute respiratory failure.

In summary, it is essential to administer NIV support in infants and children, including high-performance ventilators with inspiratory and expiratory lines able to correct gas inflation in the presence of leaks. Furthermore, it is essential that different modalities of ventilation, such as pressure time or flow cycled, can be delivered, together with the possibility to regulate inspiratory trigger in flow or pressure, inspiratory-expiratory triggering and pressure rise time.

References

1. Jardine E, O'Toole M, Paton JY, Wallis C (1999) Current status of long term ventilation of children in United Kingdom: a questionnaire survey. BMJ 318:295–298
2. Fauroux B, Sardet A, Foret D (1995) Home treatment for chronic respiratory failure in children: a prospective study. Eur Respir J 8:2062–2066
3. Masa J, Celli B, Riesco J et al (1997) Noninvasive positive pressure ventilation and not oxygen may prevent overt ventilatory failure in patients with chest wall disease. Chest 112:207–213
4. Gay P, Edmonds L (1995) Severe hypercapnia after low-flow oxygen therapy in patients with neuromuscular disease and diaphragmatic dysfunction. Mayo Clin Proc 70:327–330
5. Gozal D (1997) Nocturnal ventilatory support in patients with cystic fibrosis: comparison with supplemental oxygen. Eur Resp J 10:1999–2003
6. Norregaard O (2002) Non invasive ventilation in children. Eur Respir J 2002:1332–1342
7. O'Brodovich HM, Haddad G (1998) The functional basis of respiratory pathology and disease. In: Chernick V, Boat TF (eds) Kendig's disorders of the respiratory tract in children. WB Saunders, Philadelphia, pp 27–74
8. Mortola JP, Fisher JT, Smith JB et al (1982) Onset of respiration in infants delivered by caesarian section. J Appl Physiol 52: 716–724
9. Lopes J, Muller NL, Bryan MH, Bryan AC (1981) Importance of inspiratory muscle tone in the maintenance of FRC in the newborn. J Appl Physiol 51: 830–834
10. Berry FA (1985) Inhalation agents in pediatric anesthesia. Clin Anesthesiol 3:515–537
11. Halliday HL (1996) Controversies: synthetic or natural surfactant. The case for natural surfactant. J Perinat Med 24:417–426
12. Keens TG, Bryan AC, Levison H, Ianuzzo CD (1978) Developmental pattern of muscle fiber types in human ventilatory muscles. J Appl Physiol 44:909–913
13. Muller N, Gulston G, Cade D et al (1979) Diaphragmatic muscle fatigue in the newborn. J Appl Physiol 46:688–695

14. Davidson-Ward SL, Bautista DB, Keens TG (1989) Hypoxic arousal responses in normal infants. Pediatr Pulmonol 7:276 (abs)
15. Jobe AH, Ikegami M (1998) Mechanisms initiating lung injury in the preterm. Early Hum Dev 53:81–94
16. Kotecha S, Chan B, Azam N et al (1995) Increase in interleukin-8 and soluble intercellular adhesion molecule-1 in bronchoalveolar lavage fluid from premature infants who develop chronic lung disease. Arch Dis Child Fetal Neonatal 72:F90-F96
17. Manktelow BN, Draper ES, Annamalai S, Field D (2001) Factors affecting the incidence of chronic lung disease of prematurity in 1987, 1992, and 1997. Arch Dis Child Fetal Neonatal Ed 85:F33-F35
18. Furman L, Baley J, Borawski-Clark E et al (1996) Hospitalization as a measure of morbidity among very low birth weight infants with chronic lung disease. J Pediatr 128:447–452
19. Millar D, Kirpalani H (2004) Benefits of non invasive ventilation. Indian Pediatr 41(10):1008–1017
20. Krauss AN, Klain DB, Auld PA (1995) Chronic pulmonary insufficiency of prematurity (CPIP). Pediatrics 55:55–58
21. Gregory GA, Kitterman JA, Phibbs RH et al (1971) Treatment of the idiopathic respiratory distress syndrome with continuous positive airway pressyre. N Engl J Med 284:1333–1340
22. Lemyre B, Davis PG, De Paoli AG (2002) Nasal intermittent positive pressure ventilation (NIPPV) versus nasal continuous positive airway pressure (NCPAP) for apnea of prematurity. Cochrane Database Syst Rev CD002272
23. De Paoli AG, Morley C, Davis PG (2002) Nasal CPAP for neonates: what do we know in 2003? Arch Dis Child Fetal Neonatal 87:F168-F172
24. Van Marter LJ, Allred EN, Pagano M et al (2002) Do clinical markers of barotrauma and oxygen toxicity explain interhospital variation in rates of chronic lung disease? The Neonatology Committee for the Developmental Network. Pediatrics 105:1194–1201
25. Subramaniam HJJ, Henderson Smart DJ, Davis PG (2002) Continuous distending pressure for respiratory distress syndrome in preterm infants. The Cochrane Database of Systematic Reviews CD 002377
26. Guilleminault C, Pelayo R, Clerk A et al (2005) Home nasal continuous positive airway pressure in infants with sleep disordered breathing. J Pediatr 127:905–912
27. Fauroux B, Pigeot J, Polkey MI et al (2001) Chronic stridor caused by laryngomalacia in children. Work of breathing and effects of non invasive ventilatory assistance. Am J Respir Crit Care Med 164:1874–1878
28. Pieper CH, Smith J, Maree D, Pohl FC (2003) Is nCPAP of value in extreme preterms with no access to neonatal intensive care? J Trop Pediatr 49:148–152
29. Ryan CA, Finer NN, Peters KL (1989) Nasal intermittent positive-pressure ventilation offers no advantages over nasal continuous positive airway pressure in apnea of prematurity. Am J Dis Child 143:1196–1198
30. Moretti C, Gizzi C, Papoff P et al (1999) Comparing the effects of nasal synchronized intermittent positive pressure ventilation (nSIPPV) and nasal continuous positive airway pressure (nCPAP) after extubation in very low birth weight infants. Early Hum Dev 56:167–177
31. Barrington KJ, Bull D, Finer NN (2001) Randomized trial of nasal synchronized intermittent mandatory ventilation compared with continuous positive airway pressure after extubation of very low birth weight infants. Pediatrics 107:638–641
32. Davis PG, Lemyre B, De Paoli AG (2003) Nasal intermittent positive pressure ventilation (NIPPV) versus nasal continuous positive airway pressure (NCPAP) for preterm neonates after extubation. Cochrane Database Syst Rev CD0023499
33. Friedlich P, Lecart C, Posen R et al (1999) A randomized trial of nasopharyngeal-synchronized intermittent mandatory ventilation versus nasopharyngeal continuous positive airway pressure in very low birth weight infants after extubation. J Perinatol 19:413–418
34. Khalaf MN, Brodsky N, Hurley J, Bhandari V (2001) A prospective randomized, controlled trial comparing synchronized nasal intermittent positive pressure ventilation versus nasal continuous positive airway pressure as modes of extubation. Pediatrics 108:13–17

35. Soong WJ, Hwang B, Tang RB (1999) Continuous positive airway pressure by nasal prongs in bronchiolitis. Pediatr Pulmonol 16:163–166
36. Essouri S, Nicot F, Clement A et al (2005) Noninvasive positive pressure ventilation in infants with upper airway obstruction:comparison of continuous and bilevel positive pressure. Intensive Care Med 31:574–580
37. Akingbola O, Servant GM, Custer JR, Palmisano J (1993) Non invasive Bi Level positive pressure ventilation management of two pediatric patients. Respir Care 38:1092–1098
38. Marino P, Rosa G, Cogliati AA (1997) Treatment of acute respiratory failure by prolonged non invasive ventilation in a child. Can J Anaesth 44:727–731
39. Fortenberry JD, Del Toro J, Jefferson LS et al (1995) Management of pediatric acute hypoxiemic respiratory insufficiency with bi-level positive pressure (BiPAP) nasal mask ventilation. Chest 108:1059–1064
40. Akingbola O, Palmisano J, Servant GM et al (1994) BiPAP mask ventilation in pediatric patients with acute respiratory failure. Crit Care Med 22:144 (abs)
41. Teague WG, Lowe E, Dominick J, Lang D (1998) Non invasive positive pressure ventilation (NPPV) in critically ill children with status asthmaticus. Am J Respir Crit Care Med 157:542–546
42. Teague WG, Kervin L, Dawadkar V, Scott P (1991) Non invasive positive pressure ventilation improves ventilation and oxygenation in children with upper airway obstruction. Am Rev Respir Dis 143:505–509
43. Doherty MJ, Millner PA, Latham M et al (2001) Non invasive ventilation in the treatment of ventilatory failure follwing corrective spinal surgery. Anesthesia 56:235–238
44. Padman R, Lawless ST, Kettrick RG (2001) Non invasive ventilation via bi-level positive airway pressure support in clinical practice. Crit Care Med 26:169–173
45. Niranjan V, Bach JR (1998) Non invasive management of pediatric neuromuscular ventilatory failure. Crit Care Med 26:2061–2065
46. Rosen GM, Muckle RP, Mahowald MW et al (1996) Postoperative respiratory compromise in children with obstructive sleep apnea syndrome: can it be anticipated? Pediatrics 3:784–788
47. Bimkrant DJ, Pope JJ, Eiben RM (1997) Pediatric non invasive nasal ventilation. J Child neurol 12:231–236
48. Bach JR, Nirajan V, Weaver B (2000) Spinal muscular atrophy type I. A non invasive respiratory management approach. Chest 117:1100–1105
49. Padman R, Nadkarmi V, Von Nessen S (1994) Non invasive positive pressure ventilation in end stage cystic fibrosis: a report of seven cases. Respir Care 39:736–739
50. Teague WG (2003) Non invasive ventilation in pediatric intensive care unit for children with acute respiratory failure. Pediat Pulmonol 5:418–426
51. Shah PS, Ohlsson A, Shah JP (2003) Continuous negative extrathoracic pressure or continuous positive airway pressure for acute hypoxemic respiratory failure in children. The Cochrane Database of Systematic Reviews, CD00279009
52. Chernick V (1973) Continuous distending pressure in hyaline membrane disease: of devices, disadvantages, and a daring study. Pediatrics 52:114–115
53. Kopelman AE (2003) Use of oxygen cannulas in extremely low birthweight infants is associated with mucosal trauma and bleeding, and possibly with coagulase-negative staphylococcal sepsis. J Perinatol 23:94–97
54. Benveniste D, Berg O, Pedersen JE (1976) A technique for delivery of continuous positive airway pressure to the neonate. J Pediatr 88:1015–1019
55. Antonelli M, Conti G, Pelosi P et al (2002) New treatment of acute hypoxemic respiratory failure. Noninvasive pressure support ventilation delivered by helmet: A pilot controlled trial. Crit Care Med 30:602–683
56. Taccone P, Hess D, Caironi P, Bigatello L (2004) Continuous positive airway pressure delivered with a 'helmet': Effects on carbon dioxide rebreathing. Crit Care Med 32:2092–2096
57. Trevisanuto D, Grazzina N, Doglioni N (2005) A new device for administration of continuous airway pressure in preter infants: comparison with a standard nasal CPAP continuous positive airway pressure system. Intensive Care Med 31:859–864

58. Piastra M, Antonelli M (2004) Treatment of acute respiratory failure by helmet delivered noninvasive pressure support ventilation in children with acute leukemia: a clinical pilot study. Intensive Care Med 30:472–474
59. Squadrone V, Coha M, Cerutti E et al; Piedmont Intensive Care Units Network (PICUN) (2005) Continuous positive airway pressure for treatment of postoperative hypoxemia: a randomized controlled trial. JAMA 293:589–595
60. Courtney SE, Pyon KH, Saslow JG et al (2001) Lung recruitment and breathing pattern during variable versus continuous flow nasal continuous positive airway pressure in premature infants: an evaluation of three devices. Pediatrics 107:304–308
61. Jobe AH, Kramer BW, Moss TJ et al (2002) Decreased indicators of lung injury with continuous positive expiratory pressure in preterm lambs. Pediatr Res 52:387–392
62. Lindner W, Vossbeck S, Hummler H, Pohlandt F (1999) Delivery room management of extremely low birth weight infants: spontaneous breathing or intubation? Pediatrics 103:961–967
63. Bott J, Carroll MP, Conway JH (1993) Randomized controlled trial of nasal ventilation in acute ventilatory failure due to chronic obstructive airways disease. Lancet 341:1555–1557
64. Lofaso F, Brochard L, Hang T et al (1996) Home versus intensive care pressure support devices. Experimental and clinical comparison. Am J Respir Crit Care Med 153:1581–1599
65. Tassaux D, Strasser S, Fonseca S et al (2002) Comparative bench study of triggering, pressurization and cycling between the home ventilator VPAP II and three ICU ventilators. Intensive Care Med 28:1254–1261
66. Bach JR, Niranjan V, Weaver B (2000) Spinal muscular atrophy type 1. A noninvasive respiratory management approach. Chest 117:1100–1105
67. Elliott M, Moxham J (1999) Noninvasive mechanical ventilation by nasal or face mask. In: Tobin MJ, ed. Principles and Practice of Mechanical Ventilation. McGraw-Hill, New York, pp 427–454
68. Calderini E, Confalonieri M, Puccio PG et al (1999) Patient ventilator asynchrony during non invasive ventilation: the role of the expiratory trigger. Intensive Care Med 25:622–627

Subject Index